Deadly Medicines and Organised Crime

How big pharma has corrupted healthcare

PETER C GØTZSCHE

Forewords by

RICHARD SMITH
former editor-in-chief, BMJ

and

DRUMMOND RENNIE
deputy editor, *JAMA*

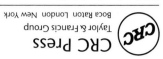

CRC Press
Taylor & Francis Group

Boca Raton London New York

CRC Press is an imprint of the
Taylor & Francis Group, an **informa** business

Radcliffe Publishing Ltd
33–41 Dallington Street
London
EC1V 0BB
United Kingdom

British Library Cataloguing in Publication Data

A catalogue record for this book is available from the British Library.

ISBN-13: 978 184619 884 7

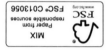

The paper used for the text pages of this book is FSC® certified. FSC (The Forest Stewardship Council®) is an international network to promote responsible management of the world's forests.

Typeset by Darkriver Design, Auckland, New Zealand

Contents

Contents

Foreword by Richard Smith

There must be plenty of people who shudder when they hear that Peter Gøtzsche will be speaking at a meeting or see his name on the contents list of a journal. He is like the young boy who could not only see that the emperor had no clothes but also said so. Most of us can either cannot see that the emperor is naked or will not announce it when we see his nakedness, which is why we badly need people like Peter. He is not a compromiser or a dissembler, and he has a taste for strong, blunt language and colourful metaphors. Some, perhaps many, people might be put off reading this book by Peter's insistence on comparing the pharmaceutical industry to the mob, but those who turn away from the book will miss an important opportunity to understand something important about the world – and to be shocked.

Peter ends his book with a story of how the Danish Society for Rheumatology asked him to speak on the theme *Collaboration with the drug industry. Is it harmful?* The original title was *Collaboration with the drug industry. Is it THAT harmful?* but the society thought that too strong. Peter started his talk by enumerating the 'crimes' of the meeting's sponsors. Roche had grown by selling heroin illegally. Abbott blocked Peter's access to drug regulators' unpublished trials that eventually showed that a slimming pill was dangerous. UCB too concealed trial data, while Pfizer had lied to the Food and Drug Administration and been fined $2.3 billion in the United States for promoting off label use of four drugs. Merck, the last sponsor, had, said Peter, caused the deaths of thousands of patients with its deceptive behaviour around a drug for arthritis. After this beginning to his talk he launched into his condemnation of the industry. You can imagine being at the meeting, with the sponsors spluttering with rage and the organisers acutely embarrassed. Peter quotes a colleague as saying that he felt 'my direct approach might have pushed some people away who were undetermined.' But most of the audience were engaged and saw legitimacy in Peter's points.

The many people who have enthusiastically supported routine mammography to prevent breast cancer deaths might empathise with the sponsors – because Peter has been critical of them and published a book on his experiences around mammography. The important point for me is that Peter was one of few people criticising routine mammography when he began his investigations but – despite intense attacks on him – has been proved largely right.

He did not have any particular view on mammography when he was asked by the Danish authorities to look at the evidence, but he quickly concluded that much of the evidence was of poor quality. His general conclusion was that routine mammography might save some lives, although far fewer than enthusiasts said was the case, but at the cost of many false positives, women undergoing invasive and anxiety-creating procedures for no benefit, and of overdiagnosis of harmless cancers. The subsequent arguments around routine mammography have been bitter and hostile, but Peter's view might now be called the orthodox view. His book on the subject shows in a detailed way how scientists have distorted evidence in order to support their beliefs.

I have long recognised that science is carried out by human beings not objective robots and will therefore be prone to the many human failings, but I was shocked by the stories in Peter's book on mammography.

Much of this book is also shocking and in a similar way: it shows how science can be corrupted in order to advance particular arguments and how money, profits, jobs and reputations are the most potent corrupters.

Peter does acknowledge that some drugs have brought great benefits. He does so in one sentence: 'My book is not about the well-known benefits of drugs such as our great successes with treating infections, heart diseases, some cancers, and hormone deficiencies like type 1 diabetes.' Some readers may think this insufficient, but Peter is very clear that this is a book about the failures of the whole system of discovering, producing, marketing and regulating drugs. It is not a book about their benefits.

Many of those who read this book will ask if Peter has over-reached himself in suggesting that the activities of the drug industry amount to organised crime. The characteristics of organised crime, racketeering, is defined in US law as the act of engaging repeatedly in certain types of offence, including extortion, fraud, federal drug offenses, bribery, embezzlement, obstruction of justice, obstruction of law enforcement, tampering with witnesses and political corruption. Peter produces evidence, most of it detailed, to support his case that pharmaceutical companies are guilty of most of these offences.

And he is not the first to compare the industry with the Mafia or mob. He quotes a former vice-president of Pfizer, who has said:

It is scary how many similarities there are between this industry and the mob. The mob makes obscene amounts of money, as does this industry. The side effects of organized crime are killings and deaths, and the side effects are the same in this industry. The mob bribes politicians and others, and so does the drug industry …

The industry has certainly fallen foul of the US Department of Justice many times in cases where companies have been fined billions. Peter describes the top 10 companies in detail, but there are many more. It's also true that they have offended repeatedly, calculating perhaps that there are large profits to be made by flouting the law and paying the fines. The fines can be thought of as 'the cost of doing business' like having to pay for heat, light and rent.

Many people are killed by the industry, many more than are killed by the mob. Indeed, hundreds of thousands are killed every year by prescription drugs. Many will see this as almost inevitable because the drugs are being used to treat diseases that themselves kill. But a counter-argument is that the benefits of drugs are exaggerated, often because of serious distortions of the evidence behind the drugs, a 'crime' that can be attributed confidently to the industry.

The great doctor William Osler famously said that it would be good for humankind and bad for the fishes if all the drugs were thrown into the sea. He was speaking before the therapeutic revolution in the middle of the 20th century that led to penicillin, other antibiotics, and many other effective drugs, but Peter comes close to agreeing with him and does speculate that we would be better off without most psychoactive drugs, where the benefits are small, the harms considerable, and the level of prescribing massive.

Most of Peter's book is devoted to building up the case that the drug industry has systematically corrupted science to play up the benefits and play down the harms of their drugs. As an epidemiologist with very high numerical literacy and a passion for detail, so that he is a world leader in critiquing clinical studies, Peter is here on very solid ground. He joins many others, including former editors of the *New England Journal of Medicine*, in showing this corruption. He shows too how the industry has bought doctors, academics, journals, professional and patient organisations, university departments, journalists, regulators, and politicians. These are the methods of the mob.

The book doesn't let doctors and academics avoid blame. Indeed, it might be argued that drug companies are doing what is expected of them in maximising financial returns for shareholders, but doctors and academics are supposed to have a higher calling. Laws that are requiring companies to declare payments to doctors are showing that very high proportions of doctors are beholden to the drug industry and that many are being paid six figure sums for advising companies or giving talks on their behalf. It's hard to escape the conclusion that these 'key opinion leaders' are being bought. They are the 'hired guns' of the industry. And, as with the mob, woe be to anybody who whistleblows or gives evidence against the industry. Peter tells several stories of whistleblowers being hounded, and John le Carré's novel describing drug company ruthlessness became a bestseller and a successful Hollywood film.

So it's not entirely fanciful to compare the drug industry to the mob, and the public, despite its enthusiasm for taking drugs, is sceptical about the drug industry. In a poll in Denmark the public ranked the drug industry second bottom of those in which they had confidence, and a US poll ranked the industry bottom with tobacco and oil companies. The doctor and author, Ben Goldacre, in his book *Bad Pharma* raises the interesting thought that doctors have come to see as 'normal' a relationship with the drug industry that the public will see as wholly unacceptable when they fully understand it. In Britain doctors might follow journalists, members of Parliament, and bankers into disgrace for failing to see how corrupt their ways have become. At the moment the public tends to trust doctors and distrust drug companies, but the trust could be rapidly lost.

Peter's book is not all about problems. He proposes solutions, some of which are more likely than others to happen. It seems most unlikely that drug companies will be nationalised, but it is likely that all the data used to license drugs will be made available. The independence of regulators should be enhanced. Some countries might be tempted to encourage more evaluation of drugs by public sector organisations, and enthusiasm is spreading for exposing the financial links between drug companies and doctors, professional and patient bodies, and journals. Certainly the management of conflicts of interest needs to be improved.

Marketing may be further constrained, and resistance to direct consumer advertising is stiffening.

Critics of the drug industry have been increasing in number, respectability, and vehemence, and Peter has surpassed them all in comparing the industry with organised crime. I hope that nobody will be put off reading this book by the boldness of his comparison, and perhaps the bluntness of the message will lead to valuable reform.

Richard Smith, MD
June 2013

Foreword by Drummond Rennie

EVIDENCE-BASED OUTRAGE

There already exist hundreds of reports of scientific studies, and many books written, about the way pharmaceutical companies pervert the scientific process and, using their massive wealth, all too often work against the interests of the patients they claim to help. I myself have contributed to the piles. So what makes this book new and worth your attention?

The answer is simple: the unique scientific abilities, research, integrity, truth-fulness, and courage of the author. Gøtzsche's experience is unequaled. He has worked in sales for drug companies either as a drug company representative pitching pills to doctors or as a product manager. He is a physician and a medi-cal researcher and has built a high reputation as head of The Nordic Cochrane Centre. So when he speaks about bias, he bases his opinions on careful research over decades, published in peer-reviewed journals. He deeply understands the statistics of bias and the techniques of analyzing reports of clinical trials. He has been in the forefront of the development of systematic review and rigorous and meta-analysis of reports of clinical trials, to winnow out, using strict criteria, the true effectiveness of drugs and tests. He is often annoyingly persistent, but he is always driven by the evidence.

So I trust Gøtzsche to have his facts right. My trust is based on solid evidence, and on my own experience over several decades struggling with the results of pharmaceutical company influence upon my clinical researcher colleagues, and upon the public. In addition, I trust Gøtzsche because I know him to be correct when he writes about events of which I have independent knowledge.

My last reason for trusting Gøtzsche's account has to do with my own job as an editor at a very large medical clinical journal. Editors are the first to be able to examine the written report as it comes from a research institution. Editors or their reviewers detect problems of bias in the papers submitted to their journals, and it is to editors that complaints and allegations are directed.

I have written repeated, and often indignant, editorials revealing unethical behavior by commercially-supported researchers and their sponsors. At least three editors whom I also know well, Drs. Jerome Kassirer and Marcia Angell (*The New England Journal of Medicine*) and Richard Smith (*British Medical Journal*) have written books in which they have expressed dismay at the magni-tude of the problem. Other editors such as Fiona Godlee of the *British Medical Journal* have written eloquently on the corrupting influence of money and the way it biases the treatment of patients and increases the costs.

I don't pretend to vouch for all Gøtzsche's facts – this is a foreword, not an audit – but the general picture he gives is only too familiar. While Gøtzsche may seem to talk in hyperbole, my own depressing experiences and that of medical editors and researchers I know personally tell me he's right.

In a lecture I gave to an audience of judges I noted that clinical researchers and the legal profession used the same word, 'trial', for two sorts of process, one legal and the other scientific. Speaking for my own profession, I had to acknowledge that legal 'trials' were set up in a way that was generally fairer, and based on a sounder ethical footing than clinical trials. (Gøtzsche quotes this on page 59.) Gøtzsche has proposals and calls for revolution. To me nothing will help unless we disconnect completely the performance and assessment of trials from the funding of trials. We base our treatments on the results of clinical trials, so the results are a matter of life and death. Patients who allow themselves to be entered into trials expect their sacrifice to benefit humanity. What they do not expect is that their results will be held, and manipulated, as trade secrets. These results are a public good and they should be financed by the government using taxes paid by the industry, and available to all. As it is, we have the ironic situation in the US where the drug companies pay the agency, the FDA, to assess their projects. Is it any surprise that the agency has been captured by the industry it is supposed to regulate?

Revolution? Gøtzsche is right. We landed in our present mess because of innumerable mistakes in the past, and he describes many of these in his detailed inventory. They include failure of clinical scientists, their institutions and the editors of the journals publishing their science to understand how thoroughly they were being caught up by the marketers who paid them. I believe it will take a revolution to sweep away decades of self-dealing by industry.

I hope you will read this book and reach your own conclusions. Mine? If Gøtzsche is angry at the behavior of academia and industry, he has a right to be. What's needed is more of Gøtzsche's evidence-based outrage.

Drummond Rennie, MD
June 2013

About the author

Professor Peter C Gøtzsche graduated as a Master of Science in biology and chemistry in 1974 and as a physician in 1984. He is a specialist in internal medicine; he worked with clinical trials and regulatory affairs in the drug industry 1975–83, and at hospitals in Copenhagen 1984–95. He co-founded The Cochrane Collaboration in 1993 and established The Nordic Cochrane Centre the same year. He became professor of Clinical Research Design and Analysis in 2010 at the University of Copenhagen.

Peter Gøtzsche has published more than 50 papers in 'the big five' (BMJ, Lancet, JAMA, Annals of Internal Medicine and New England Journal of Medicine) and his scientific works have been cited over 10 000 times.

Peter Gøtzsche has an interest in statistics and research methodology. He is a member of several groups publishing guidelines for good reporting of research and has co-authored CONSORT for randomised trials (www.consort-statement.org), STROBE for observational studies (www.strobe-statement.org), PRISMA for systematic reviews and meta-analyses (www.prisma-statement.org), and SPIRIT for trial protocols (www.spirit-statement.org). Peter Gøtzsche is an editor in the Cochrane Methodology Review Group.

BOOKS BY PETER GØTZSCHE

Gøtzsche PC. *Mammography Screening: truth, lies and controversy.* London: Radcliffe Publishing; 2012.

Gøtzsche PC. *Rational Diagnosis and Treatment: evidence-based clinical decision-making.* 4th ed. Chichester: Wiley; 2007.

Gøtzsche PC. [On safari in Kenya] [Danish]. Copenhagen: Samlerens Forlag; 1985.

Wulff HR, Gøtzsche PC. *Rationel klinik. Evidensbaserede diagnostiske og terapeutiske beslutninger.* [Rational clinical practice. Evidence-based diagnostic and therapeutic decisions] 5th ed. Copenhagen: Munksgaard Danmark; 2006.

Introduction

The big epidemics of infectious and parasitic diseases that previously took many lives are now under control in most countries. We have learned how to prevent and treat AIDS, cholera, malaria, measles, plague and tuberculosis, and we have eradicated smallpox. The death tolls of AIDS and malaria are still very high, but that's not because we don't know how to deal with them. It has more to do with income inequalities and the excessive costs of life-saving drugs for people in low-income countries.

Unfortunately, we now suffer from two man-made epidemics, tobacco and prescription drugs, both of which are hugely lethal. In the United States and Europe,

drugs are the third leading cause of death after heart disease and cancer.

I shall explain in this book why this is so and what we can do about it. If drug deaths had been an infectious disease or a heart disease or a cancer caused by environmental pollution, there would have been countless patient advocacy groups raising money to combat it and far-ranging political initiatives. I have difficulty understanding that – since it is drugs, people do nothing.

The tobacco and the drug industries have much in common. The morally repugnant disregard for human lives is the norm. The tobacco companies are proud that they have increased sales in vulnerable low-income and middle-income countries, and without a trace of irony or shame, Imperial Tobacco's management team reported to investors in 2011 that the UK-based company won a Gold Award rating in a corporate responsibility index.[1] The tobacco companies see 'many opportunities ... to develop our business', which the *Lancet* described as 'selling, addicting, and killing, surely the most cruel and corrupt business model human beings could have invented'.[1]

Tobacco executives know they are peddling death and so do drug company executives. It is no longer possible to hide the fact that tobacco is a major killer, but the drug industry has done surprisingly well in hiding that its drugs are also a major killer. I shall describe in this book how drug companies have deliberately hidden lethal harms of their drugs by fraudulent behaviour, both in research and marketing, and by firm denials when confronted with the facts. Just like the chief tobacco executives each testified at a US Congressional hearing in 1994 that nicotine wasn't addictive, although they had known for decades that this was a lie.[2] Philip Morris, the US tobacco giant, set up a research company that documented the dangers of sidestream smoke, but even though more than 800 scientific reports were produced none were published.[2]

Both industries use hired guns. When robust research has shown that a product is dangerous, numerous substandard studies are produced saying the opposite, which confuse the public because – as journalists will tell you – 'researchers disagree'. This doubt industry is very effective at distracting people into ignoring the harms; the industry buys time while people continue to die.

This is corruption. Corruption has many meanings and what I generally understand by it is defined in my own dictionary, which is moral decay. Another meaning is bribery, which may mean a secret payment, usually in cash, for a service that would otherwise not be rendered, or at least not so quickly. However, as we shall see, corruption in healthcare has many faces, including payment for a seemingly noble activity, which might be nothing else than a pretence for handing over money to a substantial part of the medical profession.

The characters in Aldous Huxley's novel from 1932, *Brave New World*, can take Soma pills every day to give them control over their lives and keep troubling thoughts away. In the United States, TV commercials urge the public to do exactly the same. They depict unhappy characters that regain control and look happy as soon as they have taken a pill.[3] We have already superseded Huxley's wildest imaginations and drug use is still increasing. In Denmark, for example, we use so many drugs that every citizen, whether sick or healthy, can be in treatment with 1.4 adult daily doses of a drug every day, from cradle to grave. Although many drugs are life-saving, one might suspect that it is harmful to medicate our societies to such an extent, and I shall document that this is indeed the case.

The main reason we take so many drugs is that drug companies don't sell drugs, they sell lies about drugs. Blatant lies that – in all the cases I have studied – have continued after the statements were proven wrong. This is what makes drugs so different from anything else in life. If we wish to buy a car or a house, we may judge for ourselves whether it's a good or a bad buy, but if we are offered a drug, we have no such possibility. Virtually everything we know about drugs is what the companies have chosen to tell us and our doctors. Perhaps I should explain what I mean by a lie. A lie is a statement that isn't true, but a person who tells a lie is not necessarily a liar. Drug salespeople tell many lies, but they have often been deceived by their superiors in the company who deliberately withhold the truth from them (and are therefore liars, as I see it). In his nice little book *On Bullshit*, moral philosopher Harry Frankfurt says that one of the salient features of our culture is that there is so much bullshit, which he considers short of lying.

My book is not about the well-known benefits of drugs such as our great successes with treating infections, heart diseases, some cancers, and hormone deficiencies like type 1 diabetes. The book addresses a general system failure caused by widespread crime, corruption and impotent drug regulation in need of radical reforms. Some readers will find my book one-sided and polemic, but there is little point in describing what goes well in a system that is out of social control. If a criminologist undertakes a study of muggers, no one expects a 'balanced' account mentioning that many muggers are good family men.[4]

If you don't think the system is out of control, please email me and explain why drugs are the third leading cause of death in the part of the world that uses most drugs. If such a hugely lethal epidemic had been caused by a new bacterium or a virus, or even one-hundredth of it, we would have done everything we could to get it under control. The tragedy is that we could easily get our drug epidemic under control, but our politicians who hold the power to make changes do virtually nothing. When they act, they usually make matters worse because they have been so heavily lobbied by the industry that they have come to believe all its luring myths, which I shall debunk in every chapter of the book.

The main problem with our healthcare system is that the financial incentives that drive it seriously impede the rational, economical and safe use of drugs. The drug industry prospers on this and exerts tight information control. The research literature on drugs is systematically distorted through trials with flawed designs and analyses, selective publication of trials and data, suppression of unwelcome results, and ghostwritten papers. Ghostwriters write manuscripts for hire without revealing their identity in the papers, which have influential doctors as 'authors', although they have contributed little or nothing to the manuscript. This scientific misconduct sells drugs.

Compared to other industries, the pharmaceutical industry is the biggest defrauder of the US federal government under the False Claims Act.[5] The general public seems to know what the drug industry stands for. In an opinion poll that asked 5000 Danes to rank 51 industries in terms of the confidence they had in them, the drug industry came second to the bottom, only superseded by automobile repair companies.[6] A US poll also ranked the drug industry at the bottom, together with tobacco and oil companies.[7] In another survey, 79% of US citizens said the drug industry was doing a good job in 1997, which fell to 21% in 2005,[8] an extraordinarily rapid decline in public trust.

On this background, it seems somewhat contradictory that patients have great confidence in the medicines their doctors prescribe for them. But I am sure the reason patients trust their medicine is that they extrapolate the trust they have in their doctors into the medicines they prescribe. The patients don't realise that, although their doctors may know a lot about diseases and human physiology and psychology, they know very, very little about drugs that hasn't been carefully concocted and dressed up by the drug industry. Furthermore, they don't know that their doctors may have self-serving motives for choosing certain drugs for them, or that many of the crimes committed by the drug industry wouldn't be possible if doctors didn't contribute to them.

It is difficult to change systems and it is not surprising that people who have to live with a faulty system try to make the most out of it, even though it often results in well-intentioned people doing bad things. However, many people at senior levels in the drug industry cannot be excused in this way, as they have deliberately told lies to doctors, patients, regulators and judges.

I dedicate this book to the many honest people working in the drug industry who are equally appalled as I am about the repetitive criminal actions of their superiors and their harmful consequences for the patients and our national economies. Some of these insiders have told me they would wish their top bosses were sent to jail, as the threat of this is the only thing that might deter them from continuing committing crimes.

REFERENCES

1 Tobacco companies expand their epidemic of death. *Lancet.* 2011; 377: 528.

2 Diethelm PA, Rielle JC, McKee M. The whole truth and nothing but the truth? The research that Philip Morris did not want you to see. *Lancet.* 2005; 366: 86–92.

3 Tanne JH. Drug advertisements in US paint a 'black and white scenario'. *BMJ.* 2007; 334: 279.

4 Braithwaite J. *Corporate Crime in the Pharmaceutical Industry.* London: Routledge & Kegan Paul; 1984.

5 Almashat S, Preston C, Waterman T, *et al.* Rapidly increasing criminal and civil monetary penalties against the pharmaceutical industry: 1991 to 2010. *Public Citizen.* 2010 Dec 16.

6 Straarup B. [Good treatment – then hotels are no. 1]. *Berlingske Tidende.* 2005 Nov 25.

7 Harris G. Drug makers seek to mend their fractured image. *New York Times.* 2004; July 8.

8 Brody H. *Hooked: ethics, the medical profession, and the pharmaceutical industry.* Lanham: Rowman & Littlefield; 2008.

2 Confessions from an insider

'You should take two vitamin pills every day, a green and a red one,' my mother said. I was only about eight years old but asked,

'Why?'

'Because they are good for you.'

'How do you know?'

'Because grandfather says so.'

End of argument. Grandfather had a lot of authority. He was a general practitioner and he was bright and therefore right. When I studied medicine, I once asked him whether he had spared some textbooks I could compare with my own to see how much progress there had been in 50 years. His reply stunned me. He had donated all his books to younger students shortly after he qualified. He felt he didn't need them because he knew what they contained!

I had great respect for my grandfather and his superb memory, but I have scepticism in my genes. How could he be so sure the pills were good for me? In addition, the pills tasted and smelled bad despite being sugar-coated; opening the bottles felt like entering a pharmacy.

I dropped the pills and my mother undoubtedly found out why they lasted for so long but didn't try to force me into eating them.

It all looked so simple back then, in the late 1950s. As vitamins are essential for our survival, it must be good to eat vitamin pills to ensure we get enough of what we need to thrive. But biology is rarely simple. Human beings have developed over millions of years into the current species, which is very well adapted to its environment. Thus, if we eat a varied diet, we can expect to get adequate amounts of vitamins and other micronutrients. If some of our ancestors had gotten too little of an essential vitamin, they would have had less chance of reproducing their genes than people who needed less of the vitamin or absorbed it better.

We also need essential minerals, e.g. zinc and copper, to make our enzymes work. But if we ingest too much, we get intoxicated. Thus, given what we know about the human body, we cannot assume that vitamin pills must be healthy. It is the earliest memory I have of a medical prophylactic intervention, and it took about 50 years before it became known whether vitamins are beneficial or harmful. A 2008 review of the placebo-controlled trials of antioxidants (beta-carotene, vitamin A and vitamin E) showed that they increase overall mortality.[1]

Another childhood memory illustrates how harmful and deceitful the marketing of drugs is. Because of our generally bad weather in Denmark, my parents, who were teachers with long vacations, migrated south every summer. In the beginning only to Germany and Switzerland, but after some heavy bouts of bad weather with pouring rain even there, which isn't great fun when you live in a tent, northern Italy became the destination. My grandfather gave us Enterovioform (clioquinol) to be used if we got diarrhoea. This drug was launched in 1934 and had been very poorly studied.[2] What my grandfather didn't know and hadn't been told by the salesman from the Swiss company Ciba was that the drug only had a possible effect on diarrhoea caused by protozoans (amoebae and *Giardia*) and *Shigella* bacteria, and that even that effect could be disputed, as no ran-domised trials had compared the drug with placebo. Furthermore, it wasn't likely we would get exposed to such organisms in Italy. Traveller's diarrhoea is almost always caused by bacteria other than *Shigella* or by viruses.

Like so many other general practitioners, even nowadays, my grandfather appreciated visits by drug salespeople, but he had been the victim of shady marketing, which had caused the drug to be very commonly used.[3] Ciba started marketing clioquinol to fight amoebic dysentery,[2] but by the time the company entered the lucrative Japanese market in 1953, it was pushing clioquinol world-wide for all forms of dysentery. The drug is neurotoxic and caused a disaster in Japan where 10000 people had developed subacute myelo-optic neuropathy (SMON) by 1970.[2] SMON victims suffered a tingling in the feet that eventually turned into total loss of sensation and then paralysis of the feet and legs. Others suffered from blindness and other serious eye disorders.

Ciba, which later became Ciba-Geigy and Novartis, knew about the harms but concealed them for many years.[4] When the catastrophe in Japan became known, the company released statements defending the drug, saying that clio-quinol couldn't be the cause of SMON because it was essentially insoluble and couldn't be absorbed into the body.[2] However, attorneys preparing a lawsuit against the company found disturbing evidence that the drug could indeed be absorbed, which the company also knew. Already in 1944, clioquinol's inventors advised in light of animal studies that the administration of the drug be strictly controlled and that treatment should not exceed 2 weeks.

In 1965, a Swiss veterinarian published findings that dogs treated with clioqui-nol developed acute epileptic convulsions and died. Guess what Ciba's response was to this. Ciba inserted a warning in the drug's packaging in England that it should not be used in animals!

In 1966, two Swedish paediatricians studied a 3-year-old boy who had been treated with clioquinol and suffered severely impaired vision. They reported their findings in the medical literature and also informed Ciba that clioquinol was absorbed and could damage the optic nerve. These events, including the catastrophe in Japan, had no visible effect on the company that continued its marketing efforts worldwide. In 1976, clioquinol was still widely available as an over-the-counter drug for the prophylaxis and treatment of travellers' diarrhoea despite the lack of evidence that it was effective.[3] Package inserts from 35 coun-tries showed wide variation in dosage, duration of treatment, contraindications for use, side effects and warnings; a complete mess.

By 1981, Ciba-Geigy had paid out over $490 million to Japanese SMON vic-tims, but the company didn't take the drug off the market until 1985, 15 years after the catastrophe struck. In contrast, the Japanese Ministry of Health banned the drug 1 month after it became known in 1970 that clioquinol was behind the SMON tragedy.

The story also illustrates an all-too-common gross failure of drug regulatory agencies, which should have taken action but did nothing.

A third of my childhood memories about the drugs my grandfather used is about corticosteroids. When the newly synthesised cortisone was first given to 14 patients with rheumatoid arthritis in 1948 at the Mayo Clinic in Rochester, Minnesota, the effect was miraculous.[5] The results were so striking that some people believed a cure for rheumatoid arthritis had been discovered. Corticosteroids are highly effective for many other diseases, including asthma and eczema, but the initial enthusiasm evaporated quickly when it was discovered that they have many serious adverse effects, too.

In the mid-1960s, my grandfather broke his hip and the fracture wouldn't heal. He spent 2 years in hospital, lying immobilised on his back with his leg in a huge plaster. It must have been some sort of a record for a hip fracture. I have difficulty remembering exactly what he told me, but the reason for his troubles was that he had abused corticosteroids for many years. It was something about the drug having so many good effects that he thought it worth taking even if you were healthy, to increase your strength and to be cheered up. As I shall explain in later chapters, it seems that the dream of a 'quick fix', whether by a legal or an illegal drug, that improves our natural physical performance, mood or intellectual capacity, never dies.

Back then, I found it very likely that my grandfather had been persuaded by a drug salesperson to take the corticosteroids, as salespeople rarely say much about the harms of their drugs while they routinely exaggerate their benefits and recommend the drugs also for non-approved indications. In terms of sales, nothing beats persuading those who are healthy to consume drugs they don't need. All my childhood memories about drugs are negative. Drugs that were supposed to be beneficial harmed me. I suffered from motion sickness and my grandfather gave me a drug against this, undoubtedly an antihistamine, which made me so drowsy and uncomfortable that I decided after a few tries that it was worse than the disease and refused to have any more of it. Instead, I asked him to stop the car when I needed to vomit.

Young people are volatile and it can be hard to choose an occupation. When I was 15, I left school to become a radio mechanic because I had been a radio amateur for some years and was fascinated by it. In the middle of the summer, I changed my mind and started in the gymnasium, now convinced I would become a graduate electrical engineer, but that didn't last long either. I switched my interest to biology, which was one of the most popular subjects in the late 1960s; the other was psychology. We knew there weren't many jobs in either discipline but didn't care about such a trivial issue. After all, we became students in 1968 when the traditions were turned upside down and the world laid at our feet. We bubbled with optimism and what was most important was to find a personal philosophy of life. After having read Sartre and Camus, I subscribed to the idea that one should not follow routines, traditions or other people's advice but should decide for oneself. I changed my mind again and now wanted to become a doctor.

As it happened, I ended up taking both educations. I spent many vacations with my grandparents, and one of these visits convinced me that I should not waste my life on being a doctor. My grandfather had invited me into his surgery during my final year at school. It was situated in a wealthy part of Copenhagen and I couldn't avoid noticing that many of the problems the patients presented with weren't really anything to bother about, but a reflection of boredom. Many women had very little to do, didn't have a job and had servants who helped them look after the house. So why not pay the gentle and handsome doctor a visit, like in the joke about the three women who met regularly in the waiting room. One day, one was missing, and one of the others asks the last one what happened.

'Oh,' she replied, 'she couldn't come as she is ill.'

The study of animals seemed more meaningful and I rushed through the education as if it were a sporting contest only to realise that I still didn't know what to do with my life. My chances of getting a job were small, as I had not done any research during my studies or had taken other initiatives that would make employers more interested in me than in 50 others.

What most people did in this situation was to become a school teacher. I tried, but it didn't work out. I had barely left school before I was back again, the only difference being that I was now on the other side of the teacher's desk. I wasn't much older than my pupils and felt I belonged more to this group than to my new tribe of teachers who, moreover, smoked to an unbelievable extent. Although I could learn to smoke a pipe, I wasn't mature for such a job and also had difficulty accepting that this was what I was going to do for the next 45 years. Like life being over before it had started.

Two things particularly annoyed me during the 6 months where I tried to learn how to teach, being supervised by another teacher. In biology, we didn't use textbooks much, although wonderful textbooks were available. We were now in the dark 1970s where our universities and academic life at large were heavily influenced by dogmas, particularly Marxism, and it was not healthy to raise too many questions that things could perhaps be done differently. My supervisor required of me that, instead of using textbooks, I should produce the educational material myself because it needed to be relevant for the time we were living in. Some have aptly called these years the history-free period. I found myself cutting newspaper articles about the oil industry and pollution and spent endless hours at the photocopying machine putting my 'breaking news' compendia together. I don't wish to imply that such issues are not interesting or relevant, but my subject was biology, which goes back billions of years, so why this restless emphasis on something that happened yesterday?

The other problem was the prevailing fashion in pedagogy, which dictated that I needed to write down a detailed plan before each lecture outlining what learning goals I wanted to achieve, subgoals at that, how I would achieve them, etc. After each lecture I was expected to analyse my performance and discuss with my supervisor whether I had achieved all these goals. Thinking through what you wish to achieve beforehand and evaluating it afterwards is very reasonable of course, but there was so much of it that it drained me, as I am not the book-keeping type. I also lectured in chemistry, and particularly in that subject the rigid template felt like overkill. To teach people why and how chemical substances react is straightforward. Like in mathematics, there are some facts and principles people need to learn, and if they don't want to learn them, or cannot learn them, there isn't much the teacher can do. Imagine if a piano teacher was expected to construct similarly elaborate schemes before every music lesson she gave and evaluated herself afterwards. I am sure she would run away quickly.

The séances with my supervisors reminded me of the Danish lessons at the gymnasium where we were asked to interpret poems. I was quite bad at this type of guesswork and was irritated that the authors hadn't written more clearly what was on their mind if they wanted to communicate with us mortals. The lecturer was in a much better position, as he possessed a gold standard, which was a handbook written by a scholar who had interpreted the poems the teachers used. This is actually amusing. I have heard art critics interpret paintings, and when the artist was later asked whether they were right, he laughed and exclaimed that he didn't mean anything with his paintings, he just painted and had fun while doing it. Pablo Picasso painted in many different styles over the years and was once asked what he was searching for. Picasso replied: 'I don't search, I find.'

I did well according to my pupils but not according to my supervisors. I was told they could let me pass but with an evaluation that could make it difficult for me to get a job as a teacher. They preferred to fail me to give me a chance of thinking about whether I really wanted to be a teacher. This is the only time I have failed an exam, but I am immensely grateful that they made this wise decision. I had invested far too little effort in my new profession. My university years had been so easy that I hadn't dreamed about working in the evenings, in contrast to those teachers who were more successful than me. I had no idea that it was considered so difficult to teach. Later, I lectured at the university in the theory of science for more than 20 years.

After having applied for and not getting a few jobs as a chemist or biologist, my grandfather suggested I went into the drug industry. I sent three applications and was called for two interviews. My first experience was really weird. I could almost smell the vitamin pills of my childhood when I entered the office. The man who interviewed me had a dusty appearance and was partly bald-headed with long whiskers that would have made him a perfect character in a Western movie, selling snake oil or whiskey – someone whose used car you wouldn't buy. He was also the type of salesman I associated with one who sold ladies' underwear or perfume. Even the name of the company was old-fashioned. It was pretty clear that we both felt uncomfortable in each other's presence.

The second company was modern and attractive. It was the Astra Group, with headquarters in Sweden. I got the job and spent 7 weeks in Södertälje and Lund on various courses, which mostly dealt with human physiology, diseases and drugs. There was also a course in 'Information technique', which I suggested to the course leader should more appropriately be called 'Sales technique'. He didn't comment on my suggestion, but the course was about manipulating doctors into promising to use the company's products rather than those of its competitors, and to use even more of the company's drugs, to new types of patients, and in increased doses. It was all about increasing the sales, which we learned through role plays where some of us played various types of doctors, ranging from the sour to the forthcoming ones, and others tried to penetrate the palisades and 'close the deal'.

When I learned about drug usage, my first thought was: 'Gosh, it's amazing that there are so many drugs around and that they are used so much, for all kinds of ailments. Can it really be true that they are so effective that it justifies such massive use?'

I toured my district as a drug salesman, officially called a drug representative, and visited general practitioners, specialists and hospital doctors. I didn't like it. I had a full academic education with high marks behind me but felt inferior when I talked to doctors who sometimes treated me badly, which I fully understand. It must have been a nuisance to spend time with salespeople and I often wondered why they didn't say no. There were so many companies that it was common for a general practitioner to have more than one visit a week.

The academic challenges were very small and I realised that my university education would wither pretty quickly if I didn't move on to another job. The job also threatened my self-esteem and identity as a person. To be an effective salesman, you need to behave like a chameleon, adapting your own personality to the person in front of you. The risk of playing so many roles and pretending to agree with doctors you disagree with is that you lose yourself. I had read some of Søren Kierkegaard's works and knew that losing yourself was the worst mistake you could make. If you deceive not only the doctors but also yourself, it becomes too painful to look in the mirror and accept what you see. It is easier to be living a lie and it moved me deeply when I saw Arthur Miller's 1949 play, *Death of a Salesman*, years later at a theatre in London. I knew exactly what this was about.

The doctors listened to my sales pitches without asking uncomfortable questions, but on a couple of occasions they told me I was wrong. Astra had developed a new type of penicillin, azidocillin, which it had given a catchy name, Globacillin, as if it were effective against everything. In one of our campaigns, we tried to sell the drug for acute sinusitis. We informed the doctors about a study that showed that the drug penetrated into the mucosa in the difficult-to-reach sinuses where the bacteria were located and indicated that this was an advantage over usual penicillin. An ear, nose and throat surgeon told me that it wasn't possible to take biopsies and measure the concentration of an antibiotic in the mucosa, as one would inadvertently include capillaries in the sample where the concentration was higher. It was very humiliating for me to be told by a specialist that my company had cheated me. Academics are trained to think for themselves, but I lacked the skills to do so in a medical context.

Another argument for using the new, more expensive drug was that its effect on a particular bacterium, *Haemophilus influenzae*, was 5–10 times better than penicillin. This claim resulted from laboratory experiments in a Petri dish. The right questions to ask would have been:

1. Were these studies performed by the company and have the results been replicated by independent researchers?
2. What is the effect of treating acute sinusitis with penicillin or azidocillin,

compared with placebo? And if there is an effect, is it then large enough to justify routine treatment of sinusitis with antibiotics, considering the adverse effects of the drugs?

3. Most important, has azidocillin been compared with penicillin in randomised trials of acute sinusitis, and was the effect any better?

Such questions would have made it clear that there was no rational basis for using azidocillin. We nevertheless succeeded to sell the drug with our doubtful arguments to some doctors for some time, but it is no longer on the market.

After only 8 months as a salesman, I left the roads and became a product manager with responsibility for written materials and for our 3-yearly sales campaigns, in collaboration with the sales manager. It doesn't make me proud to recollect what we were doing. We sold a drug against asthma, terbutaline (Bricanyl), and in one of the campaigns we tried to convince the doctors that the patients needed not only constant treatment with pills but also with a spray. Again, we didn't give the doctors the relevant information, which would have been the results of randomised trials of the combination treatment versus treatment with either spray or pills.

ASTHMA DEATHS WERE CAUSED BY ASTHMA INHALERS

Today, regular treatment with inhalers containing drugs like terbutaline is not recommended; in fact, such treatments have been proscribed in most guidelines because of safety concerns. Epidemiologist Neil Pearce from New Zealand has written a most disturbing account of the powers of the drug industry and its paid allies among doctors in relation to asthma.[6] When the inhalers came on the market in the 1960s, asthma death rates went up in the same way the sales did, and after the regulators had warned about overuse, they both went down again. Pearce wanted to study one of the drugs in detail, isoprenaline from Riker, and received data from the company that expected his research would show that the theory about the drugs causing the deaths was wrong. However, he confirmed the theory and when he sent his manuscript to the company (which one should *never* do), they told him he would be sued. His university promised to make its lawyers available in case of litigation and he published the paper, but now became fiercely attacked by asthma specialists.

Doctors tend to become very angry if you tell them they have harmed their patients, even when they have done that in good faith. I have written a whole book about my experiences after I demonstrated in 1999 the harmful consequences of mammography screening, which converts many healthy women to cancer patients unnecessarily.[7]

This was in 1972. But, although Pearce's findings were supported at the time, asthma experts told him 16 years later when he entered asthma research again that the theory had been proven wrong. No one was able to tell him how or what the explanation then was for the increase and fall in asthma deaths in the 1960s. The misconception seemed to have been created and fuelled by the doubt industry, i.e. drug companies commissioning substandard research to their hired consultants among the asthma specialists. 'Doubt is our product' a tobacco executive once said,[8] and this smokescreen always seems to work. Create a lot of paid noise and confuse people into disbelieving the original, rigorous study and believing the noise instead.

In 1976, a new epidemic of asthma deaths began in New Zealand. When Pearce's colleagues suggested it might be caused by overtreatment, they were met by extremely hostile reactions from the official Asthma Task Force that believed the problem was undertreatment. This is a standard industry position, and indeed the major funder of asthma research in New Zealand was Boehringer Ingelheim, the maker of fenoterol (Berotec).

When Pearce et al. found out that the new epidemic mirrored the sales curve for fenoterol, all hell broke loose. They met resistance from all quarters and demands that others should carefully scrutinise their data, not only people with amicable relations to the company; the company itself also requested the data. A lawyer prudently advised them to ignore all legal threats and not show the paper to the company before it was accepted for publication.

Pressures mounted, also from the Medical Research Council, although it hadn't funded the study, and the university. They didn't understand, or chose to ignore, that they had no right whatsoever to interfere with the research. The only way out was therefore to go to the top, the Department of Health, where the researchers learned, however, that Boehringer Ingelheim had been there first. All sorts of false rumours were spread, including false allegations that there was no protocol for the study, although this protocol had been seen by the Asthma Foundation and the Medical Research Council that refused to fund the study. Boehringer Ingelheim succeeded in postponing – and almost preventing – publication in the *Lancet*, which got cold feet after having accepted the paper because of the immense pressure. *Lancet* received several lengthy faxes every day from the company and had to ask them to stop.

Boehringer Ingelheim had invested a lot in the physicians and it paid off. Their sympathy was on the company's side, being concerned that its New Zealand branch might close down; they were not thinking of their patients. The Department of Health also sided with the company and broke the confidentiality by giving the company a copy of the manuscript it had requested from the researchers.

It was as bad as it could be. The researchers' first study was unfunded and so was the next one, and Dunedin Hospital refused to allow them access to its records. The Department of Health would not give the researchers any assurance that it would not also show the manuscript from the second study to the company, and when it didn't get it in the first place from the researchers, it requested it from their university under the Freedom of Information Act. Boehringer gave the researchers' data to its paid friends so that they could come up with other results even before the original data appeared in print.

This was an outrageous transgression of the ethical ground rules for science, but despite its dirty methods, Boehringer lost the battle. The market share for fenoterol dropped from 30% to less than 3% in just 3 years and asthma deaths plummeted simultaneously, vindicating the research by Pearce et al.

SHADY MARKETING AND RESEARCH

At one time, we visited chest physicians and showed them a film of small white particles that had been placed in the mucus in the windpipe. The movement of these particles towards the mouth was recorded with and without giving the patients terbutaline, and the story was that the cilia moved the particles faster when patients were treated. The idea was to convince the doctors that they should not only use the drug for asthma, but also for smoker's lungs (chronic bronchitis). These patients cough a lot, which is why a quicker transport of irritants out of the lungs was speculated to be beneficial. But yet again, a simple question would have revealed that the emperor had no clothes. There were no randomised trials that had shown that terbutaline was effective in patients with chronic bronchitis. Even today, terbutaline is only approved for asthma and other bronchospasm, not for chronic bronchitis.

It is illegal to market a drug for non-approved indications, so-called off-label use. As we shall see in the next chapter, illegal marketing is very common, and it is also routine that the companies circumvent the law. It is not illegal to discuss research results with doctors, and we could therefore show the film without breaking the law as long as we did not suggest to the doctors to use the drug for chronic bronchitis. If they had asked, we could say that we weren't allowed to recommend the drug for this indication but that the results were interesting, and that the doctors were free to use drugs for whatever purpose they found reasonable. Absurdly, such indirect recommendations are not illegal. In my opinion, they should be. There is no good reason to present preliminary research results to practising clinicians; it is only reasonable to discuss them with academic researchers with the purpose of embarking on a definitive clinical trial hoping the new indication will be approved by the drug regulators.

We also balanced on the edge of the law with another indication, but before I come to this, I need to explain what The Cochrane Collaboration is. It is a non-profit organisation that was started in 1993 by Iain Chalmers in Oxford, United Kingdom. It built on a common frustration among researchers and others that most medical research is of poor quality and biased, and a realisation that we needed rigorous systematic reviews of the randomised trials that could tell us more clearly what the benefits and harms of our interventions are. Once established, The Cochrane Collaboration grew quickly and currently engages about 30 000 people. The reviews are published electronically in The Cochrane Library, and there are more than 5000 such reviews, which are regularly updated. Half of the world's population have free access to the full reviews through national subscriptions usually financed by governments; the other half have access to the abstracts.

Coughing is very common and there is a huge market for over-the-counter cough medicines. A Cochrane systematic review of the randomised trials shows that none of them are effective,[9] which means that the huge market is also a huge waste of money. Drugs like terbutaline don't appear to work either,[10] but someone in Astra coined the idea that we should suggest to doctors that terbutaline had an effect on cough, with reference to the study illustrated in the mucosa film.

I didn't believe this. Why should a drug used for dilating the airways in patients with asthma work for cough that was not caused by bronchospasm? Whatever the legal technicalities, I regard this as off-label promotion, and there were no witnesses that could testify to which degree the doctors were directly encouraged to try the drug for cough, as most encounters were on a one-to-one basis where only the doctor and the salesperson were present.

We also did something good. We produced an illustrated guidance for patients with asthma in eight steps about how to use the spray, which also showed how one could estimate the remaining number of doses by immersing the container in water and see whether it floated or went to the bottom.

During my 2 years with Astra, from 1975 to 1977, we launched a new product, zinc lozenges, which was approved for treatment of venous and ischaemic leg ulcers and a very rare zinc deficiency disease, acrodermatitis enteropathica, which affected the uptake of zinc. I still have the 20-page brochure I wrote for the launch, which was based on a similar brochure in Swedish.

It is revealing to compare the brochure with the Cochrane review on zinc for leg ulcers.[11] The first study in the brochure is also the biggest and it was published in a prestigious journal, the *Lancet*, which is very attractive for marketing purposes. The results were impressive.[12] According to the brochure, the ulcers in the 52 patients treated with zinc were healed after 32 days whereas it took 77 days for the 52 placebo-treated patients. However, the trial was unreliable. The brochure stated that because the results for the first 16 patients clearly showed which group was treated with zinc, it was not possible to continue the study in a double-blind fashion. The study was excluded from the Cochrane review because it wasn't randomised, which we usually expect blinded studies to be.

The brochure reported positive effects from the randomised trials, but the Cochrane authors interpreted the same trials differently. They included six small trials of mediocre quality and found no evidence of a beneficial effect of zinc. Like Globacillin, zinc disappeared from the market.

In 1977, I was offered a job at Astra-Syntex, a new joint-venture company between Astra and the California-based Syntex. My task was to establish a medical department and to be responsible for clinical trials and registration applications for new drugs and indications. I was very happy to leave marketing but also had concerns about the research the industry did and wanted to leave. I chose the most arduous way out and started to study medicine in 1978 while I continued to work for the company. I qualified 6 years later and left the company to work at different hospitals in Copenhagen.

Astra-Syntex's survival hinged on just one drug, naproxen (Naprosyn), a nonsteroidal anti-inflammatory drug (NSAID) used for arthritis. I performed several trials with the drug and discovered along the way that I wasn't immune to company influence. There were many NSAIDs on the market, but somehow you get so used to the idea that *your* drug *might* be better than the others that you end thinking it *is* better, just as if it had been your child. One of the reasons why marketing of medicines is so effective is that the salespeople believe they are selling a very good drug.

A clear indication of my naïvety was that I asked the European headquarters in London why we didn't perform a trial comparing naproxen with a simple analgesic such as paracetamol, for example in sports injuries. The medical director kindly explained that they were not interested in such a trial but never said why, although I asked on more than one occasion. The reason was of course that such a trial might show that a much cheaper analgesic was equally effective, and on top of that we already knew that paracetamol was much safer than naproxen. In order to lure people into preferring naproxen for paracetamol, it was therefore necessary to give the doctors the impression – without having any data to support it – that naproxen was more effective.

The trick was done using theoretical arguments. This is a very powerful marketing tool, although the arguments rarely hold water. In textbooks of pharmacology, naproxen is described as having anti-inflammatory properties and the hyped argument goes somewhat like this: When you have a sports injury, there is tissue injury and inflammation with oedema, and it is important to dampen the inflammation to speed up the recovery.

It is very easy to lure doctors into doing wrong things by making them listen to the songs of the sirens while paying many of them, both for singing and for listening (*see* Chapter 8). As I shall explain in detail later, NSAIDs are dangerous drugs and many thousands of people are killed every year because of bleeding stomach ulcers and heart attacks, to mention just the two worst harms. But marketing is all that is needed. A couple of years ago, Danish TV focused on the liberal use of NSAIDs in professional football clubs for all sorts of pain. The prescription status of the drugs wasn't a hindrance, as the sports doctors provided large supplies of the drugs, letting the footballers take as many as they wanted without even asking. There was a scandal, but as is usual with scandals, it quickly died out and I suppose it is now business as usual.

Around 1980, I was approached by a rheumatologist who looked after the Danish national football team. He wanted to find out whether naproxen was better than aspirin for sports injuries. Aspirin is also an NSAID – the oldest one in existence and very cheap – but it is often used in low doses where it is assumed to have no anti-inflammatory effects, only an analgesic effect. We did the trial, using low-dose aspirin despite the concerns of my superiors in London, and just as they had predicted, there were no significant differences between the two drugs. However, the results were analysed by our statistics department in Sweden, which went on a 'fishing expedition' that eventually found something that could lessen the company's pains that naproxen wasn't any better than aspirin. The abstract of the published paper says:[13]

'Fresh injuries were over-represented in the acetylsalicylic acid group (p<0.01), and when all patients were analyzed together [i.e. from both treatment arms], a significantly better treatment result was obtained the shorter the interval between injury and start of treatment. This might have influenced the results from this study.'

Oh boy. I have contributed to this as an author. In principle, there is nothing wrong with reservations in an abstract, but imagine if naproxen had been significantly better than aspirin and there had been more fresh injuries in the naproxen group. Would this reservation about the good news for the company then have made it into the abstract? Hardly, and I doubt there would have been anything about this in the main text of the article either.

We first submitted our paper to *British Journal of Sports Medicine*. The editor was keenly aware of the commercial priorities in the industry; he said he was surprised that we posted our study from Syntex, as our work contradicted the claims the company had made about naproxen being more effective than paracetamol and aspirin. We were startled that an editor so frankly sided with a company's commercial interests and his next remark made us laugh. He noted that 18 patients received aspirin during the first 3 days of injury compared to only 2 on naproxen. He then suggested that a more fair comparison could be made if we were to treat another group of patients, at least 16 in number, with naproxen during the first 3 days following the injury. If we were willing to do this, he would reconsider our paper seriously. My goodness! How did he imagine we could include another 16 patients on only one of the drugs in a randomised double-blind trial? It cannot be done. We effectively buried the trial – although it wasn't our intention – by publishing it in a fairly unknown journal that stopped coming out 5 years later.[13]

I always wondered how it was possible to say that NSAIDs have anti-inflammatory effects, or whether it was only a marketing ploy. If a drug has an analgesic effect, it will lead to faster mobilisation, which would be expected to decrease the oedema. How could one then postulate that there was also a separate anti-inflammatory effect? NSAIDs had some effect in rats that had been treated in such a way that their paws were swollen and tender, but what did that prove? I often raised this issue with rheumatologists, but I never received a satisfactory answer.

However, one day I was contacted by a group of orthopaedic surgeons who wanted to study the effect of naproxen in ankle distorsions. I grabbed the opportunity to study also the effect on the oedema, which we measured by immersing the foot in water and comparing its volume with that of the other foot. It was a highly interesting study. We randomised 173 patients twice: to crutches or no crutches (mobilisation), and to naproxen or placebo. This so-called factorial design is much underused despite its elegance, which is that it can provide answers to two questions without needing more patients than if only one question was asked. The results surprised us.[14] The patients recovered faster when they were mobilised, which also decreased the oedema, whereas naproxen had no effect on the oedema. Our marketing-oriented bosses in Sweden interfered again with our research, and there were no numerical data on either of these outcomes in our published paper. However, I have kept the more comprehensive internal study report and the effect of mobilisation was dramatic. At the first follow-up visit after 2–4 days, 30 of 68 patients had recovered, compared to only 10 of 63 patients in the group using crutches, and the difference in volume between the two feet was only 28 mL when the patients were mobilised, compared to 71 mL when crutches were used.

It was a beautiful study that had implications for practice. Years later, after a serious ankle distorsion, I stumbled along in great pain during a trip to London to attend the *British Medical Journal*'s *(BMJ)* advisory board meeting and I moved with immense difficulty. One of the other members of the board asked me why I didn't use crutches and I replied that I had shown in a trial that patients recover faster if they don't. Our trial inspired him to do a systematic review of bed rest for all diseases and he identified 39 trials (5777 patients) with 15 different conditions.[15] He found that it is harmful to immobilise people in a bed; not a single outcome improved significantly whereas several outcomes worsened.

We submitted our trial to *Acta Orthopaedica*, a humble Nordic journal, but its editors didn't understand how important it was and rejected it. We had also tried the *BMJ* and my co-authors now just wanted to get the trial out. I couldn't convince them that it was too important to publish in Danish, but that's what happened after we had translated the paper. Years later, I was approached by a researcher working on a systematic review of treatment of soft tissue injuries, and he told me that our study was not only the largest but also the best, so he asked me to translate our Danish paper into English!

In 1990, I defended my doctoral thesis, *Bias in Double-Blind Trials*,[16] which consisted of six papers. I had analysed 244 reports of trials in depth that had compared one NSAID with another. It was the first time a whole therapeutic area had been so thoroughly investigated and I uncovered an overwhelming amount of bias favouring the sponsoring company's drug over the control drug. The trial reports were generally so unreliable that they should be seen not as scientific publications but as advertisements for the drugs.

I had also assembled trials that compared an NSAID with placebo, which I used to study whether there is any anti-inflammatory effect with NSAIDs. In some trials, the researchers had used jeweller rings to measure if the drugs had an effect on swollen finger joints in patients with rheumatoid arthritis. They hadn't.[17] I therefore believe the idea of an anti-inflammatory effect of NSAIDs is a hoax, like so many other myths about drugs that the drug companies have invented and marketed.

It is highly unfortunate that the drug companies define for us how we should think about drugs, as their manipulations are so massive. For example, it is common to talk about second-generation or even third-generation drugs, e.g. second-generation antipsychotics. This gives you the impression that they are better than old drugs, which is rarely what independent, publicly funded researchers find when they compare them in large randomised trials.

Like Astra, Astra-Syntex also engaged in unethical marketing. The standard dose of naproxen was 500 mg daily, but the salespeople were asked to persuade the doctors to use 1000 mg, equipped with dose-response studies that had been written up by the company. I reviewed such studies as part of my thesis,[18] and they were terribly flawed. In the naproxen studies, the patients received placebo and two or three different doses of naproxen in a crossover design where all patients tried each treatment in random order. The doses varied between 250 mg and 1500 mg daily. Many of the outcomes were not reported and with a British understatement I called the statistical methods 'rather unusual'.[18]

None of the papers presented any graphs that could tell the readers what was gained by using a higher dose. Instead, a significant linear relationship between dose and response was claimed, which gives the readers the clear message that by doubling the dose, they double the effect. This comes close to fraud. I presented nine dose-response curves in my review of NSAIDs and an example is shown in Figure 2.1. There is nothing to be gained by using higher doses. The difference between 250 mg and 1500 mg naproxen is six times in terms of money but only 1.0 cm on a 10 cm pain scale, and the least difference in pain patients can perceive is about 1.3 cm.[19] The difference of 1.0 cm therefore makes no difference for the patients. The smallest clinically relevant effect, i.e. an effect that might make it worthwhile to take a drug or increase the dose, is larger than what the patients can barely perceive. In contrast, the harms actually *do* increase in a linear fashion so that twice the dose means twice the amount of harms.[20] As some harms are serious, e.g. bleeding ulcers and death, these drugs should be used at the lowest possible dose.

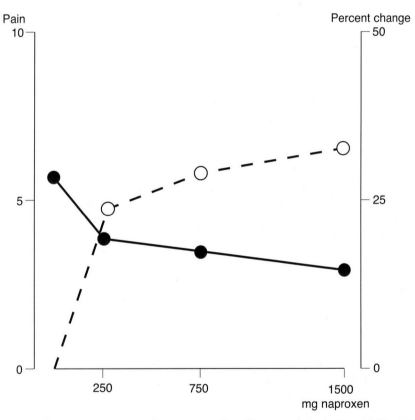

Figure 2.1 Dose-response curve for naproxen. The effect on pain is shown with black dots (10 is the highest pain possible) and the mean percentage improvement for all the reported outcomes is shown with open circles

Such manipulations with the science have the intended effect, to increase sales. Few doctors are able to read research reports critically and they might have forgotten what they learned in clinical pharmacology. The dose-response curves for drugs virtually always have the shape of a hyperbola and standard doses are quite high, corresponding to the uppermost part of the curve where the effect levels off and approaches a ceiling (*see* Figure 2.1).

The marketing of naproxen is an unequivocal example that drug companies put profits before patients and don't care that their actions increase deaths. The worst company was not Astra-Syntex, however, it was Pfizer. There was general agreement in other companies that Pfizer's marketing was particularly aggressive and ruthless.[21] Pfizer's NSAID, piroxicam (Feldene), was also touted at a very high dose.[18] Piroxicam has a long half-life and we therefore felt it was inappropriate to use it in the elderly, as their impaired elimination mechanisms lead to accumulation of the drug and increased toxicity.

Pfizer's marketing was very successful and completely untruthful, stating that piroxicam was more effective than aspirin and had a lower rate of gastrointestinal side effects than many other NSAIDs.[22] The truth was the opposite: piroxicam had more fatal reactions and more fatal gastrointestinal side effects than other drugs. Nonetheless, the US and UK drug regulators protected Pfizer all along instead of protecting the patients, and Pfizer tried to dissuade the editors of the *BMJ* to publish a paper that concluded about the high incidence of severe ulcer disease with piroxicam.[23] Pfizer even denied indisputable facts, e.g. that greater concentrations of an NSAID in the blood increase the risk of harms, and the company tried to get away with a ludicrous statement that the gastrointestinal toxicity to a large part was due to a local effect on the stomach rather than a systemic effect. Even if it had been correct, the harms inflicted on the patients would be the same. It is telling in relation to whether good or bad manners pay off that Pfizer became the largest drug company in the world.

Another company, Eli Lilly, also continued its aggressive marketing of its NSAID, benoxaprofen (Opren or Oraflex), undisturbed by the terrible harms they knew their drug caused.[22] The company touted that, based on laboratory experiments, the drug was different from other NSAIDs in having an effect on the disease process, but this wasn't true. Lilly presented a series of 39 patients that experienced a worsening of their joint damage, but the company concluded exactly the opposite.

Lilly ignored or trivialised the harms and failed to inform the authorities of liver failure and deaths, which a subsequent court case described as 'standard practice in the industry'.[24,25] Lilly published a paper in the *BMJ* that claimed that no cases of jaundice or deaths had been reported, but this wasn't true.[22] Furthermore, benoxaprofen causes other horrible harms, e.g. photosensitivity in 10% of patients and loosening of the nails from the nailbed in 10%, but it was approved despite this and despite insufficient animal toxicology studies, in violation of the Food and Drug Administration's (FDA's) own rules. When independent researchers found that benoxaprofen accumulated in the elderly, Lilly tried to prevent the study from being published and, as always, the UK drug regulator's action was grossly inadequate and allowed Lilly to trivialise the problem. These omissions proved fatal for some elderly patients, and the drug was withdrawn after only 2 years on the market.

I doubt any drug regulator can convince the patients that it was a good idea to approve a drug that harms at least one in five patients pretty badly when there were many less harmful NSAIDs on the market.

The FDA violated its own rules for several other NSAIDs, which, for example, had shown troubling carcinogenicity in animals and should therefore not have been approved, or drugs for which the animal studies were either insufficient or fraudulent, as many of the rats had never existed. The FDA even downplayed highly statistically significant findings in two rodent species and called them marginal or benign although they were malignant.[22]

The NSAID area is a horror story filled with extravagant claims, bending of the rules, regulatory inaction, and complacency with what the industry wants even though statements from industry scientists were often logically inconsistent or plainly wrong.[22] Several drugs that were so kindly treated by the FDA were later withdrawn from the market because of their toxicity despite claims to the contrary, e.g. 'Excellent gastrointestinal tolerance' (benoxaprofen), 'superior tolerance' (indoprofen), 'proven gastrointestinal safety' (rofecoxib), 'hurts the pain not the patient' (ketorolac) and 'least possible side effect profile' (tolmetin).[24] Sheer nonsense, as a least possible side-effect profile can only occur if you don't take a drug at all. Other withdrawn drugs are, for example, zomepirac, suprofen and valdecoxib.[22,26]

The NSAID story illustrates that drug regulators are consistently willing to award the benefit of scientific doubt to manufacturers rather than patients and also that the regulators became even more permissive during the 1980s.[22] As I shall show in later chapters, and illustrate with newer NSAIDs and other drugs, this decline in drug safety has continued.

REFERENCES

1 Bjelakovic G, Nikolova D, Gluud LL, *et al*. Antioxidant supplements for prevention of mortality in healthy participants and patients with various diseases. *Cochrane Database Syst Rev*. 2008; 2: CD007176.

2 Knaus H. Corporate profile, Ciba Geigy: pushing pills and pesticides. *Multinational Monitor*. 1993. Available online at: http://multinationalmonitor.org/hyper/issues/1993/04/mm0493_11.html (accessed 10 July 2012).

3 Dunne M, Flood M, Herxheimer A. Clioquinol: availability and instructions for use. *J Antimicrob Chemother*. 1976; 2: 21–9.

4 Hansson O. *Arzneimittel-Multis und der SMON-Skandal*. Berlin: Arzneimittel-Informations-Dienst GmbH; 1979.

5 Hench PS, Kendall EC, Slocumb CH, *et al*. The effect of a hormone of the adrenal cortex (17-hydroxy-11-dehydrocorticosterone; compound E) and of pituitary adrenocorticotropic hormone on rheumatoid arthritis. *Proc Staff Meet Mayo Clin*. 1949; 24: 181–97.

6 Pearce N. *Adverse Reactions: the fenoterol story*. Auckland: Auckland University Press; 2007.

7 Gøtzsche PC. *Mammography Screening: truth, lies and controversy*. London: Radcliffe Publishing; 2012.

8 Michaels D. *Doubt is their Product*. Oxford: Oxford University Press; 2008.

9 Smith SM, SchroederK, Fahey T. Over-the-counter (OTC) medications for acute cough in children and adults in ambulatory settings. *Cochrane Database Syst Rev*. 2008; 1: CD001831.

10 Tomerak AAT, Vyas HHV, Lakhanpaul M, *et al*. Inhaled beta2-agonists for non-specific chronic cough in children. *Cochrane Database Syst Rev*. 2005; 3: CD005373.

11 Wilkinson EAJ, Hawke CC. Oral zinc for arterial and venous leg ulcers. *Cochrane Database Syst Rev*. 1998; 4: CD001273 (updated in 2010).

12 Husain SL. Oral zinc sulphate in leg ulcers. *Lancet*. 1969; 1: 1069–71.

13 Andersen LA, Gøtzsche PC. Naproxen and aspirin in acute musculoskeletal disorders: a double-blind, parallel study in sportsmen. *Pharmatherapeutica*. 1984; 3: 535–41.

14 Jørgensen FR, Gøtzsche PC, Hein P, *et al*. [Naproxen (Naprosyn) and mobilization in the treatment of acute ankle sprains]. *Ugeskr Læger*. 1986; 148: 1266–8.

15 Allen C, Glasziou P, Del Mar C. Bed rest: a potentially harmful treatment needing more careful evaluation. *Lancet*. 1999; 354: 1229–33.

16 Gøtzsche PC. Bias in double-blind trials. *Dan Med Bull*. 1990; 37: 329–36.

17 Gøtzsche PC. Sensitivity of effect variables in rheumatoid arthritis: a meta-analysis of 130 placebo controlled NSAID trials. *J Clin Epidemiol.* 1990; **43**: 1313–18.

18 Gøtzsche PC. Review of dose-response studies of NSAIDs in rheumatoid arthritis. *Dan Med Bull.* 1989; **36**: 395–9.

19 Lopez BL, Flenders P, Davis-Moon L. Clinically significant differences in the visual analog pain scale in acute vasoocclusive sickle cell crisis. *Hemoglobin.* 2007; **31**: 427–32.

20 Gøtzsche PC. Non-steroidal anti-inflammatory drugs. *Clinical Evidence.* 2004; **12**: 1702–10.

21 Rost P. *The Whistleblower: confessions of a healthcare hitman.* New York: Soft Skull Press; 2006.

22 Abraham J. *Science, Politics and the Pharmaceutical Industry.* London: UCL Press; 1995.

23 Henry D, Lim LL, Garcia Rodriguez LA, *et al.* Variability in risk of gastrointestinal complications with individual non-steroidal anti-inflammatory drugs: results of a collaborative meta-analysis. *BMJ.* 1996; **312**: 1563–6.

24 Virapen J. *Side Effects: death.* College Station: Virtualbookworm.com Publishing; 2010.

25 Joyce C, Lesser F. Opren deaths kept secret, admits Lilly. *New Sci.* 1985; **107**: 15–16.

26 Cotter J. New restrictions on celecoxib (Celebrex) use and the withdrawal of valdecoxib (Bextra). *CMAJ.* 2005; **172**: 1299.

Organised crime, the business model of big pharma

Drug companies never talk about the benefits and harms of their drugs but about their efficacy and safety. Words create what they describe and the preferred semantics is seductive. It makes you think it can only be good for you to take drugs, as they are both efficacious and safe. Another reason why patients and doctors generally trust their drugs as being both efficacious and safe is that they think they have been carefully tested by the drug industry and carefully scrutinised by the drug regulatory agencies using high standards before they are allowed onto the market.

It's the other way round. In contrast to food and water, which are not only pretty harmless but something we need to survive, drugs are generally neither efficacious nor safe. Paracelsus stated 500 years ago that all drugs are poisons and that the right dose differentiates a poison from a remedy. Drugs always cause harm. If they didn't, they would be inert and therefore unable to give any benefit. For all drugs, it is therefore essential to find a dose that causes more good than harm in most patients. Even when we succeed with this, most patients will still not achieve any benefit from the drugs they take (*see* Chapter 4).

Although it is rather obvious that drugs can kill you, this is often forgotten, both by patients and doctors. People trust their medicines to such a degree that the Canadian physician Sir William Osler (1849–1919) wrote that 'the desire to take medicine is perhaps the greatest feature which distinguishes man from animals'.[1] A particularly amusing example is botulinum toxin, which is a neurotoxin produced by the bacterium *Clostridium botulinum*. It is one of the strongest poisons in nature, and a dose of only 50 ng killed half of the monkeys in a toxicity study (which means that 1 g can kill 10 million monkeys). I wonder who needed this information so badly that it was worth killing our animal relatives to get it. And yet, what is this amazing killer drug used for? For treating wrinkles between the eyebrows! This comes with age, but you shouldn't be too old and have too much tremor when you inject the toxin, as it can be absorbed from the mucous membranes in the eye and kill you. The package insert warns that deaths have occurred. Is it really worth running a risk of dying, however small it might be, just because you have wrinkles? Other questions that pop up are: Can the drug be used for suicide or murder? Why was it ever approved?

The fact that drugs are dangerous and should be used with caution means that the ethical standards for those who do research on drugs and market them should be very high. I have talked to many people in the drug industry to find out what the companies think of themselves, and the replies have ranged from very positive ones from people who were proud of the clinical trials they carried out to very negative ones. What is perhaps more interesting is to see which impression the drug companies want to give of themselves to the public and to compare this with what they actually do. The Pharmaceutical Research and Manufacturers of America (PhRMA) claims its members are 'committed to following the highest ethical standards as well as all legal requirements'.[2] Its *Code on Interactions with Healthcare Professionals* states that:[3]

> Ethical relationships with healthcare professionals are critical to our mission of helping patients ... An important part of achieving this mission is ensuring that healthcare professionals have the latest, most accurate information available regarding prescription medicines.

Here is another quotation. Under the heading, FOCUS ENGAGEMENT HONESTY, came this text: 'Our goal is to be the world's most successful, respected and socially responsible consumer ware producer.'[4] As you'll see shortly, the drug industry's actions have very little to do with honesty, respect and social responsibility. How could they then write this about themselves? Well, they didn't. They could have, but the quotation comes from a newspaper advertisement for Philip Morris that shows a portrait of a smiling young woman who won't continue to look so good if she smokes.

I tell you this to illustrate that not even the most deadly industry on the planet can resist the temptation of spreading bullshit while they increase the total consumption of tobacco because their marketing is directly targeted towards teenagers in the developing countries who have not yet started smoking. This marketing more than compensates for the decline in smoking in developed countries. How can it be socially responsible to deliberately kill millions of people every year who didn't need the product in the first place? People who have tried to smoke a cigarette know what I'm talking about. Aged 15, I only succeeded in smoking half a cigarette before I became so intoxicated that I vomited and left school to go directly to bed, as white as my sheets. My mother wondered what terrible disease had hit me so hard and told me later that she'd found half a cigarette in my shirt pocket.

The disconnect between the drug industry's proclamations of 'highest ethical standards', 'following ... all legal requirements' and 'most accurate information available regarding prescription medicines' and the reality of big pharma's conduct is also vast. The top executives' views of themselves – or rather the impression they try to convey about their activities – are not even shared by their own employees. An internal 2001 survey of Pfizer employees, which is not available to the public, showed that about 30% didn't agree with the statement, 'Senior management demonstrates honest, ethical behavior.'[5]

In 2012, Pfizer agreed to pay $60 million to settle a US federal investigation into bribery overseas. Pfizer wasn't only accused of bribing doctors, but also hospital administrators and drug regulators in several countries in Europe and Asia.[6] The investigators said Pfizer units sought to hide the bribery by listing the payments in accounting records as legitimate expenses, such as training, freight and entertainment. According to court papers, the company wired monthly payments for what it described as 'consultancy services' to a doctor in Croatia who helped decide what drugs the government would register for sale and reimbursement. Pfizer didn't admit or deny the allegations, which is routine practice when drug companies settle accusations of fraud.

HOFFMAN–LA ROCHE, THE BIGGEST DRUG PUSHER

The 10 largest drug companies[7] are all signatories to the US PhRMA code, apart from Hoffman-La Roche, Switzerland,[3] which was the largest corporate fraudster worldwide in the 1990s according to a 1999 listing of all industries, including banks and oil.[8] High-level Roche executives led a cartel that, according to the US Justice Department's antitrust division, was the most pervasive and harmful criminal antitrust conspiracy ever uncovered.[9] Top executives at some of the world's biggest drug companies, largely from Europe and Asia, met secretly in hotel suites and at conferences. Working together in a coalition they brazenly called 'Vitamins Inc.', they carved up world markets and carefully orchestrated price increases, in the process defrauding some of the world's biggest food companies. Roche alone had revenues of $3.3 billion in the United States while the conspiracy was running, and during that time, the conspirators gradually and artfully raised the prices of raw vitamins, so as not to attract notice; they also rigged the bidding process.[9]

The Justice Department charged Kuno Sommer, former Director of Worldwide Marketing, Hoffmann-La Roche Vitamins and Fine Chemicals Division, with participating in the vitamin cartel and for lying to Department investigators in 1997 in an attempt to cover up the conspiracy.[10] Sommer pleaded guilty and got a 4-month prison term. After the conspiracy collapsed, those involved agreed to pay nearly $1 billion to settle federal antitrust charges, and virtually every big vitamin maker in the world was on the brink of agreeing to pay an additional $1 billion. Roche agreed to pay $500 million, equivalent to about 1 year's revenue from its vitamin business in the United States, and two executives were sentenced to prison terms of a few months. In Europe, the European Commission fined some of the world's biggest drug companies, including Roche, a record £523 million in 2001.[11] It is surprising that the cartel could exist for so long, as a Roche insider blew the whistle already in 1973, which the European Commission acted on (see Chapter 19).

Between the two world wars, Roche supplied morphine to the underworld. Other drug companies in the United Kingdom, Germany, Japan, Switzerland and the United States also participated in the trade with opium, morphine and heroin.[12-14] The CEO of Roche in the United States, Elmer Bobst, had great difficulty persuading his superiors in Basel that they should stop their unethical business practice.[13] Roche continued to ship narcotics to the United States behind Bobst's back, but he came across a cryptic telegram while visiting the headquarters, which left no doubt that it came from US criminals. It spoke about a shipment of sodium bicarbonate, which is used for baking cakes!

Roche agreed to stop the trade when Bobst reported that the US government had threatened to exclude Roche from doing business in the United States if the company didn't stop. However, Roche took up the habit again, and again without telling Bobst. In his book,[13] Bobst mentions that the man who was responsible for this wasn't at heart an immoral man, but utterly amoral in business. Bobst couldn't understand how it was possible to have two ethical standards, one for private life and one for business. He also describes how Roche avoided Swiss taxes by setting up a company in the tax refuge, Lichtenstein.

Pushing drugs that people don't need is a highly lucrative business, particularly when the drugs affect brain functions. Roche pushed Valium (diazepam) to become the top-selling drug in the world, although many indications for its use were highly doubtful and the wholesale price was 25 times the price of gold.[12] In the early 1970s, Roche was fined by antitrust officials in Europe for engaging in anticompetitive behaviour in the sale of Valium and another best-selling tranquilliser, Librium (chlordiazepoxide).[9]

It took 27 years after the first report about dependence had been published before the drug regulators fully acknowledged that tranquillisers are strongly addictive,[15] just like heroin and other narcotics. I believe that the fact that some drugs affecting the brain are legal and others are illegal is irrelevant from an ethical perspective, if we try to understand what the drug industry is doing to the population. Another reason why the distinction is irrelevant is that the drug industry doesn't really bother whether their actions are legal or not, as illustrated by the pervasive use of illegal, off-label marketing. Furthermore, what is legal isn't static, but can change with country, fashion and prevailing beliefs. For example, narcotics haven't always been illegal, and although it's illegal to sell hash in most countries, it's legal to smoke hash in the Netherlands. It is sold in so-called coffee shops, and this funny name once fooled me. Breakfasts at hotels are exceedingly expensive compared to how little most of us eat in the morning, so I went into a coffee shop one morning in Amsterdam. The owner was very amused when I asked for coffee, which he didn't have. Shortly afterwards, three lovely girls from the Middle East entered the shop and told me that Black Lebanon was the best and that they were going to smoke just that.

As another example of legal inconsistency for substances affecting the brain, it is illegal to produce your own brandy but legal to buy it in a shop.

Whatever the legal status of brain active substances, drugs are being pushed in both cases. After having examined the drug industry in great detail, John Braithwaite published his observations in the book *Corporate Crime in the Pharmaceutical Industry*. In it he said:[12]

> *People who foster dependence on illicit drugs such as heroin are regarded as among the most unscrupulous pariahs of modern civilisation. In contrast, pushers of licit drugs tend to be viewed as altruistically motivated purveyors of a social good.*

HALL OF SHAME FOR BIG PHARMA

The *BMJ* comes out weekly and most issues describe one or more scandals related to the drug industry in its News section or elsewhere. The *New York Times* also publishes many stories about drug industry misconduct, and most of the documentation I have collected over the years comes from these two highly respected sources. In recent years, numerous articles and books have described serious cases of research misconduct and marketing fraud committed by big pharma,[2,5,6,16-22] but although the facts are overwhelming, the standard response from the drug industry when a company has been caught is that there are a few bad apples in any enterprise.

The interesting question is whether we are seeing a lone bad apple now and then, which might be excusable, or whether pretty much the whole basket is rotten, i.e. whether most companies routinely break the law.

To find out, I did 10 Google searches in 2012 combining the names of the 10 largest drug companies[7] with 'fraud'. There were between 0.5 and 27 million hits for each company. I selected the most prominent case described in the 10 hits on the first Google page and supplied the information with additional sources.

The 10 cases were all recent (2007–2012) and were all related to the United States.[23,24] The most common criminal offences were illegal marketing recommending drugs for off-label uses, misrepresentation of research results, hiding data on harms, and Medicaid and Medicare fraud. I describe the cases in descending order according to the size of the company.

1 Pfizer agreed to pay $2.3 billion in 2009

This was the largest healthcare fraud settlement in the history of the US Department of Justice at the time.[25] A subsidiary of the firm pleaded guilty to misbranding drugs 'with the intent to defraud or mislead', and the firm was found to have illegally promoted four drugs: Bextra (valdecoxib, an anti-arthritis drug, withdrawn from the market in 2005), Geodon (ziprasidone, an antipsychotic drug), Zyvox (linezolid, an antibiotic) and Lyrica (pregabalin, an epilepsy drug).

An amount of $1 billion was levied to resolve the allegations that Pfizer paid bribes and offered lavish hospitality to healthcare providers to encourage them to prescribe the four drugs, and six whistle-blowers would receive $102 million. Pfizer entered a Corporate Integrity Agreement with the US Department of Health and Human Services, which means that good behaviour is required for the next 5 years. Pfizer had previously entered into three such agreements,[26] and when Pfizer promised the federal prosecutors not to market drugs illegally again in 2004, Pfizer was busily doing exactly this while they signed the agreement.[27]

Pfizer's antibiotic, Zyvox, cost eight times as much as vancomycin, which even Pfizer admitted in its own fact book is a better drug, but Pfizer lied to the doctors, telling them Zyvox was best. Even after the FDA had told Pfizer to stop its unsubstantiated claims because they posed serious safety concerns, as vancomycin is used for life-threatening conditions, Pfizer continued to tell hospitals and doctors that Zyvox would save more lives than vancomycin.[27]

2 Novartis agreed to pay $423 million in 2010

The payment concerned criminal and civil liability arising from the illegal marketing of Trileptal (oxcarbazepine, an epilepsy drug approved for the treatment of partial seizures, but not for any psychiatric, pain or other uses).[28] The company unlawfully marketed Trileptal and five other drugs, causing false claims to be submitted to government healthcare programmes. The agreement resolved allegations that the company paid kickbacks to healthcare professionals to induce them to prescribe Trileptal and five other drugs, Diovan (valsartan, for hypertension), Zelnorm (tegaserod, a drug for irritable bowel syndrome and constipation, which was removed from the market by the FDA in 2007 because of cardiovascular toxicity), Sandostatin (octreotide, a drug that mimics a natural hormone), Exforge (amlodipine + valsartan, for hypertension) and Tekturna (aliskiren, for hypertension).

The whistle-blowers, all former employees of Novartis, would receive payments of more than $25 million, and Novartis signed a Corporate Integrity Agreement.

3 Sanofi-Aventis to pay more than $95 million to settle fraud charge in 2009

According to the settlement, Aventis had overcharged US and local health agencies for medications destined for indigent patients.[29,30] The Justice Department said they would ensure that programmes for the most vulnerable parts of the population did not pay any more for drugs than they should under the law. Aventis acknowledged that it misreported drug prices for patients in the Medicaid Drug Rebate programme for poor patients. The firm deliberately misquoted the prices, underpaying rebates to Medicaid and overcharging some public health agencies for the medications. The fraud occurred between 1995 and 2000 and concerned steroid-based nasal sprays containing triamcinolone.

4 GlaxoSmithKline to pay $3 billion in 2011

This is the largest healthcare fraud settlement in US history.[31–33] GlaxoSmithKline pleaded guilty to having marketed a number of drugs illegally for off-label use, including Wellbutrin (bupropion, an antidepressant), Paxil (paroxetine, an antidepressant), Advair (fluticasone + salmeterol, an asthma drug), Avandia (rosiglitazone, a diabetes drug) and Lamictal (lamotrigine, an epilepsy drug).

The Justice Department charged a former vice president and top lawyer for Glaxo a year earlier with making false statements and obstructing a federal investigation into illegal marketing of Wellbutrin for weight loss.[34] The indictment accused the vice president of lying to the FDA, denying that doctors speaking at company events had promoted Wellbutrin for uses not approved by the agency, and of withholding incriminating documents.

The company paid kickbacks to doctors, failed to include certain safety data about rosiglitazone in reports to the FDA, and its sponsored programmes suggested cardiovascular *benefits* from Avandia despite warnings on the FDA-approved label regarding cardiovascular *risks*. Avandia was withdrawn in Europe in 2010 because it increases cardiovascular deaths.

Allegations of Medicaid fraud by misreported prices were also covered by the agreement. The whistle-blowers were four employees of GlaxoSmithKline, including a former senior marketing development manager and a regional vice president. The company entered into a Corporate Integrity Agreement.

5 AstraZeneca to pay $520 million in 2010 to settle fraud case

The charges were that AstraZeneca illegally marketed one of its best-selling drugs, the antipsychotic drug Seroquel (quetiapine), to children, the elderly, veterans and inmates for uses not approved by the FDA, including aggression, Alzheimer's, anger management, anxiety, attention-deficit hyperactivity disorder (ADHD), dementia, depression, mood disorder, post-traumatic stress disorder and sleeplessness.[35] Further, the company targeted its illegal marketing towards doctors who do not typically treat psychotic patients and paid kickbacks to some of them. Other doctors were sent to lavish resorts to encourage them to market and prescribe the drug for unapproved uses. The whistle-blower would get more than $45 million.

The fine was small, as the drug sold for $4.9 billion in 2009.[36] AstraZeneca denied wrongdoing although its misdeeds were obvious. The US Attorney General said about them:[35]

'These were not victimless crimes – illegal acts by pharmaceutical companies and false claims against Medicare and Medicaid can put the public health at risk, corrupt medical decisions by healthcare providers, and take billions of dollars directly out of taxpayers' pockets.'

6 Roche convinces governments to stockpile Tamiflu

Roche has committed what to me looks like the biggest theft in history,[37–47] but no one has yet dragged the company to court. In preparation for the mild 2009 influenza epidemic, the European and US governments spent billions of Euros and dollars on the purchase of Tamiflu (oseltamivir).

Roche has omitted publishing most of their clinical trial data and has refused to share them with independent Cochrane researchers. Based on unpublished trials, Roche has claimed that Tamiflu reduces hospital admissions by 61%, secondary complications by 67%, and lower respiratory tract infections requiring antibiotics by 55%.[38] Curiously, the company convinced the European Medicines Agency (EMA) to approve the drug for prevention of influenza complications, and the agency's summary of product characteristics stated that lower respiratory tract complications were reduced from 12.7% to 8.6% ($P = 0.001$).[38]

In contrast, the FDA sent Roche a warning letter that the company should stop claiming that Tamiflu reduces the severity and incidence of secondary infections, and it required Roche to print a disclaimer on the labels: 'Tamiflu has not been proven to have a positive impact on the potential consequences (such as hospitalizations, mortality, or economic impact) of seasonal, avian, or pandemic influenza.'[37,47]

When the FDA first reviewed a similar drug, zanamivir (Relenza) from GlaxoSmithKline, the advisory committee recommended by a vote of 13 to 4 that the drug should not be approved.[39] In analysis after analysis, zanamivir was no better than placebo when the patients were taking other drugs such as para-cetamol.[39] Within days after this decision, Glaxo sent a fiery letter to the FDA stating that the decision was 'completely at odds with the will of Congress that drug development and approval proceed swiftly and surely'.[40] This threat made the FDA's leadership overrule the committee and criticise its reviewer, biostat-istician Michael Elashoff, for giving negative testimony. Elashoff was originally assigned also the oseltamivir application, but this was taken away from him[39] and he left the agency after its demonstration of how an ineffective drug gets approved. When zanamivir was approved, the FDA also had to approve osel-tamivir later the same year.[41]

There is no convincing evidence that Tamiflu prevents influenza complica-tions or reduces the spread of influenza to other people. However, Roche used ghostwriters, and one of the ghosts said: 'The Tamiflu accounts had a list of key messages that you had to get in. It was run by the marketing department and you were answerable to them.'[38] At best, Tamiflu reduces the duration of influenza by 21 hours,[42] which can likely be obtained with far cheaper drugs like aspirin and paracetamol.[44] Furthermore, Tamiflu has important harms, but they were concealed to such an extent that the Cochrane researchers could not report on them in their Cochrane review. Even so, the Cochrane researchers found that cases of hallucination and weird accidents have been fairly commonly reported in Roche's post-marketing surveillance of Tamiflu,[41] in accordance with case series from Japan and experiments in rats that exhibited many of the same symptoms. A journal article signed by a group of Roche authors claimed that rats and mice given a very high dose of Tamiflu showed no ill effect, but according to docu-ments submitted to the Japanese Ministry of Health, Labor, and Welfare by Chugai, the Japanese Roche subsidiary, the exact same dose of Tamiflu killed more than half of the animals![41]

If Roche's unpublished data had really shown what the company purports they have, Roche would hardly have hesitated to share them with Cochrane researchers or to publish them. Stunningly, however, Roche has stated that the additional studies 'provided little new information and would therefore be unlikely to be accepted for publication by most reputable journals'.[38] These claims are ridiculous. I cannot abstain at this point from quoting Drummond Rennie, editor of *JAMA*, who, in his announcement for the first peer review congress, stated:[43]

> *'There seems to be no study too fragmented, no hypothesis too trivial, no literature citation too biased or too egoistical, no design too warped, no methodology too bungled, no presentation of results too inaccurate, too obscure, and too contradictory, no analysis too self-serving, no argument too circular, no conclusions too trifling or too unjustified, and no grammar and syntax too offensive for a paper to end up in print.'*

After much media attention, Roche promised in 2009 to make the full study reports of the unpublished trials available on its website, but this hasn't happened.

Another curiosity is that Roche sent one of the Cochrane researchers a draft agreement, which stipulated that if signed, he could not even mention that such an agreement existed![38] Apparently, Roche intended not only to keep its data concealed but also the fact that it silenced people who asked for the data. The Cochrane researcher asked for clarification the next day but never received a reply.

The Council of Europe has criticised national governments, the World Health Organization (WHO) and the EU agencies for being guilty of actions that led to a waste of large sums of money.[45] Many people have wondered why the WHO selected people to write guidance about influenza drugs who were paid by the companies marketing the drugs, and who didn't disclose this in their guidance reports, and why there was so much secrecy around it that it wasn't even possible for outsiders to get information on who were on the WHO committee.[39]

WHO has been an ideal partner for Roche's excesses and Roche has boasted that it works as 'a responsible partner with governments to assist in their pandemic planning'.[39] Roche's actions belie this statement, and in 2012 I suggested that the European governments should sue Roche to get the billions of Euros back they had spent on needlessly stockpiling Tamiflu, which might also have the effect that the hidden trial results came out in the open.[46] Furthermore, I suggested we should boycott Roche's products until they publish the missing Tamiflu data.

7 Johnson & Johnson fined more than $1.1 billion in 2012

A jury found that the company and its subsidiary Janssen had downplayed and hidden risks associated with its antipsychotic drug Risperdal (risperidone).[48] The judge found nearly 240 000 violations under Arkansas' Medicaid-fraud law. Jurors returned a quick verdict in favour of the state, which had argued that Janssen lied about the potentially life-threatening side effects of Risperdal which, like other antipsychotic drugs, include death, strokes, seizures, weight gain and diabetes. The FDA had ordered Janssen to issue a letter to doctors correcting an earlier letter saying the drug didn't increase the risk of developing diabetes. Janssen continued to maintain after the verdict that it didn't break the law. Previous verdicts against the company a few months earlier included a $327 million civil penalty in South Carolina and a $158 million settlement in Texas.

The worst of all this was that the crimes hit hard also on children.[49] More than a quarter of Risperdal's use was in children and adolescents, including non-approved indications, and a panel of federal drug experts concluded that the drug was used far too much. A world-renowned child psychiatrist, Joseph Biederman from Harvard, pushed the drug heavily to children and also extorted the company. Internal emails released for use in court cases revealed that Biederman was furious after Johnson & Johnson rejected a request he had made to receive a $280 000 research grant. A company spokesperson wrote: 'I have never seen someone so angry ... Since that time, our business became non-existant [sic] within his area of control.'

The fraud case could become even bigger. In April 2012, the US government stated in a motion in a potential multibillion-dollar healthcare fraud case against Johnson & Johnson that Alex Gorsky, Vice President of Marketing, who was set to become Johnson & Johnson's next chief executive officer, was actively involved and had firsthand knowledge of the alleged fraud.[50] The allegations were that Johnson & Johnson paid kickbacks to induce Omnicare, the nation's largest nursing home pharmacy, to purchase and recommend Risperdal and other of the company's drugs. The company didn't inform Omnicare or members of Janssen's sales staff that the FDA had warned the company that marketing Risperdal as safe and effective in the elderly would be false and misleading because the drug had not been adequately studied in that population, or that the FDA had rejected the company's attempt to get approval to market Risperdal for treatment of psychotic and behavioural disturbances in dementia (by far the most prevalent use of Risperdal in Omnicare-served nursing facilities) because of inadequate safety data. Despite the weight of federal and state investigations of the Risperdal allegations, Johnson & Johnson's board of directors rewarded Gorsky by selecting him to be the next CEO. It's like in the mob: the greater the crime, the greater the advancement.

8 Merck to pay $670 million over Medicaid fraud in 2007

Merck had failed to pay the appropriate rebates to Medicaid and other government healthcare programmes, and had also paid kickbacks to doctors and hospitals to induce them to prescribe various drugs.[51] The allegations were brought in two separate lawsuits filed by whistle-blowers, and one of them would receive $68 million. From 1997 to 2001, Merck's sales force used approximately 15 different programmes to induce doctors to prescribe its drugs. These programmes primarily consisted of excess payments to doctors disguised as fees for 'training', 'consultation' or 'market research'. The government alleged that these fees were illegal kickbacks intended to induce the purchase of Merck drugs. Merck agreed to a Corporate Integrity Agreement.

9 Eli Lilly to pay more than $1.4 billion for illegal marketing in 2009

Eli Lilly entered into a settlement with the Department of Justice concerning a wide-ranging, off-label marketing scheme for its top-selling antipsychotic drug, Zyprexa (olanzapine), with worldwide sales of nearly $40 billion between 1996 and 2009.[52] In the settlement, Eli Lilly would pay $800 million in civil penalties and pleaded guilty to criminal charges, paying an additional $600 million fine. The allegations were raised by six whistle-blowers from Lilly who would share in approximately 18% of the federal and qualifying states' recoveries. All whistle-blowers were fired or forced to resign by the company. According to the complaint, one sales representative had contacted the company hotline regarding unethical sales practices but received no response.

Lilly successfully marketed Zyprexa for numerous off-label uses including Alzheimer's, depression and dementia, particularly in children and the elderly, although the harms of the drug are substantial, inducing heart failure, pneumonia, considerable weight gain and diabetes. Lilly salespeople were posed as persons in the audience who were interested in Zyprexa's expanded use and asked 'planted questions' during off-label lectures and audio conferences for physicians. Another tactic was that, while knowing the substantial risk for weight gain posed by Zyprexa, the company minimised the connection between Zyprexa and weight gain in a widely disseminated videotape called *The Myth of Diabetes* that used 'scientific studies of questionable integrity as well as the haphazard reporting of adverse events'. The settlement agreement included a Corporate Integrity Agreement.

10 Abbott to pay $1.5 billion for Medicaid fraud in 2012

Abbott settled allegations of Medicaid fraud for the company's illegal marketing of the epilepsy drug Depakote (valproate); $84 million would be paid to the whistle-blowers.[53,54] Abbott would pay $800 million in civil damages and penalties to compensate Medicaid, Medicare and various federal healthcare programmes for harm suffered as a result of its conduct. Abbott also pleaded guilty to a violation of the Food, Drug, and Cosmetic Act and agreed to pay a criminal fine and forfeiture of $700 million.

The states alleged that Abbott promoted the sale and use of Depakote for uses that were not approved by the FDA as safe and effective; that Abbott Laboratories made false and misleading statements about the safety, efficacy, dosing and cost-effectiveness of Depakote for some unapproved uses; improperly marketed the product in nursing homes for demented patients while the company had halted a trial in such patients that showed increased adverse effects; and paid kickbacks to induce doctors and others to prescribe or promote the drug. Abbott entered into a Corporate Integrity Agreement.

THE CRIMES ARE REPETITIVE

My survey showed that corporate crime is common and that the crimes are ruthlessly carried out, with blatant disregard for the deaths and other serious harms they cause. You'll see in the rest of this book that corporate crime kills people[12] and it also involves huge thefts of taxpayers' money.

It was easy to find additional crimes committed by the same top 10 companies,[24] crimes committed outside the United States and crimes committed by other companies. I used 'fraud' in my searches, but I could also have used 'criminal', 'illegal', 'FBI', 'kickback', 'misconduct', 'settlement', 'bribery', 'guilty' and 'felony', which would have uncovered many additional, recent crimes. I shall describe here some other crimes and will give more examples later.

In 2007, the FDA slammed Sanofi-Aventis over its failure to act on known instances of fraud during a pivotal trial of its antibiotic Ketek (telithromycin).[55] The FDA had required this trial after its first review of the drug, and the company enrolled over 24 000 patients in just 5 months by recruiting more than 1800 physicians, many of whom were new to clinical trials.[56]

Sanofi-Aventis continued to deny the accusations, although, according to company records and testimony by a former employee, the company was aware of fraudulent data but didn't take any action. One of the physician investigators was convicted of fraud over the enrolment of patients and faking consent forms and was sentenced to 57 months in prison. The convict had enrolled over 400 patients, at a payment of $400 per patient, and no patients had withdrawn from the study or were lost to follow-up, which is clearly too good to be true.

After having inspected nine other sites enrolling many patients, the FDA referred three of them for criminal investigations.[56] However, although the FDA knew about the misconduct, it didn't mention any problems with the data at its advisory committee meeting, with the excuse that they were legally barred from this because there was a criminal investigation.[56] This is not a valid excuse, as they could have decided not to present any data from this trial or postponed the meeting till the issues had been resolved.

Unaware of the problems, the committee voted 11 to 1 to recommend approval. The FDA furthermore accepted foreign post-marketing reports as evidence of safety, although such uncontrolled data are unreliable and although the criminal investigators recommended the FDA to examine whether Sanofi-Aventis had been involved in systematic fraud. The FDA didn't follow the advice and it exerted internal pressures on its scientists to alter their conclusions in favour of the drug, which, as we shall see later, seems to be standard practice at the FDA.

Sanofi-Aventis boasted that the launch of Ketek was the most successful launch of any antibiotic in history. However, already 7 months after the launch, the first death in liver failure was reported, and more cases followed. The FDA held an emergency meeting among 'senior managers' – which do not include the safety officers – and announced that the drug was safe, with reference to the study the FDA knew was fraudulent![56] One month later, one of the reviewers for Ketek alerted FDA senior management to the irregularities, but no substantive actions were taken, and some months later, when 23 cases of severe liver injury and four deaths had been reported, the FDA's Commissioner Andrew von Eschenbach prohibited the scientists to discuss Ketek outside the agency. The FDA didn't relabel Ketek to indicate its hepatotoxicity until 16 months after the first case became public. The agency's defence to all this is an embarrassing read, very similar to when the drug industry tries to defend the indefensible.[57]

Amazingly, Ketek is still available in the United States, but carries a black box warning, and it's no longer approved for mild respiratory illnesses such as sinusitis. The official FDA information about Ketek is such that I don't understand that any doctor would dare use the drug, but the likely explanation is that doctors don't read 26-page accounts of individual drugs and don't know the history behind Ketek.[58]

AstraZeneca paid $355 million in 2003 after pleading guilty to charges that it encouraged physicians to illegally request Medicare reimbursements for its drug against prostate cancer, Zoladex (goserelin), and bribed doctors to buy it.[35]

Johnson & Johnson was to pay more than $75 million to UK and US authorities in 2009 to settle corruption charges spanning three European countries and Iraq.[59] The charges related to alleged payment of bribes to doctors in Greece, Poland and Romania to encourage them to use the company's products and to hospital administrators in Poland to award the company contracts.

Eli Lilly agreed to pay $36 million in 2005 to settle criminal and civil charges related to the illegal marketing of Evista (raloxifene, a drug against osteoporosis) for the prevention of breast cancer and heart disease in letters salespeople sent to doctors.[60] The company had also concealed data that showed an increased risk of ovarian cancer. Eli Lilly entered into a Corporate Integrity Agreement.

In 2001, TAP Pharmaceuticals, a joint venture of Abbott and Takeda, paid $875 million, pleading guilty to criminal charges of fraud for inducing physicians to bill the government for drugs that the company gave them for free or at a reduced price.[18,61,62] In 2003, Abbott paid $622 million to settle an investigation into sales practices for liquids to feed the seriously ill.[61] Abbott gave tubes and pumps to deliver the liquid food directly into the patient's digestive tracts in exchange for large orders of the liquids.

Sometimes many crimes were listed in the first 10 hits in my Google searches for the same company. GlaxoSmithKline, for example, had a manufacturing plant in Puerto Rico closed down in 2009 because it produced defective drugs.[63] The plant had sent out batches of Paxil (paroxetine) containing two different doses and had mixed different drugs, e.g. Avandia (rosiglitazone) with Tagamet (cimetidine) and Paxil. Glaxo pleaded guilty to felony fraud and was fined $750 million, $96 million of which would go to the whistle-blower, the company's global quality assurance manager, whose documented concerns were ignored by senior management that fired her.[64] Glaxo also lied to federal investigators about the problems, despite pharmacists calling the plant directly when patients showed up with different coloured pills in their medicine. In pleading guilty to the felony, Glaxo admitted that it had distributed adulterated drugs, but the company lied to the public when it indicated that it went voluntarily to the FDA in 2002 out of safety concerns about the plant and when it said that 'The plant was closed in 2009 due to a declining demand for the medicines made there.' Blockbusters such as Avandia, Paxil and Tagamet could hardly be said to be in declining demand.

In 2003, Glaxo signed a Corporate Integrity Agreement and paid $88 million in a civil fine for overcharging Medicaid for Paxil and the nasal-allergy spray Flonase (fluticasone);[65] in 2003, the company faced a demand for $7.8 billion in backdated taxes and interest, the highest in the history of the US Internal Revenue Service;[65] in 2004, the Italian finance police accused over 4000 doctors and 73 employees in Glaxo of corruption, a €228 million scheme involving cash and other benefits to induce doctors to use the company's products, most seriously in relation to cancer drugs;[66] and in 2006, the company settled a tax dispute agreeing to pay $3.1 billion in a case that concerned intracompany 'transfer pricing'.[65]

Some crimes are about keeping manufacturers of generics out of the market when the patent has run out, and GlaxoSmithKline has also been involved in such activities.[67] The company agreed in 2004 to pay $175 million to settle a lawsuit contending that it blocked cheaper generic forms of Relafen (nabumetone, an NSAID), in violation of antitrust laws, and the company expected to pay $406 million to cover settled and pending Relafen claims. In 2006, Glaxo would pay $14 million to resolve allegations that state-government programmes paid inflated prices for Paxil because the firm engaged in patent fraud, antitrust violations and frivolous litigation to maintain a monopoly and block generic versions from entering the market.[65]

In the United States, generics can be kept out of the market for years, even legally. A company can file a lawsuit against a generics competitor claiming it has broken some other patent, and no matter how ridiculous the claim is, FDA approval of the generic drug is automatically delayed for 30 months. In a course programme for senior executives and lawyers in the industry, one of the agenda items was: 'How to use one 30 month stay per generic challenge.'[68] In this way, Glaxo succeeded in extending its exclusivity for its best-selling antidepressant drug Paxil by over 5 years![69]

Lawyers' tricks are also a big problem in Europe. In 2008, a report from the European Commission estimated that the companies' legal tactics to keep generics out of the market had cost the EU €3 billion in just 8 years.[70] An illustration of how sick our patent laws are was provided by a case where a company had filed 1300 patents for a single drug.

I shall mention also some recent examples from drug and device companies that are not among the top 10. Bristol-Myers Squibb agreed in 2007 to pay more than $515 million to settle illegal marketing and fraudulent pricing practices involving payments to doctors to induce them to use the company's drugs, also for off-label use.[71] In 2003, Bristol-Myers Squibb paid $670 million to settle antitrust charges that had involved forcing cancer patients and others to overpay by hundreds of millions of dollars for important and often life-saving medications.[72,73] The Federal Trade Commission accused the company of a decade-long pattern of illegally blocking the entry of generic competitors, deceiving the patent office by submitting fraudulent claims and offering a competitor a bribe of $72 million not to market its generic drug.[73]

In 2013, the European Commission imposed a fine of €94 million on Lundbeck and fines totalling €52 million on several producers of generic citalopram (Cipramil), which, in return for cash, had agreed with Lundbeck in 2002 to delay market entry of the antidepressant in violation of EU antitrust rules.[74] Lundbeck had also purchased generics' stock for the sole purpose of destroying it.

In 2006, it was reported in a whistle-blower lawsuit that Medtronic had spent at least $50 million on payments to prominent back surgeons over some 4 years.[75] According to the US Justice Department, Medtronic paid physicians $1000 to $2000 for each patient who was implanted with one of the company's devices.[76] One surgeon, who earned nearly $700 000 in consulting fees from Medtronic for 9 months, stated that his fees were compensation for his time spent away from his family and his practice.[75] The lawsuit said that Medtronic hosted medical conferences where the principal objective was to 'induce the physician, through any financial means necessary' to use its devices.

Medtronic closely tracked the use of its devices by the doctors who attended the conferences, choosing some for 'special attention'. A former president of the American Academy of Orthopedic Surgeons noted that the amount of money was astronomical (the cost of the components involved in typical fusion surgery for the lower back was around $13 000), and that the device makers knew the volumes these surgeons have. The bribery programme involved colourful activities like taking the doctors to PlatinumPlus, a strip club in Memphis, disguising the expenses as an evening at the ballet.

In 2007, five manufacturers of hip and knee replacements, Zimmer, DePuy Orthopaedics, Biomet, Smith & Nephew and Stryker Orthopedics, settled with the US federal government after having admitted that they paid surgeons tens to hundreds of thousands of dollars per year in 'consulting fees' to use their devices.[77]

In 2006, Serono Laboratories pleaded guilty to two counts of conspiracy and agreed to pay $704 million to settle criminal charges that it engaged in an elaborate kickback scheme to encourage sales of its AIDS drug, Serostim (recombinant DNA somatropin).[78]

In 2004, Schering-Plough accepted a settlement of $346 million for kickbacks; Bayer paid $257 million and GlaxoSmithKline $87 million to settle similar allegations.[79] Other involved companies were AstraZeneca, Dey, Pfizer and TAP Pharmaceuticals.[80]

In 2007, Purdue Pharma and its president, top lawyer and former chief medical officer were to pay a total of $635 million in fines for claiming that OxyContin (oxycodone, a morphine-like drug) was less addictive, less subject to abuse and less likely to cause withdrawal symptoms than other opiates. The company admitted that it lied to doctors and patients about the risks to boost sales.[81] The drug became very popular among drug abusers and became a leading drug of abuse under the nickname 'hillbilly heroin'.[82] It has killed a huge number of people. In Australia, most of the people who died were not drug abusers but people accidentally overdosing.[83] The head of the US Center on Addiction and Substance Abuse stated:[84]

'I think these people are drug pushers, just like street drug pushers ... It is outrageous that these people pushed this drug, addictive as they knew it was, onto the market and in effect damaged millions of innocent people.'

Three top executives were excluded from government business for 12 years.[83] Purdue trained its salespeople to tell doctors that the risk of addiction was less than 1%, which isn't true, as the risk is similar to that of other opiods.[82]

Purdue gave Massachusetts General Hospital in Boston $3 million to have its pain centre renamed as 'MGH Purdue Pharma Pain Center'.[18] The agreement also involved that the pain specialists at the hospital should use 'Purdue-designed curriculum written, in part, to encourage wary doctors and pharmacists to prescribe pain-killers such as OxyContin.' Total corruption.

In Denmark, OxyContin was also extremely aggressively pushed, to such an extent that it became a common conversation subject even among doctors who rarely use morphine-like drugs. The salespeople were like tsetse flies going after everything that moved in a white coat. The drug is highly expensive and provides no advantage over far cheaper alternatives, but even so, it proved necessary for the drug committee at my own hospital to ban the drug altogether, so that the clinicians could no longer order it from the pharmacy.

The crimes are so widespread, repetitive and varied that the inescapable conclusion is that they are committed deliberately because crime pays. The companies see the fines as a marketing expense and carry on with their illegal activities, as if nothing had happened.

It is also important to note that many of the crimes would have been impossible to carry out, if doctors had not been willing to participate in them. Doctors are complicit in the crimes when they accept kickbacks and engage in other types of corruption, often in relation to illegal marketing. It is curious that doctors can get away with getting paid by the companies for doing exactly this without being punished. When drugs are marketed for non-approved uses, we don't know whether they are effective or whether they are too harmful, e.g. if used in children. This practice has therefore been described as using the citizens as guinea pigs[85] on a large scale without their informed consent.

Even when doctors use drugs only for approved indications, the crimes have consequences for their patients. Doctors only have access to selected and manipulated information[16–22,42] and therefore believe drugs are far more effective and safe than they really are. Thus, both legal and illegal marketing lead to massive overtreatment of the population and a lot of harm that could have been avoided.

Many crimes involve large-scale corruption of doctors who receive money to induce them to prescribe drugs that are often 10 or 20 times more expensive than older drugs that are equally good and sometimes even better. The US Office of the Inspector General of the Department of Health and Human Services has warned that, as many of the existing practices involving gifts and payments to doctors are intended to influence their prescribing, they might potentially violate federal anti-kickback laws.[69] Unfortunately, the only organisation that seems to have taken the writing on the wall seriously is the American Medical Student Association, which voted for a total ban on the acceptance of all gifts and favours to medical students.[69]

IT'S ORGANISED CRIME

In 2004–5, the Health Committee in the British House of Commons examined the drug industry in detail[17] and found that its influence was enormous and out of control.[86] They found an industry that buys influence over doctors, charities, patient groups, journalists and politicians, and whose regulation is sometimes weak or ambiguous.[87] Furthermore, the Department of Health is not only responsible for the national health service but also for representing the interests of the drug industry. The committee's report made it clear that reducing the influence of industry would be good for everybody, including the industry itself, which could concentrate on developing new drugs rather than on corrupting doctors, patient organisations, and others.[88] The report also said that we need an industry that is led by the values of its scientists, not those of its marketing force, and the committee was particularly worried about the increasing medicalisation, i.e. the belief that every problem requires a pill.

Nevertheless, the British government did nothing in response to the Health Committee's damning report, likely because the British drug industry is the third most profitable activity, after tourism and finance.[88] After having been shown unequivocal and massive evidence of unhealthy industry influence on public health, government officials declared that there was no evidence of unhealthy industry influence on public health![89]

The Department of Health defended the industry, citing its trade surplus of more than £3 billion and argued that drug company representatives were giving doctors good information. It even defended the rising numbers of prescriptions for antidepressants although this is pretty indefensible, as I shall explain in Chapter 17. Alleged promotional excesses were dismissed with the argument that appropriate mechanisms were in place. This is what Ben Goldacre calls 'fake fixes'.[90] The public is repeatedly given false reassurances that the problem has been fixed.

When asked directly about whether the department understood that there was a fundamental conflict between the industry's drive for profit and the government's responsibility for public health, the reply was that the 'stakeholder relationship' between government and industry 'brings many gains and many innovative medicines … with huge impacts on health outcomes'.

I'm speechless. With a governmental attitude of total denial it's no great wonder that crime flourishes in the drug industry and spreads like weeds.

The centrepiece of the US Organized Crime Control Act from 1970 is the Racketeer Influenced and Corrupt Organizations Act (RICO).[91] Racketeering is the act of engaging in a certain type of offence more than once. The list of offences that constitute racketeering include extortion, fraud, federal drug offences, bribery, embezzlement, obstruction of justice, obstruction of law enforcement, tampering with witnesses, and political corruption. Big pharma does so much of this all the time that there can be no doubt that its business model fulfils the criteria for organised crime.

A previous global vice president of marketing for Pfizer turned whistle-blower when the company wouldn't listen to his complaints about illegal marketing[5] holds a similar view:[92]

> *It is scary how many similarities there are between this industry and the mob. The mob makes obscene amounts of money, as does this industry. The side effects of organized crime are killings and deaths, and the side effects are the same in this industry. The mob bribes politicians and others, and so does the drug industry … The difference is, all these people in the drug industry look upon themselves – well, I'd say 99 percent, anyway – look upon themselves as law-abiding citizens, not as citizens who would ever rob a bank … However, when they get together as a group and manage these corporations, something seems to happen … to otherwise good citizens when they are part of a corporation. It's almost like when you have war atrocities; people do things they don't think they're capable of. When you're in a group, people can do things they otherwise wouldn't, because the group can validate what you're doing as okay.*

When a crime has led to the deaths of thousands of people, we should see it as a crime against humanity. Whether they are killed by arms or by pills should make no difference for our perception of the misdeed. But, until recently, there was a remarkable complacency with even lethal crimes. This may be about to change, at least in the United States. In 2010, the Justice Department charged a former vice president for GlaxoSmithKline.[34]

One of the pharmaceutical industry's standard responses when scandals are revealed in the media is that its practices have changed radically since the crimes were committed. This isn't true; in fact, the crimes are steeply *increasing*. According to Public Citizen's Health Research Group, three-quarters of the 165 settlements comprising $20 billion in penalties during the 20-year interval from 1991 to 2010 occurred in just the past 5 years of that period.[93] An update showed that in just 21 months, till July 2012, an additional $10 billion in settlements were reached.[94]

In contrast to the drug industry, doctors don't harm their patients deliberately. And when they do cause harm, either accidentally, by lack of knowledge, or by negligence, they harm only one patient at a time. As the actions of senior executives in the drug industry have the potential to harm thousands or millions of people, their ethical standards should be much higher than those of doctors, and the information they give about their drugs should be as truthful as possible after meticulous and honest scrutiny of the data. None of this is the case, and when journalists ask me what I think of the ethical standards of the drug industry, I often joke about it and say I have no answer as I cannot describe what doesn't exist. The only industry standard is money, and the amount of money you earn to the firm decides how good you are. There are many decent and honest people in the drug industry, but those who make it to the top have been described as 'ruthless bastards' by criminologist John Braithwaite who interviewed many of them.[12] In the United States, big pharma beat all other industries in terms of crimes. They have more than three times as many serious or moderately serious law violations as other companies, and this record holds also after adjustment for company size.[12,61] Big pharma also has a worse record than other companies for international bribery and corruption and for criminal negligence in the unsafe manufacture of drugs.[12] In a 5-year period, from 1966 to 1971, the FDA recalled 1935 drug products, 806 because of contamination or adulteration, 752 because of sub- or superpotency and 377 because of label mix-ups.[61]

Bribery is routine and involves large amounts of money. Almost every type of person who can affect the interests of the industry has been bribed: doctors, hospital administrators, cabinet ministers, health inspectors, customs officers, tax assessors, drug registration officials, factory inspectors, pricing officials and political parties. In Latin America, posts as ministers of health are avidly sought, as these ministers are almost invariably rich with wealth coming from the drug industry.[12]

In the beginning of this chapter, I asked the question whether we are seeing a lone bad apple now and then, or whether pretty much the whole basket is rotten. What we are seeing is organised crime in an industry that is completely rotten.

REFERENCES

1 Available online at: http://en.wikiquote.org/wiki/William_Osler (accessed 30 August 2012).
2 Kelton E. More drug companies to pay billions for fraud, join the 'dishonor roll' after Abbott settlement. *Forbes*. 2012 May 10.
3 *PhRMA Code on Interactions with Healthcare Professionals – Signatory Companies*. Available online at: www.phrma.org/sites/default/files/108/signatory_companies_phrma_code_061112.pdf (accessed 25 June 2012).

4 Advertisement for Philip Morris International. *Berlingske.* 2004 Mar 14.

5 Rost P. *The Whistleblower: confessions of a healthcare hitman.* New York: Soft Skull Press; 2006.

6 Rockoff JD, Matthews CM. Pfizer settles federal bribery investigation. *Wall Street Journal.* 2012 Aug 7.

7 Reuters. *Factbox – The 20 largest pharmaceutical companies.* 2010 Mar 26.

8 Corporate Crime in the '90s: the top 100 corporate criminals of the 1990s. *Multinational Monitor.* 1999 July/August; **20**(7, 8).

9 Barboza D. Tearing down the facade of 'Vitamins Inc.'. *New York Times.* 1999 Oct 10.

10 *F. Hoffmann-La Roche and BASF Agree to Pay Record Criminal Fines for Participating in International Vitamin Cartel.* US Department of Justice. 1999 May 20.

11 Mathiason N. Blowing the final whistle. *The Guardian.* 2001 Nov 25.

12 Braithwaite J. *Corporate Crime in the Pharmaceutical Industry.* London: Routledge & Kegan Paul; 1984.

13 Bobst EH. *Bobst: the autobiography of a pharmaceutical pioneer.* New York: David McKay Company; 1973.

14 Bruun K. International drug control and the pharmaceutical industry. In: Cooperstock R, editor. *Social Aspects of the Medical Use of Psychotropic Drugs.* Toronto: Addiction Research Foundation of Ontario. Papers presented at the International Symposium on Alcohol and Drug Research; 1973. Department of National Health and Welfare; 1974.

15 Nielsen M, Hansen EH, Gøtzsche PC. What is the difference between dependence and withdrawal reactions? A comparison of benzodiazepines and selective serotonin re-uptake inhibitors. *Addiction.* 2012; **107**: 900–8.

16 Healy D. *Let Them Eat Prozac.* New York: New York University Press; 2004.

17 House of Commons Health Committee. *The Influence of the Pharmaceutical Industry. Fourth Report of Session 2004–05.* Available online at: www.publications.parliament.uk/pa/cm200405/cmselect/cmhealth/42/42.pdf (accessed 26 April 2005).

18 Abramson J. *Overdo$ed America: the broken promise of American medicine.* New York: HarperCollins; 2004.

19 Angell M. *The Truth about the Drug Companies: how they deceive us and what to do about it.* New York: Random House; 2004.

20 Kassirer JP. *On the Take: how medicine's complicity with big business can endanger your health.* Oxford: Oxford University Press; 2005.

21 Mundy A. *Dispensing with the Truth.* New York: St. Martin's Press; 2001.

22 Petersen M. *Our Daily Meds.* New York: Sarah Crichton Books; 2008.

23 Gøtzsche PC. Big pharma often commits corporate crime, and this must be stopped. *BMJ.* 2012; **345**: e8462.

24 Gøtzsche PC. Corporate crime in the pharmaceutical industry is common, serious and repetitive. Available online at: www.cochrane.dk/research/corporatecrime/Corporate-crime-long-version.pdf (accessed 20 December 2012).

25 Pfizer agrees record fraud fine. BBC News. 2009 Sept 2.

26 Tanne JH. Pfizer pays record fine for off-label promotion of four drugs. *BMJ.* 2009; **339**: b3657.

27 Evans D. Big pharma's crime spree. *Bloomberg Markets.* 2009 Dec: 72–86.

28 United States Department of Justice. *Novartis Pharmaceuticals Corp. to Pay More than $420 million to Resolve Off-Label Promotion and Kickback Allegations.* 2010 Sept 30.

29 SourceWatch. *Sanofi-Aventis.* 2011 Jan 23. Available online at: www.sourcewatch.org/index.php?title=Sanofi-Aventis (accessed 19 June 2012).

30 Aventis to pay $95 million to settle fraud charge. AFP. 2009 May 28.

31 Rabiner S. Glaxo $3B fine largest healthcare fraud settlement in history? *FindLaw.* 2011 Nov 10.

32 United States Department of Justice. *GlaxoSmithKline to Plead Guilty and Pay $3 billion to Resolve Fraud Allegations and Failure to Report Safety Data.* 2012 July 2.

33 Thomas K, Schmidt MS. Glaxo agrees to pay $3 billion in fraud settlement. *New York Times.* 2012 July 2.

34 Wilson D. Ex-Glaxo executive is charged in drug fraud. *New York Times.* 2010 Nov 9.

35 Khan H, Thomas P. Drug giant AstraZeneca to pay $520 million to settle fraud case. *ABC News*. 2010 April 27.

36 Tanne JH. AstraZeneca pays $520m fine for off-label marketing. *BMJ*. 2010; **340**: c2380.

37 Doshi P. Neuraminidase inhibitors: the story behind the Cochrane review. *BMJ*. 2009; **339**: b5164.

38 Cohen D. Complications: tracking down the data on oseltamivir. *BMJ*. 2009; **339**: b5387.

39 Cohen D, Carter P. WHO and the pandemic flu 'conspiracies'. *BMJ*. 2012; **340**: c2912.

40 Willman D. Relenza: official asks if one day less of flu is worth it. *Los Angeles Times*. 2000 Dec 20.

41 Epstein H. Flu warning: beware the drug companies! *New York Review of Books*. 2001 Apr 11.

42 Jefferson T, Jones MA, Doshi P, *et al*. Neuraminidase inhibitors for preventing and treating influenza in healthy adults and children. *Cochrane Database Syst Rev*. 2012; **1**: CD008965.

43 Rennie D. Guarding the guardians: a conference on editorial peer review. *JAMA*. 1986; **256**: 2391–2.

44 Doshi P, Jefferson T, Del Mar C. The imperative to share clinical study reports: recommendations from the Tamiflu experience. *PLoS Med*. 2012; **9**: e1001201.

45 O'Dowd A. Response to swine flu was 'unjustified', says Council of Europe. *BMJ*. 2012; **340**: c3033.

46 Gøtzsche PC. European governments should sue Roche and prescribers should boycott its drugs. *BMJ*. 2012; **345**: e7689.

47 Cohen D. Search for evidence goes on. *BMJ*. 2012; **344**: e458.

48 Ark. judge fines Johnson & Johnson more than $1.1B in Risperdal case. *CBS/AP*. 2012 April 11.

49 Harris G. Research center tied to drug company. *New York Times*. 2008 Nov 25.

50 Kelton E. J&J needs a cure: new CEO allegedly had links to fraud. *Forbes*. 2012 17 April.

51 Silverman E. Merck to pay $670 million over Medicaid fraud. *Pharmalot*. 2008 Feb 7.

52 Reuters. The largest pharma fraud whistleblower case in U.S. history totaling $1.4 billion. 2009 Jan 15.

53 Anonymous. Abbott Labs to pay $1.5 billion more for Medicaid fraud. 2012 May 8. Available online at: http://somd.com/news/headlines/2012/15451.shtml (accessed 19 June 2012).

54 Roehr B. Abbott pays $1.6bn for promoting off label use of valproic acid. *BMJ*. 2012; **344**: e3343.

55 Barnes K. Sanofi slammed by FDA over failure to act on Ketek fraud. *Outsourcing*. 2007 Oct 25.

56 Ross DB. The FDA and the case of Ketek. *N Engl J Med*. 2007; **356**: 1601–4.

57 Soreth J, Cox E, Kweder S, *et al*. Ketek – the FDA perspective. *N Engl J Med*. 2007; **356**: 1675–6.

58 Ketek Official FDA information, side effects and uses. Available online at: www.drugs.com/pro/ketek.html (accessed 18 Nov 2012).

59 Russell J. Johnson & Johnson feels pain of $75m bribery fines. *The Telegraph*. 2011 9 April.

60 Pringle E. Eli Lilly hides data: Zyprexa, Evista, Prozac risk. *Conspiracy Planet*. Available online at: www.conspiracyplanet.com/channel.cfm?channelid=55&contentid=4181&page=2 (accessed 28 June 2012).

61 Clinard MB, Yeager PC. *Corporate Crime*. New Brunswick: Transaction Publishers; 2006.

62 Harris G. As doctors write prescriptions, drug company writes a check. *New York Times*. 2004 June 27.

63 Lane C. Bad medicine: GlaxoSmithKline's fraud and gross negligence. *Psychology Today*. 2011 Jan 7.

64 Silverman E. Glaxo to pay $750M for manufacturing fraud. *Pharmalot*. 2010 Oct 26.

65 Wikipedia. GlaxoSmithKline. Available online at: http://en.wikipedia.org/wiki/GlaxoSmithKline (accessed 20 June 2012).

66 Carpenter G. Italian doctors face charges over GSK incentive scheme. Over 4000 doctors are alleged to have received cash, gifts, and prizes to encourage them to prescribe GSK products. *Lancet*. 2004; **363**: 1873.

67 Company news; drug maker agrees to pay $175 million in lawsuit. *New York Times*. 2004 Feb 7.

68 Prescription generics & patent management. *Strategies in the Pharmaceutical Industry 2004*. 2004 Nov 29.

69 Relman AS, Angell M. America's other drug problem: how the drug industry distorts medicine and politics. *The New Republic.* 2002 Dec 16: 27–41.

70 Jack A. Legal tactics to delay launch of generic drugs cost Europe €3bn. *BMJ.* 2008; 337: 1311.

71 Tanne JH. Bristol-Myers Squibb made to pay $515 m to settle US law suits. *BMJ.* 2007; 335: 742–3.

72 Anonymous. Bristol-Myers will settle antitrust charges by U.S. *New York Times.* 2003 March 8.

73 Avorn J. *Powerful Medicines: the benefits, risks, and costs of prescription drugs.* New York: Vintage Books; 2005.

74 European Commission. *Antitrust: Commission fines Lundbeck and other pharma companies for delaying market entry of generic medicines.* Press release. 2013 June 19.

75 Abelson R. Whistle-blower suit says device maker generously rewards doctors. *New York Times.* 2006 Jan 24.

76 Poses RM. Medtronic settles, yet again. Blog post. *Health Care Renewal.* 2011 Dec 15. Available online at: http://hcrenewal.blogspot.co.nz/2011/12/medtronic-settles-yet-again.html (accessed 10 July 2013).

77 Tanne JH. US companies are fined for payments to surgeons. *BMJ.* 2007; 335: 1065.

78 Harris G, Pear R. Drug maker's efforts to compete in lucrative insulin market are under scrutiny. *New York Times.* 2006 Jan 28.

79 Abelson R. How Schering manipulated drug prices and Medicaid. *New York Times.* 2004 July 31.

80 Harris G. Drug makers settled 7 suits by whistle-blowers, group says. *New York Times.* 2003 Nov 6.

81 OxyContin's deception costs firm $634M. CBS News. 2007 May 10.

82 Zee A van. The promotion and marketing of OxyContin: commercial triumph, public health tragedy. *Am J Publ Health.* 2009; 99: 221–7.

83 Wordsworth M. Deadly epidemic fears over common painkiller. ABC News. 2012 Nov 14.

84 Kendall B. Court backs crackdown on drug officials. *Wall Street Journal.* 2010 July 27.

85 Tansey B. Huge penalty in drug fraud: Pfizer settles felony case in Neurontin off-label promotion. *San Francisco Chronicle.* 2004 May 14.

86 Collier J. Big pharma and the UK government. *Lancet.* 2006; 367: 97–8.

87 Ferner RE. The influence of big pharma. *BMJ.* 2005; 330: 857–8.

88 Smith R. Curbing the influence of the drug industry: a British view. *PLoS Med.* 2005; 2: e241.

89 Moynihan R. Officials reject claims of drug industry's influence. *BMJ.* 2004; 329: 641.

90 Goldacre B. *Bad Pharma.* London: Fourth Estate; 2012.

91 Free Online Law Dictionary. Organized crime. Available online at: http://legal-dictionary.thefreedictionary.com/Organized+Crime (accessed 2 December 2012).

92 *Peter Rost.* Blog. Available online at: http://peterrost.blogspot.dk (accessed 26 June 2012).

93 Almashat S, Preston C, Waterman T, *et al.* Rapidly increasing criminal and civil monetary penalties against the pharmaceutical industry: 1991 to 2010. *Public Citizen.* 2010 Dec 16.

94 Almashat S, Wolfe S. Pharmaceutical industry criminal and civil penalties: an update. *Public Citizen.* 2012 Sept 27.

Very few patients benefit from the drugs they take

I am sure this statement will surprise many patients who faithfully take their drugs every day, and I shall therefore explain in some detail why it is correct, using depression as an example.

If we treat patients with depression in primary care with an antidepressant drug for 6 weeks, about 60% of them will improve.[1] This seems like a good effect. However, if we treat the patients with a blinded placebo that looks just the same as the active pill, 50% of them will improve. Most doctors interpret this as a large placebo effect, but it isn't possible to interpret the result in this way. If we don't treat the patients at all, but just see them again after 6 weeks, many of them will also have improved. We call this the spontaneous remission of the disease or its natural course.

It is important to be aware of these issues. At my centre, we do research on antidepressant drugs, and I have often explained to the media that most patients don't benefit from their treatment. Leading psychiatrists have counter-argued that, although the effect is modest, the patients will benefit from what they erroneously call the 'placebo effect', which they exaggerated to be about 70%.

Thus, there are three main reasons why a patient may feel better after having been treated with a drug: the drug effect, the placebo effect and the natural course of the disease. If we wish to study the effect of giving patients placebo, we will need to look at trials where some of the patients are randomised to placebo and others to no treatment. One of my co-workers, Asbjørn Hróbjartsson, identified 130 such trials in 2001, most of which had a third group of patients that received an active intervention, often similar in appearance to the placebo. Contrary to the prevailing belief that placebos have large effects, we found – much to our surprise – that placebo might have a possible small effect on pain, but we couldn't exclude the possibility that this result was caused by bias and not by the placebo.[2]

The bias we mentioned occurs because it isn't possible to blind patients to the fact that they don't get any treatment. These patients may therefore become disappointed and tend to report less improvement than what actually occurred, e.g. in their depression or pain. Conversely, patients on placebo may tend to exaggerate the improvement, particularly in three-armed trials where they don't know what they get but hope they receive active treatment rather than placebo.

We have updated our results with recent trials and now have 234 trials investigating 60 different clinical conditions in our Cochrane review.[3] We confirmed our original findings that placebo interventions do not seem to have important clinical effects in general and that it is difficult to distinguish a true effect of placebo from biased reporting.

You may wonder why I tell you so much about the effects of placebos and not of drugs, but that's because drug effects are determined relative to placebo in placebo-controlled trials. And if the intended blinding is not impeccable, we would expect the reported effect of a drug to be exaggerated when the outcome is subjective, such as general mood or pain.

So how often is the blinding not working? Quite often, for two reasons. First, trials called double-blind may not have been effectively blinded at the outset. As an example, researchers that performed six double-blind studies of antidepressants or tranquillisers noted that in all cases, the placebo was different from the active drug in physical properties such as texture, colour and thickness.[4] Second, even when drug and placebo are indistinguishable in their physical properties, it is usually difficult to maintain the blind during trial conduct because drugs have side effects, e.g. antidepressant drugs cause dryness of the mouth.

Because of these inherent problems in testing drugs, the true difference in the improvement rates of 60% and 50% on an antidepressant drug and placebo, respectively, in these trials is likely considerably smaller than 10%. But let's first assume, for the sake of the argument, that these rates are true and construct a trial with such improvement rates (see Table 4.1). We have randomised 400 patients into two groups, and 121 of 200 patients (60.5%) improved on active drug and 100 of 200 patients (50.0%) on placebo. Should we then believe that the drug is better than placebo or could the difference we observed have arisen by chance? We may address this question by asking how often we will see a difference of 21 improved patients or more, if we repeat the trial many times, if the truth is that the drug has no effect.

Table 4.1 Results of a randomised trial that compared an antidepressant drug with placebo

	Improved	Not improved	Total
Drug	121	79	200
Placebo	100	100	200

This is where statistics is so helpful. A statistical test calculates a P value, which is the probability that we will observe a difference of 21 patients or more if the drug doesn't work. In this case, $P = 0.04$. The medical literature is full of P values, and the tradition is that if P is less than 0.05, we say that the difference is statistically significant and choose to believe that the difference we found is real. $P = 0.04$ means that we would only observe a difference of 21 patients or more four times in a hundred if the drug didn't work and we repeated our trial many times.

If two fewer patients had improved on active drug, i.e. 119 rather than 121, the difference would still be very much the same, 19 patients instead of 21, but the difference would not have been statistically significant ($P = 0.07$).

What this illustrates is that, quite often, a 'proof' that a treatment works hinges on a few patients even though, as in the example, 400 patients were randomised, which is a fairly large trial for depression. It usually doesn't take much bias to convert a non-significant result into a significant one. Sometimes, investigators or companies reinterpret or reanalyse the data after they have found a P value above 0.05 until they come up with one below 0.05 instead, for example by deciding that a few more patients had improved on active drug, or a few less on placebo, or by excluding some of the randomised patients from the analysis.[5] This is not an honest approach to science, but as we shall see in Chapters 5 and 9, violations of good scientific practice are very common.

Apart from such scientific misconduct, insufficient blinding can also make us believe that ineffective drugs are effective. Blinding is not only important when the patients evaluate themselves, but also when their doctors evaluate them. Depression is evaluated on elaborate scales with many subjective items, and it's clear that knowledge about which treatment the patient receives can influence the doctor's assessments in a positive direction.

This was shown convincingly by Hróbjartsson and colleagues in 2012 using trials in a variety of disease areas that had both blinded and nonblinded outcome assessors. A review of 21 such trials, which had mostly used subjective outcomes, found that the effect was exaggerated by 36% on average (measured as odds ratio) when nonblinded observers rather than blinded ones evaluated the effect.[6] This is a disturbingly large bias considering that the claimed effect of most of the treatments we use is much less than 36%.

Thus, a double-blind trial that is not effectively blinded may exaggerate the effect quite substantially. We can try this out on our antidepressant example, assuming for simplicity that the blinding is broken for all patients. To calculate the odds ratio, we rearrange the numbers so that a low odds ratio means a beneficial effect, which is the convention (*see* Table 4.2). The odds ratio for the significant effect is $(79 \cdot 100)/(121 \cdot 100) = 0.65$. As we expect this effect to be exaggerated by 36%, we may estimate what the true effect is. A bias of 36% means that the ratio between the biased and the true odds ratio is 0.64. Thus, the true result is 0.65/0.64, or an odds ratio of 1.02. As the odds ratio is now about 1, it means that the antidepressant drug didn't work.

Table 4.2 Same results as in Table 4.1, but rearranged

	Not improved	Improved	Total
Drug	79	121	200
Placebo	100	100	200

My example was too simplified, as the blinding is rarely broken for all the patients, but the exercise was nevertheless very sobering. Even if the blinding is broken for only a few patients, it can be enough to render a nonsignificant result significant. In fact, Hróbjartsson and colleagues noted in their review that the 36% exaggeration of treatment effects associated with nonblinded assessors was induced by the misclassification of the trial outcome in a median of only 3% of the assessed patients per trial (corresponding to 12 of the total of 400 patients in the example).

Thus, it takes very little unblinding to turn a totally ineffective drug into one that seems to be quite effective.

The importance of this finding for patients cannot be overstated. Most drugs have conspicuous side effects, so there can be no doubt that the blinding is broken for many patients in most placebo-controlled trials. When we use drugs to save people from dying, it doesn't matter that the blinding is broken, as we can say with certainty whether a patient is alive or not. However, we are rarely in that situation. Most of the time, we use drugs to reduce the patients' symptoms or to reduce the risk of complications to their disease, and the outcomes are very often subjective, e.g. degree of depression or schizophrenia, anxiety, dementia, pain, quality of life, functional ability (often called activities of daily living), nausea, insomnia, cough and dyspnoea. Even to decide whether a patient has had a heart attack can be rather subjective (*see* Chapter 5).

The randomised clinical trial is the most reliable design we have for evaluating treatments. But we have accepted much too readily that what comes out of these experiments should be believed if the trial was blinded and the main result is accompanied by a significant P value.

What is so disturbing about this is that all drugs cause harms whereas many of the drugs we use aren't effective at all. We are therefore harming immense numbers of patients in good faith, as our randomised trials don't allow us to say which of the drugs that don't work.

On this background, it is easy to understand why companies that have shown that their drug works for a disease that the drug was supposed to influence through its mechanism of action can later study the drug in many, completely unrelated diseases and find that their drug also works for these. The unblinding is a major reason why it is so much easier to invent new diseases than to invent new drugs.[7,8] It is easy to show some effect on a simple or more elaborated scale that, on top of this, may have little clinical relevance and let the marketing machine do the rest.

An older member of my golf club once told me that he was uncertain whether the pills he took for his dementia had any effect. He wondered whether he should stop taking them and asked for my advice. I rarely give advice to patients, as I am not their doctor, not a specialist in the area in question, and don't have any knowledge about their medical histories and preferences. He also told me, however, that he was bothered by the drug's side effects and its high price. Given that the effect of antidementia drugs isn't impressive and has been established in industry sponsored trials with highly subjective outcomes, and given the many other biases in industry trials, I made an exception. I told him that if I were him, I wouldn't take the drug. As he was pretty demented, I doubt he followed my advice, which he likely forgot.

The lack of effective blinding should make doctors much more cautious than they are; they should wait and see, think twice before they prescribe drugs to patients, write in their notes exactly what they want to obtain by using a drug and when, and remember to stop the drug if the goal is not obtained.

A convenient way to see that few patients will be helped by the drugs we give them – even if we choose to believe the results from trials at face value – is to convert improvement rates into the Number Needed to Treat (NNT). This is the inverse of the risk difference. Thus, if we believe that 60% of patients receiving an antidepressant become better and 50% of those on placebo improve, the NNT is 1/(60% − 50%) = 10.

This means that for every 10 patients we treat with an antidepressant, only one will achieve any benefit. If we accept that any possible placebo effect is so small that we can disregard it,[3] it furthermore means that it made no difference for the other nine patients that they received a drug, apart from its side effects and cost. Even if we don't accept the findings that placebos are generally pretty ineffective, it would still be true that very few patients benefit from an antidepressant drug. It is actually much worse than this, not only because of the lack of effective blinding, but also because the 10% difference is derived from industry trials that were carefully designed to recruit those types of patients that are most likely to respond (*see* Chapter 17).[9] In actual practice, the NNT is much higher than 10.

If we turn our attention to prophylaxis, i.e. to healthy citizens rather than patients with a disease, the NNT becomes much larger. Statins are very popular drugs, as they lower cholesterol, and a trial from 1994 showed that if patients at very high risk for a coronary attack received simvastatin for 5 years, 30 patients would need to be treated to avoid one death.[10] This is impressive, but simvastatin was very expensive in the 1990s when it was a patented drug. I therefore looked at Table 1 in the paper, which describes the enrolled patients. Although 80% of them had already had a heart attack before they entered the study, only one-third were in treatment with aspirin, although it is a life-saver. Furthermore, one-quarter were smokers although all of them suffered from either angina or had had a heart attack. Thus, we could have saved many lives very cheaply by reminding the physicians that their patients should receive aspirin, and also that they needed to talk to them a bit more about quitting smoking; even brief conversations have an effect on smokers.[11]

Statins are currently intensively marketed to the healthy population, both by the industry and some enthusiastic doctors, but the benefit is very small when statins are used for primary prevention of cardiovascular disease. When the data from eight trials were combined in a Cochrane review, the researchers found that statins reduced all-cause mortality by 16%.[12] This looks like an impressive effect, and this is also how the drug industry advertises their findings. However, it says virtually nothing about the benefit of the prophylaxis, as we don't know what the death rate was in those who didn't take a statin. The authors reported that 2.8% of the trial participants died (note that I don't call healthy people patients, as they are not patients). What was missing in this review was the NNT. A 16% reduction from a rate of 2.8% gives a rate of 2.35% and an NNT of 1/(2.8% − 2.35%) = 222.

To understand what this result means, one needs to read the whole review carefully. It turns out that the average age of the participants was 57 years and that they weren't that healthy to begin with. Some trials only recruited patients with diabetes, hypertension or increased lipids, and some included in addition some patients with previous cardiovascular disease. Further, the rate of smokers ranged from 10% to 44% in the trials that provided such data. One also needs to know after how long the benefit was obtained, and most trials ran for several years. Finally, what I always look for is whether the trials were funded by industry or by public funds, as many industry trials never get published if the results are disappointing. Only one of the trials that provided data on all-cause mortality was publicly funded. It seems to me, which the authors of the review confirmed in the Discussion section, that the 16% reduction in all-cause mortality is much exaggerated. For example, a large, publicly funded trial, the ALLHAT-LLT trial, which was not included in the review because more than 10% of the patients had pre-existing cardiovascular disease, didn't find a reduction in mortality, risk ratio 0.99 (95% confidence interval 0.89 to 1.11, which means that we are 95% certain that the true effect lies somewhere between an 11% reduction and an 11% increase in total mortality).

The authors advised caution in using statins for primary prevention arguing that some trials were stopped early when the benefit was large, and that selective reporting of outcomes was common. They further noted that many trials didn't report any adverse events, although it's unlikely there weren't any. Unfortunately, the abstract of the review, which is the only part most people read, gives a different impression. It notes that there was a reduction in all-cause mortality and that there was no clear evidence of any significant harm caused by statin prescription or of effects on the quality of life, and that there was no excess of muscle pain.

This information is not reliable. Statins cause muscle pain and weakness, and I shall again draw on my experience from the golf course. One of my partners, a physicist scientist, told me that he needed to take a statin for the rest of his life because he had had a heart attack. It bothered him a great deal and his muscle pain made it difficult for him to walk 18 holes. He also remarked that everybody else he knew who were on a statin suffered from muscle pain or weakness, or both. He had looked in the research literature and was perplexed to find that few people in the trials had reported muscle pain. At this point, I revealed that I am a medical researcher, and he asked why there was such a huge discrepancy between what the patients experienced and what the literature said. I explained how tremendously the drug industry manipulates their trials, particularly when it comes to the harms of their drugs. He wasn't the least surprised.

Actually, my golf partner's experience was more truthful than the randomised trials. In 2012, I found a paper about the impact of statins on energy and exertional fatigue.[13] It said that, although many observational reports had cited fatigue and exertional fatigue with statin use, no randomised trials had addressed this issue. The paper reported the results of such a trial that found that 20% of the men and 40% of the women experienced a worsening in either energy or exertional fatigue. I have never heard any of my enthusiastic colleagues who advocate that most of us should take a statin for the rest of our lives, no matter what our cholesterol is, say anything about this. In fact, their arguments for irrigating the population with statins are that they work and have no side effects.

For many drugs, it's relatively easy to overcome the fundamental problem with breaking of the blind through side effects by using so called 'active placebos'. The term is somewhat misleading, as the idea is not that the placebo should contain a substance that is active against the disease, only a substance that gives a similar side effect as the active drug. For antidepressants, trials have been performed where the placebo contained atropine, which causes dryness in the mouth like the active drugs. As expected, such trials showed a considerably smaller difference between drug and placebo than trials that didn't use an 'active placebo'.[14]

The bias introduced by insufficient blinding can be aggravated by the fact that doctors and patients don't always do what is expected of them. Psychiatrists are usually paid per patient enrolled and may not bother to go through all the items on Hamilton's depression scale with the patient, as it takes time, but may use their overall impression to score some of the items without having asked, or to score later based on memory.[9]

Some patients participate in depression trials without being depressed just to cash the money, as a healthy person told a doctor on a train ride:[15]

'I'm not depressed ... the trials are advertised, the best pay about £100 a day to volunteers. For a 20 day trial that's £2000 ... it's nice to see your regular friends.'

The atropine trials were performed a long time ago, and 'active placebos' are no longer used. The reason for this is clear. By far most placebo-controlled trials are performed by drug companies and they have no interest in showing that their drugs don't work. I believe we should require active placebos and flatly refuse to approve drugs based on trials with conventional placebos, at least in areas where the expected effects are modest and the outcomes are subjective.

The companies go further than this. They often refuse to provide inactive placebos to independent researchers who wish to do their own studies.[16] When Novo Nordisk did this, the researcher had no other option than do to the study without placebo, which was criticised as a great weakness when the study was published. In another case, Novo required that the authors dropped their idea of studying whether liraglutide (Victoza, a diabetes drug) reduced overweight, and the company also required changes to the part of their study that concerned a possible beneficial effect on psoriasis. It might have played a role that Novo was trying to get Victoza approved for treatment of overweight, and if independent researchers found other results, or more harms, than Novo reported, it wouldn't be to Novo's advantage.

Drug companies may try to avoid to be seen as uncooperative by demanding ludicrous sums for the placebos, although the cost for producing them is close to zero, knowing that academic researchers would not be supported by a public funder for such excesses. On one occasion, the largest drug company in the world said that the placebos would cost about €40000, which was enough to block an otherwise well-motivated trial.

Please consider this: doctors and patients help the companies with their trials but companies won't help doctors and patients with their trials. This asymmetry is immoral, just as it was immoral when the imperial powers exploited the colonies. We should make it obligatory for companies to deliver placebos for independent research at low cost, i.e. the manufacturing cost, as a condition for having a product on the market.

Drug companies may abort important studies that threaten their income in other ways. Ciprofloxacin is an antibiotic that is prone to develop resistance. In 2000, when a bacteriologist asked Bayer for a supply of pure ciprofloxacin for his research into antibiotic resistance, he was asked to sign a document stating that he would not publish without written permission from Bayer. He wrote to the European Commission but was told that the only thing the Commission could do was to remind companies of 'the potential public interest of this type of research'.[17] Again, we should not accept this state of affairs but make it obligatory for companies to deliver the pure drug to independent research at the manufacturing cost. I have heard many stories of blank refusals to give away or sell a pure drug sample.

REFERENCES

1 Arroll B, Elley CR, Fishman T, *et al*. Antidepressants versus placebo for depression in primary care. *Cochrane Database Syst Rev.* 2009; 3: CD007954.

2 Hróbjartsson A, Gøtzsche PC. Is the placebo powerless? An analysis of clinical trials comparing placebo with no treatment. *N Engl J Med.* 2001; 344: 1594–602.

3 Hróbjartsson A, Gøtzsche PC. Placebo interventions for all clinical conditions. *Cochrane Database Syst Rev.* 2010; 1: CD003974.

4 Blumenthal DS, Burke R, Shapiro AK. The validity of 'identical matching placebos'. *Arch Gen Psychiatry.* 1974; 31: 214–15.

5 Gøtzsche PC. Believability of relative risks and odds ratios in abstracts: cross-sectional study. *BMJ.* 2006; 333: 231–4.

6 Hróbjartsson A, Thomsen AS, Emanuelsson F, *et al*. Observer bias in randomised clinical trials with binary outcomes: systematic review of trials with both blinded and non-blinded outcome assessors. *BMJ.* 2012; 344: e1119.

7 Angell M. *The Truth about the Drug Companies: how they deceive us and what to do about it.* New York: Random House; 2004.

8 Moynihan R, Cassels A. *Selling Sickness: how the world's biggest pharmaceutical companies are turning us all into patients.* New York: Nation Books; 2005.

9 Healy D. *Let Them Eat Prozac.* New York: New York University Press; 2004.

10 Randomised trial of cholesterol lowering in 4444 patients with coronary heart disease: the Scandinavian Simvastatin Survival Study (4S). *Lancet.* 1994; 344: 1383–9.

11 Stead LF, Bergson G, Lancaster T. Physician advice for smoking cessation. *Cochrane Database Syst Rev.* 2008; 2: CD000165.

12 Taylor F, Ward K, Moore THM, *et al*. Statins for the primary prevention of cardiovascular disease. *Cochrane Database Syst Rev.* 2011; 1: CD004816.

13 Golomb BA, Evans MA, Dimsdale JE, *et al*. Effects of statins on energy and fatigue with exertion: results from a randomized controlled trial. *Arch Intern Med.* 2012; 172: 1180–2.

14 Moncrieff J, Wessely S, Hardy R. Active placebos versus antidepressants for depression. *Cochrane Database Syst Rev.* 2004; 1: CD003012.

15 Boyd R. A view from the man in the seat opposite. *BMJ.* 1998; 317: 410.

16 Villesen K, Rottbøll E. [Drug industry blocks free research]. *Information.* 2012 Feb 3.

17 The tightening grip of big pharma. *Lancet.* 2001; 357: 1141.

Clinical trials, a broken social contract with patients

If clinical trials become a commercial venture in which self-interest overrules public interest and desire overrules science, then the social contract which allows research on human subjects in return for medical advances is broke.

Jonathan Quick, WHO, director of essential drugs and medicines policy[1]

The social contract between researchers and patients was broken long before the WHO director warned against this in 2002. Epidemiologist Jan Vandenbroucke has described why industry-sponsored drug trials are not research but marketing:[2]

> In usual clinical or epidemiologic research, studies are repeated by others, in different settings and by different means, looking for biases, flaws, and ways of remedying them, endlessly arguing whether the biases are remedied or not. That is the essence of open scientific debate and criticism, which is the only guarantee for progress. That is no longer possible with pharmaceutical products because the monopoly of the pharmaceutical industry of studies of its own products leads to persistently one-sided studies that can no longer be questioned by studies from other sides. Moreover, the one-sidedness cannot be seen from the public record, that is the published papers. Without the possibility of open debate, science simply ceases to exist ... all data submitted to drug regulatory authorities should become public because these data are different from the published papers. Even better would be independent funds for clinical research.

Science philosopher Karl Popper would have come to the same conclusion.[3] In *The Open Society and Its Enemies*, he depicts the totalitarian, closed society as a rigidly ordered state in which freedom of expression and discussion of crucial issues are ruthlessly suppressed.

Most of the time, when I have tried to publish unwelcome truths about the drug industry, I have been exposed to the journal's lawyers, and even after I have documented that everything I say is correct and have been said before by others, I have often experienced that important bits have been removed or that my paper was rejected for no other reason than fear of litigation. This is one of the reasons I decided to write this book, as I have discovered that I have much more freedom when I write books.

Popper would have viewed the pharmaceutical industry as an enemy of the open society.[3] Rigorous science should put itself at risk of being falsified and this practice should be protected against those who try to impede scientific understanding, as when the industry intimidates those who discover harms of its drugs (*see* Chapter 19). Protecting the hypotheses by ad hoc modifications, such as undeclared changes to the measured outcomes or the analysis plan once the sponsor has seen the results, or by designing trials that make them immune to refutation, puts the hypotheses in the same category as pseudoscience.[3]

In healthcare, the open democratic society has become an oligarchy of corporations whose interests serve the profit motive of the industry and shape public policy, including that of weakened regulatory agencies. Our governments have failed to regulate an industry, which has become more and more powerful and almighty, and failed to protect scientific objectivity and academic curiosity from commercial forces.

In the first half of the 20th century, drugs were very poorly researched before they were allowed onto the market. There weren't any demands that they should have been demonstrated to have a therapeutic or prophylactic effect. What was most important was that they were not unduly harmful and not even that was adequately investigated. As a result, a number of drug catastrophes emerged and many dangerous drugs were withdrawn from the market after having harmed or killed many people.

The thalidomide disaster marked a watershed in drug regulation. The drug, which was produced by the German drug maker Grünenthal, was marketed for a broad range of indications including pregnancy-induced nausea, although it hadn't been adequately tested in pregnant animals.[4] Before long, the first reports of children being born with an extremely rare condition, phocomelia, which means lack of arms or legs, were submitted to Grünenthal. The company ignored the reports and didn't take any action, although the reports continued to flow in. It was a classical case of profits before patients. It didn't matter how seriously malformed the children were and how many they were, as long as the company managed to keep the reports secret.

In the United States, an astute FDA scientist had concerns about the drug and refused to recommend approval. Because of her well-placed stubbornness, the drug never made it to the US market, but its citizens weren't totally spared, as the company had distributed samples of the drug all over the country even though it had not been approved. Thalidomide was withdrawn worldwide in 1962 and the disaster led to demands of extensive animal experiments and also that new drugs needed to have demonstrated their efficacy in randomised trials. These requirements had a major impact on the efficacy and safety of new drugs. Patients could now be more confident that the drugs their doctor prescribed were good for them. However, there was a huge backlog of drugs that had not been adequately tested and were still widely used. It took decades before most of these drugs disappeared and some of them are still with us today, although we don't know whether they are effective and what their harms are.

Armed with its new powers, the FDA actually did nothing that could raise eyebrows in the drug industry. It came up with a new categorisation of drugs and required manufacturers to list in small print in their promotional materials:

'The Food and Drug Administration has determined that this product is "possibly effective".' It would surely have been more honest to say that the old products were likely to be ineffective than to pull the wool over the public's eyes. Drug epidemiologist Jerry Avorn has explained what this really meant:[5]

> There is not a shred of solid evidence on the entire planet Earth that this drug is of any use whatsoever for any purpose known to man or beast, but the manufacturer has successfully demanded additional years to study it, and we don't have the political clout to take it off the market until that unbearably lengthy foot-dragging process has run its course.

The main purpose of requiring randomised trials was to ensure that useless drugs didn't make it onto the market. However, there was a problem with the regulatory requirements, which is still with us today, 50 years later. All that is required to demonstrate that a drug is effective is that a statistically significant effect has been found in two placebo-controlled trials. As I showed in the previous chapter, this can often be accomplished for drugs that have no beneficial effects.

The drug companies give the impression that they play by the rules, seemingly following Good Clinical Practice guidelines and other requirements for randomised trials, e.g. using adequate randomisation procedures and blinding, and monitoring the trial sites to ensure that what is reported to the company is correct.

However, there are numerous ways in which a drug company can manipulate its clinical trials to ensure that the results become useful for its salespeople, no matter what an honest approach to science would have shown. The manipulations are so common and serious that one of my colleagues said that we should see published reports of industry trials as nothing else than advertisements for its drugs. To which I dryly remarked that industry trials do not even live up to EU requirements for advertising:[6]

'No person shall issue an advertisement relating to a relevant medicinal product unless that advertisement encourages the rational use of that product by presenting it objectively and without exaggerating its properties.'

It is not surprising that the drug industry manipulates its results. The difference between an honest and a not-so-honest data analysis can be worth billions of Euros on the world market (see the CLASS study in Chapter 14). It is therefore naïve to expect the industry will perform disinterested research on its own products, with the aim of finding out whether its new drug is any better than placebo or much cheaper alternatives. If the industry truly had this aim, it would put its drugs at risk by comparing them with 'active placebos' and it would let independent researchers perform its trials.

The 'best' drugs may simply be those with the most shamelessly biased data. Bias is often introduced already in the design of the trial, but independent physicians who challenge the design can be fired and may acquire a negative reputation among other drug companies as well for not being 'cooperative'.[7]

One of the best safeguards we have against biased results is to establish a central adjudication committee, blinded for the drugs, which decides whether an adverse event occurred or not. However, if such a committee is fed biased and selected information from the sponsor, it will end up putting its quality stamp on a deceitful trial. This seems to have occurred for three major cardiovascular trials that were all published in the drug industry's preferred journal, the *New England Journal of Medicine*.[8–10] Independent investigators compared the number of heart attacks as reported by a central adjudication committee in the publications with those reported to the FDA for the same trials.[11] It turned out that what was published was seriously misleading and favoured the sponsor's drug over the control drug in all three cases.

The names of the drugs, trials and sponsors were prasugrel (TRITON, Daiichi Sankyo and Eli Lilly),[8] rosiglitazone (RECORD, GlaxoSmithKline),[9] and ticagrelor (PLATO, AstraZeneca).[10] Compared to the FDA records for the individual study sites, the committee more than doubled the difference between the sponsor's drug and the comparator in the TRITON and PLATO trials, from 72 to 145 and from 44 to 89 heart attacks, respectively, whereas in the RECORD trial, heart attacks went down from 24 to 8, which was also beneficial for the sponsor.[11]

These differences are really remarkable. The probability that the larger difference in the PLATO trial had occurred by chance is so low that it will happen in only one of five trillion trials,[11] or about once in 20 billion years, which is longer than the universe has existed. In the TRITON trial, the definition of heart attack was changed to a very liberal one towards the end of the trial, raising the heart attack rate to an unprecedented 10% on the control drug, which is also highly suspicious. Finally, an FDA scientist showed that the adjudication of the events in the RECORD trial was also seriously flawed (*see* Chapter 16).

In the not so distant past, the situation was better. Academic, independent clinical investigators were key players in design, patient recruitment, and data interpretation in clinical trials.[12] Twenty-five years ago, I led the Nordic Coordination Office for AIDS trials, and after we had conducted a trial sponsored by the Nordic Medical Research Councils,[13] we negotiated with a drug company about performing a trial with the company's product, sponsored by the company. During a meeting with company representatives and academic investigators from all over the world, I suggested a change to the trial protocol, which was in the patients' interest, as it addressed the – undoubtedly negative – impact of the drugs on the patients' quality of life. To my big surprise, an Australian professor remarked that my proposal was not in the company's best interest. I was so baffled to discover that an academic investigator who was going to enrol patients behaved like this that I still recall his name: David Cooper. In the coffee break, I discussed the event with some of my colleagues who were equally appalled as I was that Cooper seemed to put profits before patients, and one guessed on the amount of money he received by 'consulting' for the company.

In the end, we decided to perform another large AIDS trial in the Nordic countries alone, funded by Bristol-Myers Squibb that respected that our academic freedom was not for sale. We did everything ourselves. We wrote the protocol, monitored the trial, analysed it and wrote the report for publication, after which I visited the company's headquarters in Connecticut and told them about our results.[14] The company never interfered with anything we did. It was a rare example of what I consider the ideal way of collaborating with a drug company.

Today, academic investigators have little or no input into trial design, no access to the raw data and limited participation in data interpretation.[12] A saying commonly attributed to Josef Stalin is that those who cast the votes decide nothing whereas those who count the votes decide everything. The drug industry has hijacked clinical trials for marketing purposes, thereby making a mockery of clinical investigation, misusing a powerful tool, and betraying the trust and altruism patients exhibit when they volunteer to participate in trials.[12]

We have investigated the lack of academic freedom and honest scientific inquiry. In 1994–95, the research ethics committees in Copenhagen approved 44 industry-sponsored trials, which were subsequently carried out and published. It was stated explicitly in 22 of the 44 trial protocols that the sponsor owned the data or needed to approve the manuscript or both.[15] Not a single one of the 44 trial reports mentioned anything about that the clinical investigators had participated in the trials with tied hands and had effectively accepted that if the results or their interpretation didn't please the sponsor, they might never be published.

When we submitted our results to *JAMA*, we were met with the usual industry excuse that these were old trials and it's much better now. In agreement with the editor, we therefore sampled a new set of protocols, from 2004, for studies that were ongoing. The industry's practice had not improved; it had become worse. There were 27 protocols out of 44 that stated ownership to data or control over the publication, similar to 1994–95, but it seemed that the industry now tried to hide what it was doing. Thirteen of the new protocols mentioned separate publication agreements with the investigators, in contrast to none of the protocols from 1994–95, and none of these secret agreements were available in any documents filed with the research ethics committees.

For confidentiality reasons, we were only allowed to see those pages in the new protocols that addressed publication rights. For the old protocols, we had access to everything and it was clear that the sponsors had tight control over their trials. It was stated in 16 protocols that the sponsor had access to accumulating data, e.g. through interim analyses and participation in data and safety-monitoring committees. Such access was disclosed in only one corresponding trial article. An additional 16 protocols noted that the sponsor had the right to stop the trial at any time, for any reason; this was not noted in any of the trial publications. The sponsor therefore had potential control over a trial in progress in 32 (73%) of these studies. When the sponsor can peep repeatedly at the data as they accumulate, there is a risk that the trial will be stopped when it is favourable to the sponsor. Trials reported as having stopped early for benefit exaggerated the effect by 39% compared to trials of the same intervention that had not stopped early.[16]

None of the protocols or trial publications stated that the investigators had access to all of the data generated from the trial or had final responsibility for the decision to submit for publication without requiring approval from the sponsor.

These findings are deeply worrying. Among the protocols we examined, a sponsor had the potential to prevent publication in half of the trials and had recourse to practical or legal obstacles in most of the others. Surveys of US medical schools[17,18] have shown that they frequently engage in industry-sponsored research that fails to adhere to editorial guidelines regarding trial design, access to data, and publication rights.[19]

A survey from 2005 was particularly shocking. It showed that 80% of the medical schools would allow a multicentre trial agreement that granted data ownership to the sponsor, and 50% would allow the sponsor to write up the results for publication and let the investigators review the manuscript and suggest revisions.[18] Ownership of the data was a tough issue; 25% replied that the negotiations were very difficult.

Even *after* the contract had been signed, 82% of the medical schools had experienced difficulties in a 5-year period, and in one case, the sponsor refused to send the final payment because they didn't like the results!

The researchers could not study the trial agreements directly because sponsors generally require that institutions keep them confidential. It is likely that the extent of the problems was underestimated, as it is uncomfortable to admit in an audiotaped telephone interview that your institution accepts highly dubious practices. Nonetheless, 69% of the administrators said that competition for research funds created pressures on them to compromise the conditions in the contract.

This study shows that academic drug research in the United States has been almost totally corrupted by industry. The companies shop between the various academic centres and choose those who are least willing to raise uncomfortable questions. The Association of American Medical Colleges held talks with drug company officials to explore the development of standardised contract terms, but the discussions fell apart when drug company executives baulked.[19]

Here is an example of the consequences of the corruption. In 2003, the FDA was reviewing unpublished data from studies in its possession on the use of selective serotonin reuptake inhibitors (SSRIs) in children and adolescents to see if the drugs increased the suicide risk. The academics at the medical schools who had published positive results of these drugs were worried and issued a report in January 2004 defending the effectiveness of the drugs and disputing evidence that their use increased suicidal behaviour. Subsequently, however, the FDA determined that such a risk existed (*see* Chapter 18). The academic researchers had contacted the companies to get access to the data they had themselves generated, but some drug companies refused to turn over the data. This decision could not be disputed because the medical schools, in agreeing to run the trials, had signed agreements with the drug makers that kept the data confidential.[19]

According to the voluntary principles of the Pharmaceutical Research and Manufacturers of America, sponsors own the study database and

> have discretion to determine who will have access to the database ... Sponsors will make a summary of the study results available to the investigators. In addition, any investigators who participated in the conduct of a multi-site clinical trial will be able to review relevant statistical tables, figures and reports for the entire study at the sponsor's facilities, or other mutually agreeable location.[20]

Don't you find it scary that the only people in the world who have seen the entire dataset in industry trials are company employees? I do.

If, despite all the precautions, disaster strikes and the results show that the competitor's drug is best, the easiest way out is to bury the trial. An industry insider once told me that in such a predicament the investigators were informed that, most unfortunately, the company had screwed up the randomisation so it wasn't possible to say which patients had received which of the two cancer drugs being compared. That ended any discussion about publication before it even started.

The situation has deteriorated substantially. In 1980, 32% of biomedical research in the United States was financed by the industry, and in 2000, it was 62%.[21] Currently, most trials are industry sponsored, both in the EU and in the United States.[18,22] However, the proportion of the industry's projects that go to academic medical centres has decreased dramatically, from 63% in 1994 to 26% in 2004.[20] It is now mainly private companies, so-called contract research organisations (CROs), that run trials and some of them also work with marketing and advertising; yet another sign that industry trials are marketing ploys.

In order to compete with the CROs, academic medical centres have set up clinical trials offices and openly court the industry, offering the services of their clinical faculties and easy access to patients.[23] Thus, instead of fighting the corruption of academic integrity, the academics participate in a race to the ethical bottom, making it less and less likely that any outsiders will ever get to see the data.

Doctors have accepted that they are no longer partners in the clinical research enterprise, but merely provide patients for the trials, in return for publications and various benefits, above all financial support that can be used for other research at the clinic or as a supply to the doctor's private economy. Specialists may receive as much as $42 000 for enrolment of one patient in a trial, which the US Department of Health and Human Services described in a report with the telling title, *Recruiting Human Subjects: pressures in industry-sponsored clinical research*.[24] With such copious amounts of money at stake, it is difficult to believe that patients are never coerced into participating.

When I started to work in the drug industry in 1975, there was still a good deal of respect for doctors among industry employees and there were limits as to what one could get away with. There was a reasonable degree of academic freedom for industry investigators and it was more prestigious to work in a clinical trials department than in a marketing department.

In the 1980s, this changed quickly. Marketing people became louder and more aggressive, both internally and towards doctors, and clinical trials became integrated in marketing. Modern business managers or salespersons with little or no sense for science or medicine – sometimes with a background of selling refrigerators or cars, or a lower rank in the military – replaced research heads and took over control not only of clinical research but also basic research, with disastrous consequences for innovation. An industry insider has explained how highly useful drugs like acyclovir for herpes, zidovudine for AIDS, and cimetidine for stomach ulcers hardly made it to the market because the managers couldn't see the need for them.[25] The merger mania created stiff and bureaucratic corporate cultures with milestones, flowcharts and decision trees – which is not how scientists work – and the blockbuster mania changed the focus from innovation to me-too drugs.

In his autobiography, the grand old man in Swedish medicine, cardiologist

Lars Werkö, tells a similar story. Werkö spent many successful years at Astra and became the head of its pharmaceutical division, but the company deteriorated when a salesman took over as CEO and started to focus on cough medicines and other useless bazaar products, instead of continuing saving people's lives with drugs against heart attacks and stroke.[26] Werkö was thrown out of the board of directors after he had pointed out on several occasions that the proposals about research put forward by the CEO – who knew virtually nothing about medical research – were based on erroneous assumptions. Werkö explains that to argue methodologically with scientific facts is difficult and takes too much time; what mattered was to sell an idea and have the right supporters. In the academic world you could discuss, demonstrate your preferences, and try to argue your case even if it involved criticism of other participants' views – which it often did – whereas anything of this kind was unthinkable in Astra's board of directors where the decisions had been made before the meetings. Objections were not welcomed even when the facts as well as the decisions were obviously erroneous; saving face was more important.

I knew Werkö, who accepted to be on the advisory board for The Nordic Cochrane Centre when I founded it in 1993, and it is very disheartening to read his book about these events. In the past, several drug companies were founded by visionary and idealistic scientists who genuinely wanted to help the patients, e.g. George Merck said in a speech in 1950 that Merck tried never to forget that medicine is for the people and not for the profits.

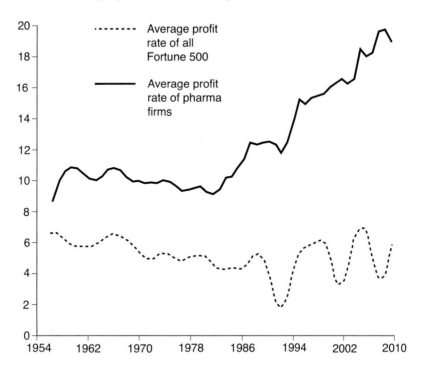

Figure 5.1 Average profit rate (in percent) for Fortune 500 companies (including drug companies) and for drug companies alone

The science shaded into marketing and the professors ended up as promoters while some industry scientists were sickened by the process they had become involved in,[27] but there was nothing they could do. Good manners were gone forever and greed became the norm that trumped everything else. The profit per unit sold has always been much higher in the drug industry than in other industries, e.g. 11% in 1960 compared to 6% in all the Fortune 500 companies, big pharma included.[28] But in the 1980s, when the marketers took over, the drug industry's profits skyrocketed and was 19% in 2011 (*see* Figure 5.1). In 2002, the combined profits for the 10 drug companies in Fortune 500 exceeded the profits for all the other 490 businesses put together.[29]

Marketing drugs is so prosperous that the US sales force doubled in just 5 years, from 1996 to 2001, and a paper with the telling title 'The drug pushers' described that the average return for each dollar spent on detailing was 10 dollars![30]

Randomised trials were introduced in order to protect us from the many useless treatments on the market, but oddly enough, they have given the ultimate power of knowledge production to big pharma that now use them for getting approval for treatments of little or no value and which are often too harmful.

Marcia Angell, former editor of the *New England Journal of Medicine*, said in 2010 that 'It is simply no longer possible to believe much of the clinical research that is published, or to rely on the judgement of trusted physicians or authoritative medical guidelines. I take no pleasure in this conclusion, which I reached slowly and reluctantly over my two decades as an editor.'[31]

Curt Furberg, a seasoned clinical trialist, lamented the lack of academic freedom in partnerships with industry in this way: 'Companies can play hardball, and many investigators can't play hardball back. You send the paper to the company for comments, and that's the danger. Can you handle the changes the company wants? Will you give in a little, a little more, then capitulate? It's tricky for those who need money for more studies.'[32]

The most eloquent description I have found of a system that has broken its social contract with society and with patients – who volunteer for trials to advance science and not to increase commercial profits for a particular company – was given by deputy editor Drummond Rennie at *JAMA:*[33]

WHAT IS A TRIAL? The approval process starts with evidence gleaned from clinical trials. It might be instructive to compare the sort of trials with which clinical researchers are familiar with those that go on in the courts. It seems to me fundamental that the legal trial carries credibility and retains force and respect with the public because the various parties, judge, jury, opposing counsels, witnesses and police, are independent one from another.

A clinical trial can be different. In that process, it is very much in the interest of the drug's sponsor, or manufacturer, to make everyone in the process its dependent, fostering as many conflicts of interest as possible. Before the approval process, the sponsor sets up the clinical trial – the drug selected, and the dose and route of administration of the comparison drug (or placebo). Since the trial is designed to have one outcome, is it surprising that the comparison drug may be hobbled – given in the wrong dose, by the wrong method? The sponsor pays those who collect the evidence, doctors, and nurses, so is it surprising that in a dozen ways they influence results? All the results flow in to the sponsor, who analyses the evidence, drops what is inconvenient, and keeps it all secret – even from the trial physicians. The manufacturer deals out to the FDA bits of evidence, and pays the FDA (the judge) to keep it secret. Panels (the jury), usually paid consultant fees by the sponsors, decide on FDA approval, often lobbied for by paid grass-roots patients organizations who pack the court (that trick is called 'astro-turfing'). If the trial, under these conditions, shows the drug works, the sponsors pay subcontractors to write up the research and impart whatever spin they may; they pay 'distinguished' academics to add their names as 'authors' to give the enterprise credibility, and often publish in journals dependent on the sponsors for their existence. If the drug seems no good or harmful, the trial is buried and everyone reminded of their confidentiality agreements. Unless the trial is set up in this way, the sponsor will refuse to back the trial, but even if it is set up as they wish, those same sponsors may suddenly walk away from it, leaving patients and their physicians high and dry.

In short, we have a system where defendant, developers of evidence, police, judge, jury, and even court reporters are all induced to arrive at one conclusion in favour of the new drug.

Doctors know perfectly well what this means for the trustworthiness of industry trials. When physicians were presented with abstracts of hypothetical trials, they downgraded the perceived rigour of the trial when it was industry funded and were only half as willing to prescribe drugs studied in such trials as they were if they had been studied in National Institutes of Health (NIH) funded trials.[34]

The study was published in the *New England Journal of Medicine*, whose editor, Jeffrey Drazen, downgraded it in an editorial. He questioned whether the lack of trust was justified and argued that this reasoning 'has been reinforced by substantial press coverage of a few examples of industry misuse of publications, involving misrepresentation of the design or findings of clinical trials'.[35] He furthermore noted that investigators in NIH-sponsored studies also have substantial incentives, including academic promotion and recognition, to try to ensure that their studies change practice. Drazen's way of arguing is very similar to the way the industry and its apologists argue, and it is not tenable. The press is *not* to blame; we are *not* seeing a few examples but a research literature that has been systematically distorted by industry; and academic motives are *not* similarly strong distorting factors as is economic motives.

What Drazen's arguments really demonstrate is the pervasive conflict of interest at high-impact medical journals, which I shall discuss in the next chapter. Here is an example. A systematic review found that subgroup analyses in trials were more common in high-impact journals, and in those trials without statistically significant results for the primary outcome, industry-funded trials were twice as likely to report subgroup analyses as non-industry-funded trials and twice as likely not to have prespecified the subgroup hypotheses.[36] This is *really* bad. It's bad science to embark on subgroup analyses when the main analysis didn't find a statistically significant result. Such exercises in trawling the data till some of them happen to show something are called data massage or fishing expeditions. If you fish long enough, you may catch something, even an old boot.

Drazen has a point: Academics *can* be (but usually aren't) equally unforthcoming as the drug industry. Despite the Freedom of Information Act and NIH statements that data sharing is essential to improve human health, no one seems to have gotten access to data from NIH-funded trials.[37] When a study showed that children with attention deficit hyperactivity disorder (ADHD) had smaller brains than other children and critics suspected it might be a drug effect, access to the data was denied.

An example of a fishing expedition was a 1990 NIH study of high-dose steroids in 487 patients with spinal cord injury.[38] The data published in the abstract of the *New England Journal of Medicine* were a subset of those randomised and described an effect on neurological outcomes for patients treated within 8 hours after the injury. That was really fishy, as the inclusion criterion was that the patients must get treatment within 12 hours, so why create an arbitrary cut-off in addition to the 12 hours? It turned out that there were no significant effects if all patients were analysed. Researchers who were critical of this were denied access to the data, and a co-investigator told a journalist that he broke with the primary author as he 'was always trying to find something that I couldn't find'.[37]

Fourteen years later, a gigantic trial of steroids given to 10 000 people with serious brain injuries, the CRASH trial, was published in the *Lancet*, and it showed that steroids are very harmful. For every 31 patients treated with steroids rather than placebo, there was one additional death.[39] Thousands of patients with spinal cord or brain injuries have died because they were given steroids and the fishing expedition in the *New England Journal of Medicine* is to blame for many of these deaths.[40] Scientific dishonesty can kill people and it often does.

The social contract with patients who volunteer for trials has been broken. It's a fact that advertising and PR firms are now running clinical trials in Europe and North America,[41] and this is perhaps the clearest sign that the companies do not separate marketing from research. Many patient consent forms for industry trials should therefore state something like this:

I agree to participate in this trial, which I understand has no scientific value but will be helpful for the company in marketing their drug. I also understand that if the results do not please the company, they may be manipulated and distorted until they do, and that if this also fails, the results may be buried for no one to see outside the company. Finally, I understand and accept that should there be too many serious harms of the drug, these will either not be published, or they will be called something else in order not to raise concerns in patients or lower sales of the company's drug.

REFERENCES

1 Boseley S. Scandal of scientists who take money for papers ghostwritten by drug companies. *The Guardian*. 2002 Feb 7.

2 Vandenbroucke JP. Without new rules for industry-sponsored research, science will cease to exist. *BMJ*. 2005 Dec 14.

3 McHenry L. Biomedical research and corporate interests: a question of academic freedom. *Mens Sana Monographs*. 2008 Jan 1.

4 Brynner R, Stephens T. *Dark Remedy: the impact of thalidomide and its revival as a vital medicine*. New York: Perseus Publishing; 2001.

5 Avorn J. *Powerful Medicines: the benefits, risks, and costs of prescription drugs*. New York: Vintage Books; 2005.

6 Medawar C, Hardon A. *Medicines out of Control? Antidepressants and the conspiracy of goodwill*. Netherlands: Aksant Academic Publishers; 2004.

7 Kassirer JP. *On the Take: how medicine's complicity with big business can endanger your health*. Oxford: Oxford University Press; 2005.

8 Wiviott SD, Braunwald E, McCabe CH, *et al*. Prasugrel versus clopidogrel in patients with acute coronary syndromes. *N Engl J Med*. 2007; 357: 2001–15.

9 Home PD, Pocock SJ, Beck-Nielsen H, *et al*. Rosiglitazone evaluated for cardiovascular outcomes – an interim analysis. *N Engl J Med*. 2007; 357: 28–38.

10 Wallentin L, Becker RC, Budaj A, *et al*. Ticagrelor versus clopidogrel in patients with acute coronary syndromes. *N Engl J Med*. 2009; 361: 1045–57.

11 Serebruany VL, Atar D. Viewpoint: Central adjudication of myocardial infarction in outcome-driven clinical trials – common patterns in TRITON, RECORD, and PLATO? *Thromb Haemost*. 2012; 108: 412–14.

12 Davidoff F, DeAngelis CD, Drazen JM, *et al*. Sponsorship, authorship, and accountability. *JAMA*. 2001; 286: 1232–4.

13 Nordic Medical Research Councils' HIV Therapy Group. Double-blind dose-response study of zidovudine in AIDS and advanced HIV infection. *BMJ*. 1992; 304: 13–17.

14 Gerstoft J, Melander H, Bruun JN, *et al*. Alternating treatment with didanosine and zidovudine versus either drug alone for the treatment of advanced HIV infection: the ALTER study. *Scand J Infect Dis*. 1997; 29: 121–8.

15 Gøtzsche PC, Hróbjartsson A, Johansen HK, *et al*. Constraints on publication rights in industry-initiated clinical trials. *JAMA*. 2006; 295: 1645–6.

16 Bassler D, Briel M, Montori VM, *et al*. Stopping randomized trials early for benefit and estimation of treatment effects: systematic review and meta-regression analysis. *JAMA*. 2010; 303: 1180–7.

17 Schulman KA, Seils DM, Timbie JW, *et al*. A national survey of provisions in clinical-trial agreements between medical schools and industry sponsors. *N Engl J Med*. 2002; 347: 1335–41.

18 Mello MM, Clarridge BR, Studdert DM. Academic medical centers standards for clinical-trial agreements with industry. *N Engl J Med*. 2005; 352: 2202–10.

19 Meier B. Contracts keep drug research out of reach. *New York Times*. 2004 Nov 29.

20 Steinbrook R. Gag clauses in clinical-trial agreements. *N Engl J Med*. 2005; 352: 2160–2.

21 Bekelman JE, Li Y, Gross CP. Scope and impact of financial conflicts of interest in biomedical research: a systematic review. *JAMA*. 2003; 289: 454–65.

22 Statistics from the EudraCT database. EMEA/363785/2005.

23 Relman AS, Angell M. America's other drug problem: how the drug industry distorts medicine and politics. *The New Republic*. 2002 Dec 16: 27–41.

24 Department of Health and Human Services, Office of Inspector General. *Recruiting Human Subjects: pressures in industry-sponsored clinical research*. June 2000, OEI-01-97-00195 (accessed 18 February 2008).

25 Cuatrecasas P. Drug discovery in jeopardy. *J Clin Invest*. 2006; 116: 2837–42.

26 Werkö L. [It is always about the life] [Swedish]. Helsingborg: AB Boktryck; 2000.

27 Boseley S. Junket time in Munich for the medical profession – and it's all on the drug firms. *The Guardian*. 2004 Oct 5.

28 Gagnon M-A. *The Nature of Capital in the Knowledge-Based Economy: the case of the global pharmaceutical industry* [dissertation]. Toronto: York University; May 2009.

29 Angell M. *The Truth about the Drug Companies: how they deceive us and what to do about it*. New York: Random House; 2004.

30 Elliott C. The drug pushers. *The Atlantic Monthly*. 2006 April.

31 Marcovitch H. Editors, publishers, impact factors, and reprint income. *PLoS Med*. 2010; 7: e1000355.

32 Bodenheimer T. Uneasy alliance – clinical investigators and the pharmaceutical industry. *N Engl J Med*. 2000; **342**: 1539–44.

33 Rennie D. When evidence isn't: trials, drug companies and the FDA. *J Law Policy*. 2007 July: 991–1012.

34 Kesselheim AS, Robertson CT, Myers JA, *et al*. A randomized study of how physicians interpret research funding disclosures. *N Engl J Med*. 2012; **367**: 1119–27.

35 Drazen JM. Believe the data. *N Engl J Med*. 2012; **367**: 1152–3.

36 Sun X, Briel M, Busse JW, *et al*. The influence of study characteristics on reporting of subgroup analyses in randomised controlled trials: systematic review. *BMJ*. 2011; **342**: d1569.

37 Lenzer J. NIH secrets. *The New Republic*. 2006 Oct 10.

38 Bracken MB, Shepard MJ, Collins WF, *et al*. A randomized, controlled trial of methylprednisolone or naloxone in the treatment of acute spinal-cord injury. Results of the Second National Acute Spinal Cord Injury Study. *N Engl J Med*. 1990; **322**: 1405–11.

39 Roberts I, Yates D, Sandercock P, *et al*. Effect of intravenous corticosteroids on death within 14 days in 10008 adults with clinically significant head injury (MRC CRASH trial): randomised placebo-controlled trial. *Lancet*. 2004; **364**: 1321–8.

40 Lenzer J, Brownlee S. An untold story? *BMJ*. 2008; **336**: 532–4.

41 Mintzberg H. Patent nonsense: evidence tells of an industry out of social control. *CMAJ*. 2006; **175**: 374.

Conflicts of interest at medical journals

In what has been called the age of accountability, editors have continued to be as unaccountable as kings.

The whole business of medical journals is corrupt because owners are making money from restricting access to important research, most of it funded by public money.

Richard Smith, former editor, BMJ [1,2]

A conflict of interest is commonly defined as 'a set of conditions in which professional judgement concerning a primary interest (such as a patient's welfare or the validity of research) tends to be unduly influenced by a secondary interest (such as a financial gain)'.[3]

The International Committee of Medical Journal Editors has declared that 'researchers should not enter into agreements that interfere with their access to the data and their ability to analyze it independently, to prepare manuscripts, and to publish them' and that 'editors may choose not to consider an article if a sponsor has asserted control over the authors' right to publish'.[4] However, despite this well-intentioned declaration, our journals nonetheless accept the virtually complete lack of academic freedom in industry trials.

Our most prestigious journals have a serious conflict of interest when they deal with industry trials, as they might lose large incomes from sales of reprints if they are too critical. The *BMJ*'s former editor, Richard Smith, has written a paper with the informative title, 'Medical journals are an extension of the marketing arm of pharmaceutical companies',[5] and has explained that sometimes companies will ring when a paper is submitted and say they will purchase reprints if accepted.[2] An editor may face a frighteningly stark conflict of interest: Publish a trial that will bring US$100 000 of profit or meet the end-of-year budget by firing an editor.[5] Smith has suggested an attractive solution to the journals' conflict of interest problem: journals should stop publishing trials; instead, the protocols, results and the full dataset should be made available on regulated websites.[6] This would stop journals from being beholden to companies, and instead of publishing trials, journals could concentrate on critically describing them.

Advertising also creates a conflict of interest. When the *BMJ* in 2004 devoted a whole issue to conflicts of interest and had a cover page showing doctors dressed as pigs gorging at a banquet with drug salespeople as lizards, the drug industry threatened to withdraw £75 000 of advertising.[2] *Annals of Internal Medicine* lost an estimated US$1–1.5 million in advertising revenue after it published a study that was critical of industry advertisements.[7,8]

The solution to this problem is simple: drop advertisements for drugs, which is the only respectable thing to do, as they are harmful for patients (*see* Chapter 9). And let those journals die that cannot survive without advertisements. They don't deserve to survive anyway, and their death would benefit us, as it would diminish substantially the pollution of the research literature with papers of little or no value. That would make it less laborious to search the literature when we are looking for answers to pertinent questions.

The drug industry's preferred journal is the *New England Journal of Medicine*.[9] Previously, this journal had a very reasonable policy related to reviews and editorials:

'Because the essence of reviews and editorials is selection and interpretation of the literature, the Journal expects that authors of such articles will not have any financial interest in a company (or its competitor) that makes a product discussed in the article.'[10]

But alas, in 2002, the editors lamented that it was difficult to find non-conflicted authors and changed the rule so that only a *significant* financial interest was banned, which was defined as one exceeding $10 000.[10] There was no dollar limit on incomes from companies whose products were not discussed. Jerome Kassirer, a previous editor with the journal, wrote that he was disappointed with this decision and added that he had always been able to find good authors without conflicts of interest.[11] Kassirer hit the nail. My respect for the journal was gone and never came back.

The *Lancet* is the industry's second most preferred journal.[9] *Lancet*'s editor, Richard Horton, is as equally outspoken as Richard Smith and has stated that 'Journals have devolved into information laundering operations for the pharmaceutical industry.'[12] He has also described how drug companies sometimes offer journals to purchase a large number of reprints and may threaten to pull a paper if the peer review is too critical.[13] The income from reprints is very large for top journals; a 2012 study found that the cost for the median and largest reprint order for *Lancet* were £287 353 and £1 551 794, respectively.[14]

In 2001, we published a paper in the *New England Journal of Medicine* about the effect of placebos and my co-worker wanted to buy some reprints; 'once in a life-time,' as he said.[15] They carried the front page of the journal where the title of our paper was in normal print whereas everything else was toned down, in a light grey colour. There is nothing as helpful for a drug salesperson as to give a reprint of a trial report from this journal to a doctor. The only thing that is needed is to draw the doctor's attention to the last sentence in the abstract under Conclusions.

I have noticed on many occasions that these conclusions – and also often the results – in the abstracts of drug trials in the *New England Journal of Medicine* have been misleading. When I lecture doctors and tell them about this, I am usually met with hostile reactions. How dare I criticise the holy grail of medical journals, the very journal that all researchers hope to get into, if only once in a lifetime?

Of all general medical journals, this journal has the highest impact factor, which is the average number of citations in a year to papers published in the two previous years. Many doctors regard it as the most prestigious one, but I am not among the admirers. Here are a couple of examples why (more will follow later; see also the previous chapter). We did a Cochrane review of Pfizer's antifungal drug, voriconazole (Vfend),[16] and found two relevant studies, both from the *New England Journal of Medicine* and both with misleading abstracts.

In one of the trials, voriconazole was significantly inferior to the comparator drug, liposomal amphotericin B, according to the prespecified analysis plan, which staff at the FDA pointed out in a subsequent letter, but the paper concluded that voriconazole was a suitable alternative.[17] More patients died in the voriconazole group and a claimed significant reduction in 'breakthrough' fungal infections in favour of voriconazole disappeared when we included infections that had arbitrarily been excluded from analysis. The abstract described manipulated results that misleadingly claimed not only a significant benefit for voriconazole in terms of fungal infections but also in terms of less nephrotoxicity. The latter result was obtained by reporting the number of patients that experienced a 1.5-fold increase in serum creatinine. The convention is to report those with a 2-fold increase, which didn't show any difference (29 versus 32 patients).

The other trial used amphotericin B deoxycholate as comparator, but handicapped the drug by not requiring pre-medication to reduce infusion-related toxicity or substitution with electrolytes and fluid to reduce nephrotoxicity, although the planned duration of treatment was 84 days.[18] Voriconazole was given for 77 days on average, but the comparator for only 10 days, which precludes a meaningful comparison. The last sentence in the abstract was: 'In patients with invasive aspergillosis, initial therapy with voriconazole led to better responses and improved survival and resulted in fewer severe side effects than the standard approach of initial therapy with amphotericin B.' A trial that is seriously flawed by design doesn't allow any such a conclusion.

By publishing such terribly flawed trial reports, the *New England Journal of Medicine* not only earns a lot of money from selling reprints, the editors also boost the journal's impact factor, especially because companies usually orchestrate a large number of ghostwritten, secondary publications that cite the trial reports.

Indeed, in the first 3 years after publication, Pfizer's voriconazole trials were cited an astounding 192 and 344 times, respectively, much more than expected given the journal's impact factor of around 50. We selected a random sample of 25 references to each of these trials and found that the unwarranted conclusions were mostly uncritically propagated.[19] It was particularly disappointing – but not unexpected as most papers were likely ghostwritten by Pfizer – that the FDA's relevant criticism of the analysis of the first trial was only quoted once, and that *none* of the 25 articles mentioned the obvious flaws in the design of the second trial.

We have previously described how a series of trials sponsored by Pfizer of another antifungal drug, fluconazole, in cancer patients with neutropenia, handicapped the control drug, amphotericin B, by flaws in design and analysis.[20] The standard antifungal agent, intravenous amphotericin B, is highly effective, but most of the patients in Pfizer's trials were randomised to oral amphotericin B, which is poorly absorbed and not an established treatment. Three of these trials were large, and they all had a third arm where the patients received nystatin, but the results for amphotericin B were combined with those for nystatin. This doesn't make any sense because nystatin was recognised as ineffective in these circumstances, which we confirmed in a separate meta-analysis of nystatin trials.[20] Despite repeated requests, neither the trial authors nor Pfizer provided us with separate data for each of the three arms in these studies. Further, Pfizer didn't respond to our questions why they had used the two comparators the way they had, even though one of the Pfizer scientists we asked was an author of one of the trials.

Another example of a highly misleading abstract in the *New England Journal of Medicine* came from a trial aiming at finding out whether it could be beneficial to give corticosteroids to patients with smoker's lungs.[21,22] The market is huge and so was the trial. GlaxoSmithKline randomised 6184 patients to its steroid (fluticasone), or placebo, and randomised all patients again to its asthma drug, salmeterol, or placebo. This created four groups: placebo, salmeterol, fluticasone, and both drugs together. The design is factorial and the correct analysis showed that fluticasone had no effect, rate ratio 1.00 (95% CI 0.89 to 1.13; P = 0.99). However, the abstract said: 'The hazard ratio for death in the combination-therapy group, as compared with the placebo group, was 0.825 (95% confidence interval [CI], 0.681 to 1.002; P = 0.052, adjusted for the interim analyses).'

The editors allowed Glaxo to present a totally inappropriate analysis in the abstract that only included half of the patients, thereby spoiling the advantage of the factorial design. The misleading result in the abstract gives the clinicians the impression that both of Glaxo's drugs should be used, although one of them didn't work. I believe this is scientific misconduct.

Cool cash may be more important than scientific integrity for medical journals. Such problems are worst in specialty journals. Their editors often have financial conflicts of interest in relation to the companies that submit papers to them, including owning shares and being paid consultants, and some of the journals are financially supported by drug companies via the specialist societies that publish the journals.

Many specialist journals publish industry-sponsored symposia. These are the worst type of papers. The industry usually pays for getting them published, they are rarely peer reviewed, have misleading titles, use brand names instead of generic names for the drugs and praise them more highly than other types of articles.[23,24]

Despite three good peer reviews, the editor of a leading nephrology journal, *Transplantation and Dialysis*, rejected an editorial questioning the value of epoetin in end stage renal disease. The editor admitted to the author that he had been overruled by his marketing department: 'The publication of your editorial would, in fact, not be accepted in some quarters ... and apparently went beyond what our marketing department was willing to accommodate.'[8]

A US Congressional investigation of spinal device products revealed in 2009 that Thomas Zdeblick, an orthopaedic surgeon, had received more than $20 million in patent royalties and more than $2 million in consulting fees from Medtronic during his tenure as editor of the *Journal of Spinal Disorders &*

Techniques.[25] Medtronic sells spinal implants, and Zdeblick's journal published in every issue, on average, papers about Medtronic's spinal products, which were usually favourable and failed to disclose the financial ties between the authors and Medtronic.

An incestuous relationship, particularly considering that papers about Medtronic's spinal fusion device had rather consistently left out all the serious harms that the surgeons had observed. *Not a single device-associated adverse event was reported in 13 industry-sponsored publications regarding safety and efficacy in 780 patients treated with the device.*[25] FDA documents revealed internal inconsistencies in Medtronic's reports and suggested an occurrence of adverse events in 10%–50% of the patients, including some life-threatening ones.[26]

We have analysed by how much the impact factor depends on publication of trials with industry funding.[9] As expected, it had very little effect on the *BMJ*, whereas the impact factor dropped by 24% for the *New England Journal of Medicine* when we only included original research and reviews as citable papers. We also asked by how much (in relative terms, we carefully avoided asking for absolute amounts) the sales of advertisements and reprints contributed to the journal's economy. None of the four top US journals we included in our study (*Annals of Internal Medicine, Archives of Internal Medicine, JAMA* and *New England Journal of Medicine*) gave us any data, as it was their policy not to disclose financial information (which we didn't ask for, only relative amounts!). We got the data from the two top European journals, the *BMJ* and the *Lancet*; only 3% of the *BMJ*'s income was from reprints whereas it was 41% for the *Lancet*.

In agreement with these data, a drug industry insider told the *BMJ* in 2005 that it was a tough nut to crack; publishing a 'favourable' research paper was far trickier in the *BMJ* than in other journals.[27] However, if successful, the paper might be worth £200 million to the company, some of which would find its way into the 'swimming pool' funds of highly paid doctors who trotted the globe's conference venues putting a positive spin on the company's products.

What these examples, and numerous others, demonstrate is that, by buying doctors and editors, the industry has transformed medical science from a public good whose purpose is to improve health into a commodity whose primary function is to maximise financial returns.[28] Sadly, and although there are notable exceptions, our medical journals contribute substantially to the corruption of medical science.

REFERENCES

1 Smith R. A ripping yarn of editorial misconduct. *BMJ*. Group blogs. 2008 Oct 21.

2 Smith R. *The Trouble with Medical Journals*. London: Royal Society of Medicine; 2006.

3 Schafer A. Biomedical conflicts of interest: a defence of the sequestration thesis – learning from the cases of Nancy Olivieri and David Healy. *J Med Ethics*. 2004; **30**: 8–24.

4 *Uniform Requirements for Manuscripts Submitted to Biomedical Journals: writing and editing for biomedical publication*. February 2006. International Committee of Medical Journal Editors website. Available online at: www.icmje.org (accessed 23 January 2006).

5 Smith R. Medical journals are an extension of the marketing arm of pharmaceutical companies. *PLoS Med*. 2005; **2**: e138.

6 Smith R, Roberts I. Patient safety requires a new way to publish clinical trials. *PLoS Clin Trials*. 2006; 1(1): e6.

7 Wilkes MS, Doblin BH, Shapiro MF. Pharmaceutical advertisements in leading medical journals: experts' assessments. *Ann Intern Med*. 1992; 116: 912–19.

8 Lexchin J, Light DW. Commercial influence and the content of medical journals. *BMJ*. 2006; 332: 1444–7.

9 Lundh A, Barbateskovic M, Hróbjartsson A, *et al*. Conflicts of interest at medical journals: the influence of industry-supported randomised trials on journal impact factors and revenue – cohort study. *PLoS Med*. 2010; 7: e1000354.

10 Drazen JM, Curfman GD. Financial associations of authors. *N Engl J Med*. 2002; 346: 1901–2.

11 Kassirer J. What the *New England Journal of Medicine* did. *BMJ*. 2011; 343: d5665.

12 Horton R. The dawn of McScience. *New York Rev Books*. 2004; 51: 7–9.

13 Eaton L. Editor claims drug companies have a 'parasitic' relationship with journals. *BMJ*. 2005; 330: 9.

14 Handel AE, Patel SV, Pakpoor J, *et al*. High reprint orders in medical journals and pharmaceutical industry funding: case-control study. *BMJ*. 2012; 344: e4212.

15 Hróbjartsson A, Gøtzsche PC. Is the placebo powerless? An analysis of clinical trials comparing placebo with no treatment. *N Engl J Med*. 2001; 344: 1594–602.

16 Jørgensen KJ, Johansen HK, Gøtzsche PC. Voriconazole versus amphotericin B in cancer patients with neutropenia. *Cochrane Database Syst Rev*. 2006; 1: CD004707.

17 Walsh TJ, Pappas P, Winston DJ, *et al*. Voriconazole compared with liposomal amphotericin B for empirical antifungal therapy in patients with neutropenia and persistent fever. *N Engl J Med*. 2002; 346: 225–34.

18 Herbrecht R, Denning DW, Patterson TF, *et al*. Voriconazole versus amphotericin B for primary therapy of invasive aspergillosis. *N Engl J Med*. 2002; 347: 408–15.

19 Jørgensen KJ, Johansen HK, Gøtzsche PC. Flaws in design, analysis and interpretation of Pfizer's antifungal trials of voriconazole and uncritical subsequent quotations. *Trials*. 2006, 7: 3.

20 Johansen HK, Gøtzsche PC. Problems in the design and reporting of trials of antifungal agents encountered during meta-analysis. *JAMA*. 1999; 282: 1752–9.

21 Calverley PM, Anderson JA, Celli B, *et al*. Salmeterol and fluticasone propionate and survival in chronic obstructive pulmonary disease. *N Engl J Med*. 2007; 356: 775–89.

22 Suissa S, Ernst P, Vandemheen KL, *et al*. Methodological issues in therapeutic trials of COPD. *Eur Respir J*. 2008; 31: 927–33.

23 Bero LA, Galbraith A, Rennie D. The publication of sponsored symposiums in medical journals. *N Engl J Med*. 1992; 327: 1135–40.

24 Cho MK, Bero LA. The quality of drug studies published in symposium proceedings. *Ann Intern Med*. 1996; 124: 485–9.

25 Lenzer J. Editor earned over $20m in royalties and $2m in fees from device manufacturer. *BMJ*. 2010; 340: c495.

26 Carragee EJ, Hurwitz EL, Weiner BK. A critical review of recombinant human bone morphogenetic protein-2 trials in spinal surgery: emerging safety concerns and lessons learned. *Spine J*. 2011; 11: 471–91.

27 Abbasi K. Editor's choice: a tough nut to crack. *BMJ*. 2005; 330: Jan 29.

28 Abramson J. *Overdo$ed America: the broken promise of American medicine*. New York: HarperCollins; 2004.

The corruptive influence
of easy money

About 20 years ago, an incident alerted me to the way the industry buys friends. Clinical investigators from several countries had attended a planning meeting where we discussed various trials that both the company and we might be interested in. When we were on our way to a lavish dinner paid by the company, the person in charge of clinical trials in the company handed me an envelope, which I didn't open till later.

The envelope contained a letter thanking me for my contribution to the one-day meeting and a $1000 bill. I had never seen such a large bill before and realised that this is how corruption starts. Little by little. You don't get more in the beginning than you are able to justify to yourself: 'Isn't it reasonable that I get a handsome honorarium for ripping a day off my busy schedule to provide expert advice to a drug company?' Back then, $1000 was a good deal of money.

If you don't send the money back, you have signalled that you might be willing to think you are even more valuable for the company next time. Helped by flattering company people who tell you how important and indispensible you are, you go on telling yourself that the increasing payments are fully reasonable, until you no longer notice that the amounts have become obscene.

To pay cash leaves no trails. In December 2000, I lectured at a course in Bern, Switzerland, and during a lunch in town I talked with a woman who once worked for a Swiss drug company. She was asked by her boss to go to the Nordic countries with a stack of brown envelopes to be delivered to doctors who participated in trials in hypertension. She felt it was a weird assignment and asked what was in the envelopes. Dollar bills. She then asked why the company didn't simply transfer the money electronically and was told she could leave the company if she continued asking questions. She refused to deliver the envelopes and left the company. Twelve years later, we moved offices, and when cleaning up, I found a hand-written note where I had asked her to write her name. I Googled it, found her current phone number and called her, and she confirmed the story. She no longer works in the drug industry but with public health.

Other insiders have told similar stories and have described the practice as routine.[1] One of my friends in industry has confirmed that it's common to pay doctors in cash. A well-known male oncologist was nicknamed wall-to-wall H...... [first name left out by me] because he preferred to get paid in Persian rugs. By using far-fetched arguments that didn't hold water, this doctor had prevented the introduction of a far cheaper generic drug into the hospital containing the same active substance as the original cancer drug.

You may wonder what his interest could be in this, but it's simple. By being 'loyal' to the company that introduced the drug on the market in the first place, and which still charged far too much for it considering it ran out of patent years ago and much cheaper generics are available, the benefits he receives from the company will continue. It's like Pavlov's dogs. You'll be rewarded as long as you do what's expected of you.

There is a culture among doctors that allows acceptance of easy money,[2-14] and companies may offer to transfer the money in ways that cannot be traced.[15] In 2006, Transparency International focused on the healthcare sector in its Global Corruption Report, which left no doubt that there is widespread corruption in healthcare. It is usually the drug industry that takes the initiative, but doctors, ministers and other government officials have sometimes extorted the firms.[7]

UK researchers found that the Polish government's system for deciding which drugs will be paid for by the state is deeply flawed.[16] One heart drug was accepted for reimbursement even though the scientific evidence supporting it was doubtful. Later, the press discovered that the decision had been taken after the relative of a high-ranking ministerial official had a new flat 'arranged' by the drug company.

The pharmaceutical giants have many friends in high places. When a person from the Pennsylvania Office of the Inspector General had uncovered payments into an off-the-books account from Pfizer and Janssen, he was appointed lead investigator.[17] After his findings had revealed that these payments went to state employees who developed guidelines recommending expensive new drugs over older, cheaper drugs, he was escorted out of his workplace and told not to come back after being told by a manager that 'drug companies write cheques to politicians on both sides of the aisle'.

The approach from the drug industry is subtle in the beginning, but the size of the favours quickly escalates if a doctor proves useful for the company. A common method of getting friends is to pay them excessively for services, or even for services not rendered.[6]

A pizza and a penlight are like early inoculations, tiny injections of self-confidence that make a doctor think he will never be corrupted by money.[18] But let's see how obscene payments from the industry to doctors can be and how deep the corruption.

Some doctors are so influential that drug companies may tacitly accept when they pocket money given for another purpose. Finnish neurologists cashed money intended to cover research costs, e.g. laboratory examinations and assistants' salaries, which they let patients, communities and the university pay for.[19] In one case, the fraud amounted to millions of Euros, which involved 180 bank accounts, many in Switzerland. Ironically, two professors involved in the crimes were responsible for supervising the ethical status of scientific projects nationwide, but one of them and his son, who was found guilty of 23 crimes, ended up in prison, and the other professor was also likely to get a prison sentence.

Sometimes the industry's initial approach to doctors is blunt and leaves no doubt about the corruption. Sandoz offered a $30 000-a-year consulting position to a primary investigator to convince him to accept a favourable conclusion of a trial, although the company's drug, isradipine, a calcium channel blocker for hypertension, had a higher rate of complications than the comparator.[3,20] An unsolicited check of $10 000 arriving in the mail from Schering-Plough with a 'consulting' agreement requiring only the doctor's commitment to prescribe the company's drugs leaves no doubt either.[21] Schering-Plough's tactics included paying doctors large sums to prescribe its drug for hepatitis C and to take part in company-sponsored clinical trials that were little more than thinly disguised marketing efforts that required little effort on the doctors' part. The company 'flooded the market with pseudo-trials' and paid physicians $1000–$1500 per patient for prescribing interferon, which the patients or insurers paid for.[10]

One thing is the copious amount of money doctors may receive when they are entangled in the medico-industrial complex. An equally interesting issue is how widespread the corruption of academic integrity is.

Before I reveal these data, try to think for yourself. What proportion of all doctors do you think receive money from the drug industry? Including those who are retired, work in general practice, work with public health, don't prescribe drugs, or don't make important decisions on their own, e.g. the thousands of junior doctors who are required to follow guidelines written by their seniors.

In Denmark, it is required by law to get permission from the drug agency if a doctor wants to work for a drug company unless the assignment is trivial, such as giving a single lecture at an industry-sponsored meeting. These permissions are published on a public website, but until recently the compliance was poor. In June 2010, the drug agency sent a warning to 650 doctors on industry payroll without permission.[22] At that time, 1694 doctors were listed, but including the 650 who weren't approved, 12% of all Danish doctors worked for the drug industry. Some doctors had several roles in the same company and some worked for several companies, the maximum being 13.[22]

When we looked at the registry in November 2010, 4036 roles were listed, which is one for every five doctors in Denmark. This number is shocking, as Denmark is regarded as one of the least corrupt countries in the world, and a leading politician remarked that is must be difficult for the doctors to attend to their usual work when working for so many masters.[22]

Table 7.1 The 10 companies that collaborated with most doctors

1	Pfizer	586
2	AstraZeneca	334
3	Merck	245
4	Novo Nordisk	204
5	GlaxoSmithKline	197
6	Novartis	190
7	Sanofi-Aventis	177
8	Bristol-Myers Squibb	166
9	Boehringer Ingelheim	157
10	Roche	118

Table 7.1 shows the 10 companies that collaborated with most doctors. It is hardly a coincidence that seven of them are also in the top 10 as concerns sales (*see* Chapter 3).

The Danish Medical Association denied there were any problems, and it met requests for more transparency, including the nature of the hired work and the size of the honoraria, with arrogant remarks that this didn't concern others, including the patients.[23] We shall see in the next chapter whether this is a tenable position.

REFERENCES

1 Virapen J. *Side Effects: death*. College Station: Virtualbookworm.com Publishing; 2010.

2 Angell M. *The Truth about the Drug Companies: how they deceive us and what to do about it*. New York: Random House; 2004.

3 Abramson J. *Overdo$ed America: the broken promise of American medicine*. New York: HarperCollins; 2004.

4 Wilmshurst P. Academia and industry. *Lancet*. 2000; **356**: 338–44.

5 Steinman MA, Bero LA, Chren MM, *et al*. Narrative review: the promotion of gabapentin: an analysis of internal industry documents. *Ann Intern Med*. 2006; **145**: 284–93.

6 Braithwaite J. *Corporate Crime in the Pharmaceutical Industry*. London: Routledge & Kegan Paul; 1984.

7 Transparency International. *Global Corruption Report 2006*. Available online at: www.transparency.org/publications/gcr (accessed 8 February 2008).

8 House of Commons Health Committee. *The Influence of the Pharmaceutical Industry. Fourth Report of Session 2004–05*. 2005. Available online at: www.publications.parliament.uk/pa/cm200405/cmselect/cmhealth/42/42.pdf (accessed 26 April 2005).

9 Chren MM, Landefeld CS. Physicians' behavior and their interactions with drug companies. A controlled study of physicians who requested additions to a hospital drug formulary. *JAMA*. 1994; **271**: 684–9.

10 Wazana A. Physicians and the pharmaceutical industry: is a gift ever just a gift? *JAMA*. 2000; **283**: 373–80.

11 Grill M. *Kranke Geschäfte: wie die Pharmaindustrie uns manipuliert*. Hamburg: Rowohlt Verlag; 2007.

12 Mundy A. *Dispensing with the Truth*. New York: St. Martin's Press; 2001.

13 Avorn J. *Powerful Medicines: the benefits, risks, and costs of prescription drugs*. New York: Vintage Books; 2005.

14 Kassirer JP. *On the Take: how medicine's complicity with big business can endanger your health*. Oxford: Oxford University Press; 2005.

15 Gale EA. Conflicts of interest in guideline panel members. *BMJ*. 2011; **343**: d5728.

16 Boseley S. Drug firms using backdoor tactics to boost sales, report reveals. *The Guardian*. 2011 Sept 23.

17 Lenzer J. Whistleblower removed from job for talking to the press. *BMJ*. 2004; **328**: 1153.

18 Elliott C. The drug pushers. *The Atlantic Monthly*. 2006 April.

19 Palo J. Why did my colleagues turn to crime? *BMJ*. 2004; **328**: 1083.

20 Applegate WB, Furberg CD, Byington RP, *et al*. The Multicenter Isradipine Diuretic Atherosclerosis Study (MIDAS). *JAMA*. 1997; **277**: 297.

21 Harris G. As doctors write prescriptions, drug company writes a check. *New York Times*. 2004 June 27.

22 Elkjær B, Rebouh D, Jensen J, *et al*. [See if your doctor is in industry's pocket]. *Ekstra Bladet*. 2010 June 24.

23 Editorial. [The greedy doctors]. *Ekstra Bladet*. 2010 June 24.

What do thousands of doctors on industry payroll do?

We become doctors to help our patients, and some doctors do valuable work for the companies that might potentially benefit patients too, e.g. as investigators in relevant trials. But most doctors on industry payroll don't. It's simply not possible for so many doctors to do meaningful work for the companies of potential value for patients.

The truth is that by far most doctors assist the companies in marketing their products. This becomes clear if we look at the 4036 roles Danish doctors had in 2010 (*see* Table 8.1).[1] There were 1626 investigators, which was the most common role. However, true progress in drug treatment is very rare. In 2009, *Prescrire* analysed 109 new drugs or indications: 3 were considered a minor therapeutic breakthrough, 76 added nothing new, while 19 were deemed to represent a possible public health risk.[2] Others have estimated that 11%–16% of new drugs represent a therapeutic gain,[3] but that was with very generous definitions of what a gain is; if the gains and the trials behind them were scrutinised more closely, there wouldn't be much left.

Table 8.1 Roles of Danish doctors with permission to work for the drug industry. Data from 2010

Investigator	1626
Advisory Board member or consultant	1160
Lecturer	950
Stock ownership	175
Author	36
Other	89
Total	**4036**

If a company has developed a truly superior drug, it doesn't require many doctors to assist it in proving this in one or two multinational trials. Since Denmark is so small, not more than five Danish doctors would need to participate to such an extent that they needed permission from the drug agency to collaborate with the company. But as there are additional relevant projects for a superior drug, let's be generous and say that 50 doctors are needed and compare this with the 1626 doctors with permission to be clinical investigators, which is 30 times as many. What are all these other doctors doing?

We actually know a good deal about this. Because of our foolish patent system and the unlimited powers of marketing, it is highly profitable to develop so-called me-too drugs, which have a molecular structure similar to drugs already on the market. For common diseases, with a large market potential, more than 100 different drugs may have been developed within the same therapeutic class, e.g. antihistamines. As these drugs are variations of known substances, one could argue that they aren't really new discoveries, in the same way as the development of a new set of bumpers for a Volvo doesn't make it a different car.

It is very rare for me-too drugs to represent any therapeutic advance, but very common that it *looks* as if they do. The industry uses two main tricks. One is to perform a lot of entirely superfluous – and therefore by definition unethical – placebo-controlled trials long after the effect of the new drug has been proven. This may seem a foolish thing to do, but it isn't, as exemplified by the highly expensive triptans for treatment of migraine. The first such drug was sumatriptan from GlaxoSmithKline. There are at least 24 published trials with oral sumatriptan where the only comparator is placebo.[4] The large effect compared with placebo was used to convince doctors to prescribe these 'modern' drugs rather than the old ones. It is strange that this can work but it does; anything can be sold to a doctor it seems.

This ploy went on for many years after sumatriptan came on the market in 1991. In 2009, a researcher reported that Glaxo had omitted to publish several of its negative trials on sumatriptan,[5] and finally, in 2011, after our societies had wasted loads of money on these drugs for 20 years, the Danish National Board of Health tried to roll the clock back, announcing that aspirin was equally effective as the triptans and should be preferred because of its much lower price.[6] I'm sure this won't work. Nothing beats industry marketing, particularly not when it comes 20 years too late.

As already explained, the other way the industry fools us into believing new drugs are better than old ones is to manipulate the design, analysis and reporting of head-to-head trials that compare two active drugs.

Whether they have placebo or an active drug as comparator, few industry trials provide anything of value for patients. In fact, they generally impact negatively on patients, as their purpose is to provide support for the marketing of expensive drugs that have nothing to offer and sometimes turn out later to have caused serious harms.

Internal company documents obtained through litigation demonstrate why the drug industry performs clinical trials. Forget all the bullshit about helping patients. Pfizer has made it very clear and even speak of off-label marketing, which they call off-label data dissemination:[7]

- Pfizer-sponsored studies belong to Pfizer, not to any individual
- Purpose of data is to support, directly or indirectly, marketing of our product
  - Through use in label enhancements, & NDA [New Drug Application] filings
  - Through publications for field force use
  - Through publications that can be utilized to support off-label data dissemination

• Therefore commercial marketing/medical need to be involved in all data dissemination efforts.

It seems that at least 97% of the 1626 Danish doctors who help the companies as 'investigators' don't do valuable research but help the companies with marketing. The worst of these studies are seeding trials, one of the darkest sides of doctors' collaboration with the drug industry.

SEEDING TRIALS

Seeding trials usually have no scientific value and usually don't even have a control group. The doctors are given a portion of the company's new drug and are asked to try it out on their patients and note how it goes. The assembled data are pretty useless and are rarely published. The real aim of seeding trials is to lure as many doctors as possible into using the new drug. The doctors get a fee for each patient, and although the companies call it research, it has the character of bribery.

A German survey found that two-thirds of such 'studies' didn't even have a study plan or an aim for the study, and only 19% mentioned anything about publication.[8] The drugs being promoted in the seeding trials were 10 times as expensive, on average, than the drugs generally being used. When a German journalist exposed the corruption, the CEO of Novartis wrote to his employees that his company in all respects strictly lived up to the codes of honour Novartis had bound itself to follow. Bullshit on paper has the advantage that it doesn't stink, at least only indirectly.

Few physicians would knowingly enrol their patients in a study that placed them at risk in order to provide a company with a marketing advantage, and few patients would agree to participate.[9] Seeding trials can therefore occur only because the company doesn't disclose their true purpose to anyone. We need a societal consensus that it is immoral to deceive ethics committees and participants in this way about the true purpose of a trial.

A hallmark of seeding trials is that they involve huge numbers of doctors who treat few patients each. The law varies in different countries, but seeding trials rarely require approval by a research ethics committee or a drug regulatory agency because they are not regarded as research, but ordinary use of an approved drug. The irony is total because at the same time many doctors think they contribute to research. In contrast to ordinary clinical trials, seeding trials are usually run by marketing people and salespeople try to influence the prescribing practices while they collect the data in the doctors' offices.

In 2006, Danish researchers documented that their participation in a seeding trial led to a significant increase in the use of the company's drugs in their practices even though the effect was much diluted, as only 11 of the 26 general practitioners recruited patients for the study.[11,12] The rationale for the study was very thin, to compare an asthma drug with itself given in two different ways, in a nonblinded trial. AstraZeneca paid the doctors $800 for each patient. We have no idea how many doctors or patients were enrolled, as the study has never been published, although it appeared to have ended in 2002. I found an undated internal company report that mentioned 796 patients and that the data were on file.

A PhD thesis revealed AstraZeneca's purpose with the study: '[AstraZeneca] is very concerned with the production of clinical evidence both as a means of making doctors aware of upcoming products and as a prerequisite for further commercial marketing,' and 'in my view it was a much easier way to get a number of GPs aboard, instead of having to go out and convince them.'[13]

An accompanying editorial noted that when a gift or gesture of any size is bestowed, it imposes on the recipient a sense of indebtedness. The obligation to directly reciprocate, whether or not the recipient is conscious of it, tends to influence behaviour. Food, flattery and friendship are powerful tools of persuasion, particularly when combined.[12]

A final point about research is worth noting. Even when academic investigators perform so-called independent clinical research on drugs, the drug industry tries to meddle with it. Internal documents that were never meant to become publicly known, but which were released through US court proceedings, are revealing.[7] An internal AstraZeneca email says that:

> Lilly run a large and highly effective IIT [Investigator-initiated trials] program ... They offer significant financial support but want control of the data in return. They are able to spin the same data in many different ways through an effective publications team. Negative data usually remains well hidden.
>
> BMS [Bristol-Myers Squibb] IIT program is growing very fast in launched markets ... most proposals are modified by BMS. Strategic focus is unlicensed indications.
>
> Janssen have a well organized IIT plan ... no IIT data is allowed to be published without going through Janssen for approval, and communication is controlled by Janssen. High expectations are set on investigators who publish favourable results but they are well rewarded for their involvement. They seem less concerned than Lilly about negative data reaching the public domain.

It seems rather strange to me that companies can run investigator-initiated trials and even have programmes for this. And if it's correct that Janssen rewards investigators who publish favourable results, it looks like corruption.

RENT A KEY OPINION LEADER TO 'GIVE ADVICE'

No less than 1160 Danish doctors were hired by the drug industry to give advice to one or more companies, in a role described either as Advisory Board member or consultant (*see* Table 8.1). This huge number suggests that people working in the drug industry are either exceptionally dumb, as they seem to need advice every hour around the clock, or they are smart, as they buy doctors. *Pharmaceutical Marketing* has provided the answer:[14]

> The advisory process is one of the most powerful means of getting close to people and of influencing them. Not only does it help shape medical education overall, it can help in the process of evaluating how individuals can best be used, motivate them to want to work with you – and with subliminal selling of key messages ongoing all the while.

The guide for marketers was even bold enough to call opinion leaders for trainees, though many of them are professors.

Most of these consultancies can best be described as bribery, and the consultants as pseudo-consultants. In a criminal fraud case that was settled with TAP Pharmaceuticals, the report described that the 'consultants' never prepared reports or billed TAP for their time; further, the sales employees who nominated the doctors to attend the 'consulting' programmes typically had no discussions with the doctors regarding the consulting services to be provided.[15]

Consultancies very often lead to self-censorship. US general practitioner John Abramson describes a flawed trial in the *New England Journal of Medicine* that recommended a particular statin, but the cost of preventing one stroke was $1.2 million.[16] When he asked a specialist to write a criticism of the trial with him, he declined the offer explaining that he did 'some consulting for the drug companies'.

When I worked for Astra-Syntex, we had only one important drug, naproxen, an arthritis drug, and we had a consultant who was a specialist in rheumatology. His annual honorarium corresponded to what I earned in 6 months. Year after year, he was paid this huge sum and he didn't do much more than educate us for about 2 hours in rheumatology and go through brochures produced by our marketing department. He cannot have worked for more than 5 hours to earn what I earned after 900 hours of work. My experience fits well with what others have reported. Our consultant was positive towards our drug, and the marketing people must have felt they got more back than they paid, but how could they know? I had my doubts.

Our rheumatologist was a very nice man and he sometimes told us we used him too little, considering his honorarium. Whether he made the first contact and suggested himself as consultant, or whether we did, I cannot remember. But I do remember that influential opinion leaders sometimes used their power over the market to extort us, which we felt very badly about. When criticising the drug industry, we should remember that there are villains on both sides of the fence.

It is attractive for industry to buy specialists and particularly those the industry calls key opinion leaders, as they exert considerable influence on which drugs other specialists and general practitioners use. We combined the list of Danish doctors with permission to work for the drug industry with the Authorisation List from the Danish Medical Association to find out which specialists were most often working for the industry. Table 8.2 lists those specialties where more than one out of five doctors were involved. Unsurprisingly, specialties with highly expensive drugs and a large market potential came high up on the list, e.g. endocrinology, oncology, haematology and cardiology. Why dermatology tops the list I cannot say, but one reason could be that they use steroids a good deal, and many newly patented steroids are very expensive although they are not any better than the ones we have used for decades.

Table 8.2 Percentage of Danish specialists with permission to work for the drug industry. Data from 2010

Dermatology and venereal diseases	39%
Endocrinology	35%
Oncology	30%
Haematology	29%
Cardiology	27%
Infectious diseases	26%
Lung diseases	21%

An Australian survey showed that one-quarter of the specialists had been a member of a company's advisory board within the last year.[17] Most of the specialists said they received less than $4000 a year for their services, but other studies have reported that key opinion leaders may receive £50 000 a year to sit on a company's advisory board,[18] or $400 000 for just 8 days of consulting.[19]

John Bell, Regius Professor of Medicine at Oxford University, received €322 450 in 2011 for his role on the board of directors at Roche.[20] The editor of the *BMJ* wrote to Bell in 2012 and reminded him that Roche had not kept its promise of making unpublished Tamiflu studies available to Cochrane researchers (*see* Chapter 3); that Bell, as company director, was responsible for Roche's behaviour; and that, by refusing to release these data of enormous public interest, Bell had put Roche outside the circle of responsible pharmaceutical companies.[21] Bell didn't respond other than by saying he had referred the letter to Roche.

Four of the biggest hip and knee implant companies doled out *more than $800 million* in 6500 'consulting agreements' with doctors between 2002 and 2006.[22] Big money also changes hands in Europe. Some hospital doctors can earn up to €90 000 from the industry for a conference or €600 000 in 'consultancy' fees.[23]

Internal company documents have shown that the advice the companies want from their thousands of consultants or advisory boards members has little to do with research, but a lot to do with marketing.[24] At a meeting with such doctors, a regional business director said: 'We would like to develop a close business relationship with you.'[25] This is illegal in Denmark and should be banned in all countries. According to Danish law,[26] an application to get permission to work for a company will generally be rejected if the work contributes to marketing, e.g. writing marketing material, sales training, advice about sales arguments, and writing leaflets for doctors that are sponsored by a drug company and which contains ads for the company's drug.

I have no doubt that our rules are being circumvented and that most doctors help the companies with their marketing. I have seen written examples of it and overheard doctors tell other doctors how funny it was when they participated in role plays and played difficult doctors while the salespersons tried to sell the company's product. It's surprising doctors can be proud that they have participated in this.

Next, we'll have a look at doctors as drug pushers.

RENT A KEY OPINION LEADER TO 'EDUCATE'

'It is very dismaying to find academic psychiatrists that one has hitherto respected supporting one drug on a Monday and another on Tuesday.'

'I can think of a well-known British psychiatrist I met and I said, "How are you?" He said, "What day is it? I'm just working out what drug I'm supporting today."'

Robin Murray, professor at the Institute of Psychiatry,
Kings College, London[18,27]

The third major category when Danish doctors work for the drug industry is lecturing (*see* Table 8.1). Close to one thousand doctors had permission to give talks at industry-sponsored meetings or educational arrangements.

Like the huge number of doctors who are 'investigators' and the many who give 'advice' to companies, this number doesn't make sense until we learn what the doctors are used for. A thousand doctors in a country as small as Denmark means one lecturing doctor for every 20 doctors. Since permission is not needed if a doctor only lectures occasionally, most doctors give several lectures every year. Thus, an overwhelming amount of 'education' is available for doctors, and in the United States, over 60% of continuing medical education (CME) is being paid for by drug companies.[28]

It is of course the generous honoraria that attract such a large army of physician 'educators'. A 2002 survey found that American psychiatrists were paid about $3000 for a symposium lecture and some earned as much as $10 000.[27] The same year, there were 30 'free' symposia sponsored by a drug or device company at the American Heart Association meeting, and a prominent cardiologist bragged he made more than $100 000 at a single meeting for lecturing at symposia.[15] Jerome Kassirer, former editor of the *New England Journal of Medicine*, heard repeatedly from his colleagues that doctors who tour the country for drug companies, changing their talks repeatedly to hawk the products of the company sponsoring their talk, are called marketing whores.[15] Similarly, doctors who work for multiple companies are called drug whores by drug reps.[29] Such appointments are sometimes used as 'payback' for participation in trials, which allows the doctors to say that they had no financial conflicts of interest while doing the trial.[15]

The drug industry routinely says it has no influence over the content of its courses, which is decided by the organisers, but such reassurances shouldn't be believed. The course content is biased and the attendants favour the sponsor's drugs afterwards.[30,31] Leaked documents show that even when the concept of 'education' has been aggressively sold to general practitioners in brochures claiming that 'all content is independent of industry influence', the professional providers of medical education ask the drug companies to suggest speakers.[32] Conversely, companies ask the providers to ensure that the speaker positions the company's product appropriately. After the educational provider had accepted two doctors to speak at a seminar on women's health, Organon, now part of Schering-Plough, which sells hormones, wrote back: 'I would like to again sincerely thank you for the political help ... in respect of orchestrating the favourable consideration of the proposed topic and speaker.'

The level of generosity also seems to matter: 'Platinum' sponsors were routinely offered the chance to 'work with us to determine a speaker and topic for the programme'.

Amazingly, the drug industry representative bodies, both in Australia and in the UK, which otherwise routinely deny everything that doesn't look too good for them, admitted that this is how they do business. Perhaps it's just *too* obvious that no matter how it's arranged, a doctor who doesn't deliver won't be asked again.[24]

> *The medical director of the Association of the British Pharmaceutical Industry has admitted that whether it's called marketing, education, or research, it's all about marketing, and the companies evaluate the return on investment into their key opinion leaders.*

Companies go to great lengths to avoid wasting their money and they are sometimes whitewashed. Internal company documents have revealed that 'unrestricted educational grants' may be redirected to for-profit medical education companies that arrange meetings where the drug company controls the speakers and the content, where unapproved uses of drugs are discussed, and which gain credit from the US Accreditation Education Council of Continuing Medical Education, although this is not permissible for events directly sponsored by drug companies.[25] In one such case, the medical education company became anxious after having seen the abstract for a talk to be presented at the American Diabetes Association annual meeting at a satellite symposium. The company requested a copy of the speaker's slides 'for our review' and it developed prewritten questions to be planted in the audience immediately after the talk to counteract negative comments about the drug. This strategy worked, as it led the speaker to address positive aspects of Neurontin.[25]

Practical Guide to Medical Education says that potential 'product champions' in the medical fraternity are critical to influencing doctors' thinking and that 'The key is to evaluate their views and influence potential, to recruit them to specially designed relationship building activities and then provide them with a programme of appropriate communications platforms.'[33] A medical education company stated, 'Medical education is a powerful tool that can deliver your message to key audiences and get those audiences to take action that benefits your product.'[15]

Brochures tell the same story. 'Development & Management of Key Opinion Leaders' was a course in 2009 about identifying key opinion leaders, interacting with and developing them, and strategic management of them.[34] Top doctors as cute little puppies for the industry to raise! The first page of the brochure spoke about 'Linking business with information' and also informed that you could save £200 if you registered early. It took five more pages until the denominator was revealed: £1299 for the 2-day course and an additional £573.85 if you couldn't live without seeing all the lectures again on a CD ROM. This makes sense for a biologist like me. The drug industry parasitises on our societies and other parasites parasitise on the parasites. Just like in nature.

Drug reps are advised to work with key opinion leaders and turn them into 'product champions', and also to find younger people who can be nurtured and have their profile raised so that they also become key opinion leaders.[24] A bit like Hitler-Jugend, so that they can go out and terrorise common sense among those who are not yet members of the Party.

Doctors are more effective salespeople than drug reps. A slide show from Merck, which the *Wall Street Journal* got hold of, showed that for every dollar Merck invested in a lecture by a doctor, it got 3.66 dollars back, compared to only 1.96 dollars if Merck's own salespeople held the lecture.[35] The honoraria can be very large for doctors who are effective salespeople.[15,27,36] Peter Wilmshurst, a British cardiologist and whistle-blower who has exposed many examples of fraud in research involving complicit doctors and editors of specialty journals, wrote in 2000:[36]

> One pharmaceutical company employs several eminent British cardiologists to lecture to other doctors around the country to promote the company's drugs. The cardiologists, known to company employees as The Road Show, are each paid 3,000 to 5,000 [UK pounds] ... plus travelling expenses for a 1 hour evening talk in the UK ... Some members of The Road Show have spoken fortnightly for the company. As a result they receive more money each year from the company than their annual salary from their hospital or university ... Some have admitted to me that they have kept silent about adverse effects of drugs to avoid loss of lucrative research contracts with a manufacturing pharmaceutical company. Some opinion leaders involved in pharmaceutical research now command speaker fees that are so high that their engagements are negotiated by an agent.

A doctor reported how generous Wyeth was when he sold its SSRI venlafaxine (Effexor) to colleagues:[37]

> We were all handed envelopes as we left the conference room. Inside were checks for $750. It was time to enjoy ourselves in the city ... Receiving $750 checks for chatting with some doctors during a lunch break was such easy money that it left me giddy. Like an addiction, it was very hard to give up.

However, when this doctor said at a lecture that other drugs might be equally effective as Effexor, he was immediately visited by Wyeth's district manager who asked him whether he had been sick. At that moment, the doctor salesman decided that his lucrative career as an industry-sponsored speaker – on top of his private practice – was over.

The drug companies received printouts tracking local doctors' prescriptions every week so that they could see to which extent their doctor salesman paid back. Pharmacies typically will not release doctors' names to data-mining companies, but they will release their Drug Enforcement Agency numbers, and the American Medical Association makes millions by allowing its licence files of US physicians to be matched up by the data-mining companies with the Agency numbers. In 2005, database product sales, including an unknown amount from licensing Masterfile information, provided more than $44 million to the American Medical Association.[38]

That industry money corrupts the integrity patients expect of their doctors and their organisations was also shown in 1964 when the US Surgeon General released a report on smoking and health that condemned smoking. The American Medical Association was the only major health organisation to withhold its endorsement of the report. It had received a total of $18 million over 14 years from the tobacco industry.[39]

The bottom of academic prostitution occurs when doctors help companies with illegal off-label promotion activities that harm their patients.[25] This should be a criminal offence. Indeed, off-label promotion *is* generally harmful, as we don't know whether such use of a drug leads to any benefit, whereas we know that any use of any drug for anything always leads to harm in some patients.

A notorious example of off-label use of drugs that has harmed hundreds of thousands of healthy people is the so called hormone replacement therapy. The name legitimised the idea that the hormones should be taken not only around menopause but for the rest of the women's lives. They were touted as being good for virtually anything, including preventing coronary heart disease, but when a randomised trial was ultimately performed it turned out that hormones *cause* heart disease.[40] Wyeth was secretly behind many of the initiatives,[41] e.g. funded the book *Feminine Forever*, which was written by an American physician, and also funded several patient groups that looked as if they were independent.

After hormones were found to be harmful, Novo Nordisk hired a German PR firm that sent letters to doctors downplaying the harms.[42] Schering, Jenapharm and Organon also started massive marketing campaigns denigrating the findings and claiming that somehow they didn't apply in Germany. A professor sent a 'critical assessment' of the trial to all gynaecologists in Germany and the 29% significantly increased risk of heart disease became 'no decrease in cardiovascular risk'.[8] The professor was paid by big pharma and hadn't written the misinformation himself; it was written by Schering. The misinformation worked. While sales of hormones plummeted in the United States, little happened in Germany.

Once when I lectured specialists in training on these problems, a doctor told me that he belonged to a small specialty with only three professors. There were two main competing drug companies and it was depressing for him to attend lectures by two of the professors, as it was always easy to tell which company was currently their main benefactor. As it happened, these two professors were also accused of scientific misconduct and I was involved with assessing the merits of both cases, which were highly interesting, but under Danish rules, I am not allowed to reveal more.

I don't attend international congresses that focus on particular disease areas, but I did go to the annual AIDS congresses when I headed the Nordic coordination office for AIDS trials. I wondered why many of my colleagues presented slides that were so obviously not prepared by themselves but by a drug company. I couldn't understand why they hadn't at least made them look as if they were their own. Particularly when they spoke about an industry-sponsored trial they had contributed to, where a more academic look would have instilled more confidence in their work. Slides with company logos, or which smells company influence in other ways, give the listeners a bad taste, as if they were watching a commercial.

I didn't know at the time that doctors collaborating with industry work with tied hands. I have no doubt that these doctors generally don't know – or suppress any emerging feelings about it – that they are being used. When I have discussed with colleagues who lecture for the industry, they have typically argued that they believe the drugs they recommend to other doctors are good ones, and may even be used too little, and that they are therefore providing a good service to their colleagues. Whether this is rationalisation or not I cannot say, but what I miss in this argumentation is how they got the idea in the first place that those drugs are good. Unfortunately, the doctors generally don't think that far, or it is to their advantage not to think.

A rare admission that doctors' opinions are for sale to the highest bidder was provided by Canadian rheumatologist Peter Tugwell, who wrote a letter to several major companies soliciting funds for CME conferences on behalf of an organisation called OMERACT:[43]

> We think that support for such a meeting would be very profitable for a company with a worldwide interest in drugs targeted in these fields. The impact of sponsorship will be high as the individuals invited for this workshop, being opinion leaders in their field, are influential with the regulatory agencies. Currently, we are seeking major sponsors to pledge support of U.S. $5,000 and $10,000. These major sponsors will be given the opportunity to nominate participants to represent industry's interest and to participate actively in the conference.

CME ought to be the ultimate test of medicine's professionalism.[43] What could be more central than physicians educating other physicians to improve the quality of care? Yet doctors hope to obtain something of value without paying the full price for it, and a variety of commercial predators take full advantage of these hopes to line their own pockets.[43]

The drug industry supplies one-third of the American Psychiatric Association's budget, and when interviewed, a spokesperson said that without this funding, instead of meeting at the Philadelphia Convention Center, the members would be sitting in the basement at the YMCA.[43] The reporter cleverly asked: 'And what, exactly, is wrong with meeting in the basement at the YMCA?' Apart from this, the psychiatrists are rich enough to pay for themselves.

What has received little attention so far is the fact that by buying most knowledgeable experts in the field, the drug industry also corrupts the peer review system. Journal editors look to experts to tell them whether a submitted research study has been done well, and experts on industry payroll may tell them it is, even when that's not the case. Many experts have shares in companies and know perfectly well what it means for the company to have a trial published in one of our most prestigious journals.

Industry liaisons may also mean that doctors fail to notify the regulators when a drug-related death is suspected, e.g. if they ask the company before they submit the report. Some doctors prefer to send their reports to the companies instead of to the regulators because of their close relations with them, and the FDA and the EMA have found many cases where companies failed to sent them on even when the patients had died.[44,45]

REFERENCES

1 Danish National Board of Health. [List of permissions for physicians and dentists]. Available online at: http://ext.laegemiddelstyrelsen.dk/tilladelselaegertandlaeger/tilladelse_laeger_tandlaeger_full_soeg.asp?vis=hele (accessed November 2010).

2 Gagnon M-A. Corporate influence over clinical research: considering the alternatives. *Rev Prescrire*. 2012; **32**: 311–14.

3 Light DW, Lexchin JR. Pharmaceutical research and development: what do we get for all that money? *BMJ*. 2012; **344**: e4348.

4 Derry CJ, Derry S, Moore RA. Sumatriptan (oral route of administration) for acute migraine attacks in adults. *Cochrane Database Syst Rev*. 2012; **2**: CD008615.

5 Tfelt-Hansen PC. Unpublished clinical trials with sumatriptan. *Lancet*. 2009: **374**: 1501–2.

6 Tfelt-Hansen P, Hauchildt Juhl H. [Treatment of migraine with triptans – a commented foreign health technology assessment]. Copenhagen: Sundhedsstyrelsen; 2008.

7 Spielmans GI, Parry PI. From evidence-based medicine to marketing-based medicine: evidence from internal industry documents. *Bioethical Inquiry*. 2010. DOI 10.1007/s11673-010-9208-8.

8 Grill M. *Kranke Geschäfte: wie die Pharmaindustrie uns manipuliert*. Hamburg: Rowohlt Verlag; 2007.

9 Sox HC, Rennie D. Seeding trials: just say 'no'. *Ann Intern Med*. 2008; **149**: 279–80.

10 Harris G. As doctors write prescriptions, drug company writes a check. *New York Times*. 2004 June 27.

11 Andersen M, Kragstrup J, Søndergaard J. How conducting a clinical trial affects physicians' guideline adherence and drug preferences. *JAMA*. 2006; **295**: 2759–64.

12 Psaty BM, Rennie D. Clinical trial investigators and their prescribing patterns: another dimension to the relationship between physician investigators and the pharmaceutical industry. *JAMA*. 2006; **295**: 2787–90.

13 Nielsen HL. *Linking Healthcare: an inquiry into the changing performances of web-based technology for asthma monitoring* [PhD dissertation]. Copenhagen Business School, Department of Organization and Industrial Sociology; 2005.

14 Jackson T. Are you being duped? *BMJ*. 2001; **322**: 1312.

15 Kassirer JP. *On the Take: how medicine's complicity with big business can endanger your health*. Oxford: Oxford University Press; 2005.

16 Abramson J. *Overdo$ed America*. New York: HarperCollins; 2004.

17 Henry D, Doran E, Kerridge I, *et al*. Ties that bind: multiple relationships between clinical researchers and the pharmaceutical industry. *Arch Intern Med*. 2005; **165**: 2493–6.

18 Boseley S. Junket time in Munich for the medical profession – and it's all on the drug firms. *The Guardian*. 2004 Oct 5.

19 Abelson R. Whistle-blower suit says device maker generously rewards doctors. *New York Times*. 2006 Jan 24.

20 Thompson M, Heneghan C. *BMJ* open data campaign: time to move the debate forward. *BMJ* 2012; **345**: 25.

21 Godlee F. Open letter to Roche about oseltamivir trial data. *BMJ*. 2012; **345**: e7305.

22 Moore J. Medical device payments to doctors draw scrutiny. *Star Tribune*. 2008 Sept 8.

23 Lenzer J. Doctor's group files legal charges against nine French doctors over competing interests. *BMJ*. 2009; **338**: 1408.

24 Moynihan R. Key opinion leaders, independent experts of drug representatives in disguise? *BMJ*. 2008; **336**: 1402–3.

25 Steinman MA, Bero LA, Chren MM, *et al*. Narrative review: the promotion of gabapentin: an analysis of internal industry documents. *Ann Intern Med*. 2006; **145**: 284–93.

26 [Guidelines for the requirement of physicians and dentists to get permission to be connected to a drug company]. Copenhagen: Sundhedsstyrelsen; 2011 June 28.

27 Boseley S. Scandal of scientists who take money for papers ghostwritten by drug companies. *The Guardian*. 2002 Feb 7.

28 Elliott C. Pharma goes to the laundry: public relations and the business of medical education. *Hastings Cent Rep*. 2004; **34**: 18–23.

29 Brownlee S. *Overtreated: why too much medicine is making us sicker and poorer*. New York: Bloomsbury; 2007.

30 Bowman MA, Pearle DL. Changes in drug prescribing patterns related to commercial company funding of continuing medical education. *J Contin Educ Health Prof*. 1988; **8**: 13–20.

31 Bowman MA. The impact of drug company funding on the content of continuing medical education. *Möbius*. 1986; **6**: 66–9.

32 Moynihan R. Doctors' education: the invisible influence of drug company sponsorship. *BMJ*. 2008; **336**: 416–17.

33 Burton B, Rowell A. *Disease Mongering*. SpinWatch. 2003. Available online at: www.spin watch.org/component/content/article/47-pharma-industry/29-disease-mongering (accessed 11 November 2012).

34 Key Opinion Leaders Europe. Conference announcement. *SMI*. 2009 June 15–16.

35 Can I buy you a dinner? Pharmaceutical companies increasingly use doctors' talks as sales pitches. 2005 Aug. Available online at: www.worstpills.org (accessed August 2005).

36 Wilmshurst P. Academia and industry. *Lancet*. 2000; **356**: 338–44.

37 Carlat D. Dr drug rep. *New York Times*. 2007 Nov 25.

38 Fugh-Berman A, Ahari S. Following the script: how drug reps make friends and influence doctors. *PLoS Med*. 2007; **4**: e150.

39 Blum A, Solberg E, Wolinsky H. The Surgeon General's report on smoking and health 40 years later: still wandering in the desert. *Lancet*. 2004; **363**: 97–8.

40 Rossouw JE, Anderson GL, Prentice RL, *et al*. Risks and benefits of estrogen plus progestin in healthy postmenopausal women: principal results From the Women's Health Initiative randomized controlled trial. *JAMA*. 2002; **288**: 321–33.

41 Avorn J. *Powerful Medicines: the benefits, risks, and costs of prescription drugs*. New York: Vintage Books; 2005.

42 Clark J. A hot flush for big pharma. *BMJ*. 2003; **327**: 400.

43 Brody H. *Hooked: ethics, the medical profession, and the pharmaceutical industry*. Lanham: Rowman & Littlefield; 2008.

44 Petersen M. *Our Daily Meds*. New York: Sarah Crichton Books; 2008.

45 Wise J. European drug agency criticises Roche for failing to report adverse reactions and patient deaths. *BMJ*. 2012; **344**: e4344.

Hard sell

The drug industry is unique in that it can make exploitation appear a noble purpose.

Former medical director of Squibb at a US Senate hearing[1]

CLINICAL TRIALS ARE MARKETING IN DISGUISE

Whatever the industry does, whatever it calls it, and whatever it says about its noble motives, it all boils down to one thing: selling drugs.

This is done very effectively by tightly controlling the flow and type of information about its drugs, both in scientific papers and in marketing. Its clinical trials are rarely research in the true sense of this word (*see* Chapter 5); it is marketing disguised as research. The trials are often flawed by design, additional flaws are introduced during data analysis, and the misleading results are spun to make sure that whatever an honest trial might have shown, the trial concludes something that is useful for boosting sales.[2-8]

My thesis showed that what the industry publishes just *cannot* be true. I identified 196 double-blind trials where a new nonsteroidal anti-inflammatory drug (NSAID) had been compared with a control NSAID in patients with rheumatoid arthritis.[2] This is a highly variable disease, which makes it difficult to find differences between two similar drugs, but despite this, the trials were microscopically small, with a median sample size of only 27 patients in each group.[3] One would therefore expect virtually all statistically significant differences in effect to have arisen by chance, i.e. 5% of the differences would be statistically significant, 2.5% in favour of the new drug and 2.5% in favour of the control drug.

However, 14% of the differences, or three times as many as expected, were statistically significant, and in 73 trials, *all* differences favoured the new drug compared with only 8 trials that favoured the control drug.[3] It was rarely possible to check the statistical analyses, but I found 12 trials where the claimed statistically significant differences were not statistically significant and 5 trials where I strongly suspected it. In *all* 17 cases, the false significant findings favoured the new drug. The results for side effects were even more striking. In *all* 39 trials with a significant difference in side effects, this difference favoured the new drug.

Thus, the new NSAIDs appeared to be considerably better than the old ones. And the spin in the conclusion or abstract was even more formidable. In 81 cases, the biased conclusion favoured the new drug, and in only one case did the conclusion favour the control drug ($P = 3.4 \cdot 10^{-23}$).

However, when I looked at the data (presented as means in the papers), the impressive superiority of new drugs disappeared. The most common outcome was grip strength, and there was no difference between new drugs and control drugs, on average.[9]

I reasoned that the most important outcome when two NSAIDs are being compared is which drug the patients prefer in crossover trials where they try both drugs in random order. The patients are surely the best judges for weighing a certain degree of pain relief against the side effects of the drugs. Most trials had used indomethacin as comparator, an old drug marketed in 1963, which, according to industry myths and flawed trials, had many side effects. However, in indomethacin crossover trials, the patients preferred indomethacin about equally often as the new NSAID (*see* Figure 9.1).[10] The figure shows that the larger the trial, the less the variation in the difference between the two drugs. This is expected from statistical theory. When we randomise rather few patients, there will sometimes be more patients with a good prognosis in the indomethacin group than in the other group, and sometimes there will be more patients with a poor prognosis. When we randomise many patients, the groups will be very similar and the result therefore more precise than in a small trial. We expect the results from many similar trials to lie within a symmetric funnel and this is also the case, apart from two results that are so outlying that fraud must be suspected.

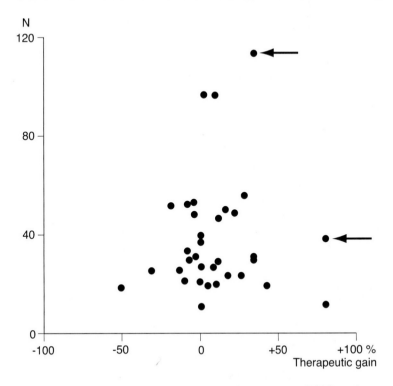

Figure 9.1 Difference in proportion of patients preferring a new NSAID and proportion preferring indomethacin (therapeutic gain) in 34 cross-over trials. Arrows mark two outlying, likely fraudulent, trials

Two of 32 trials is a high fraud rate (6%), but when I showed the graph to a colleague from industry, he laughed and said that everybody knew that about 5% of trials were fraudulent, i.e. more or less made up. Data fabrication was so widespread in the drug industry that there was slang for it: 'dry labelling' or 'graphiting' in the United States and 'making' in Japan.[11]

When I defended my thesis in 1990, the two examiners felt that NSAIDs were a particularly bad area because there was so much competition on the market. My results were *too* shocking for them to fully realise what they meant. Since then, however, we have seen similar problems in all therapeutic areas that have been thoroughly investigated.

Lipid-lowering drugs is another example of a highly competitive market. In head-to-head statin trials there is often no blinding, no concealment of treatment allocation (which means that the randomisation could have been violated), poor follow-up and no intention-to-treat analysis (where the fate of all randomised patients are accounted for, also those who drop out).[12] Funding from the test drug company rather than the comparator drug company was associated with more favourable results (odds ratio 20) and more favourable conclusions (odds ratio 35). This is not surprising considering that head-to-head statin trials are not fairly designed, as the compared doses in most of the trials are not equivalent.[13] Further, there are no trials of good quality that have compared different statins for clinically relevant outcomes such as coronary disease events. In contrast, no less than 29 placebo-controlled trials have reported on such events, which suggest that many of the trials were unethical, as patients on placebo were denied an effective drug.

Looking at it from a helicopter perspective, a Cochrane review that included 48 papers that in total comprised thousands of individual trials found that industry-sponsored studies more often had favourable efficacy results, favourable harms results and favourable conclusions for the drug or medical device of interest, compared with non-industry sponsored studies.[14]

The industry's many tricks make the impossible possible. It is very rare that the title of a paper tells you everything you need to know, but here is an example:[15]

'Why olanzapine beats risperidone, risperidone beats quetiapine, and quetiapine beats olanzapine: an exploratory analysis of head-to-head comparison studies of second-generation antipsychotics.' In a mathematical sense, this shouldn't be possible. If A is higher than B, and B is higher than C, then C cannot be higher than A.

GHOSTWRITING

The misleading information in original research papers is subsequently propagated in scores of ghostwritten reviews and other secondary articles. Ghostwriting is very harmful to public health, as it misleads doctors about the benefits and harms of drugs.[16] It is also fraud, as doctors are deceived deliberately. The very purpose of not informing the readers about who wrote the paper is to make it appear as if it came from disinterested, prominent academics and not from a corporate sponsor.

Ghostwritten papers are subsequently cited in promotional materials and in other ghost-papers, as if they provide independent verification that the drug is effective and safe and better than other drugs. Thus, marketing people produce ghost-papers that are used by the same marketing people, a perfect incestuous way of fooling unsuspecting doctors into believing what they think their own leaders have written.

If deceit wasn't intended, we would expect the company to tell us who the writer was, make it clear that the writer was paid and commissioned to do the work, and publish the paper in that writer's name. Instead, companies go to great lengths to find academics that cover up the scam with their names and omit any mentioning of the medical writer's contribution, even in the acknowledgement. The academics get paid for their non-work and may receive a letter offering them tens of thousands of dollars simply to add their names to a review they have never seen that praises the company's new drug.[17]

Ghostwriting corrupts the trust that is so essential for scientific communication. It's looks like a win–win situation for the doctors and the company that share an interest in not telling anyone about the arrangement, but lawsuits have made it possible for everyone to get a glimpse of the dirty business. I shall first describe how common the practice is.

A study of papers on the antidepressant drug sertraline (Zoloft, Pfizer) showed that in a 3-year period, 55 papers had been written by a medical writing agency, *Current Medical Directions*, whereas only 41 papers had been written by other people.[18] Only two of the 55 papers acknowledged writing support from people not listed as authors, and *all* results were favourable for Pfizer.

In 2007, the International Society of Medical Planning Professionals included a workshop at its annual meeting where a consultant warned of the dangers of regulators seeing publication plans: 'If they looked at a publication strategy that, I don't know, had, "We're going to put out 80 papers this year on one drug, all off-label. Fifty of those will be review articles where we'll pay someone to write about off-label use ..."'[19]

We had access to both the protocol and the publication for 44 industry-initiated trials and used our sample to study ghostwriting.[20] We didn't find any trial protocol or publication that stated explicitly that the clinical study report or the manuscript was to be written or was written by the clinical investigators, and none of the protocols stated that clinical investigators were to be involved with data analysis. We found evidence of ghost authorship for 75% of the trials, which increased to 91% when we included cases where a person qualifying for authorship was acknowledged rather than appearing as an author. In most trials, the ghost authors we identified were statisticians, but we likely overlooked others, as we had very limited information to identify the possible omission of other people who would have qualified as authors. The trial protocol is an important document, but only five protocols explicitly identified the author. None of these people – all of whom were company employees – were listed as authors of the publications or were thanked in the acknowledgements, even though one protocol noted that the 'author of this protocol will be included in the list of authors'. The ghosts operate in complete darkness, it seems, and shy from the light.

A good way of reducing the prevalence of ghosts and guests is to write in the paper who did what, like film credits. This idea was coined by Drummond

Rennie in 1996 and the *Lancet* was the first journal to introduce it, in 1997.[21] Here is an example:

'Ms. Yank first conceived of and designed this study; collected, analyzed, and interpreted the data; and wrote the article. Dr. Rennie assisted with refining the concept and design, assisted with data collection, and critically revised the article for important intellectual content.'

According to internationally accepted criteria for authorship, persons listed as authors are required to have made all of the following substantial contributions: (1) conceived and designed the paper or analysed and interpreted the data; (2) drafted the paper or revised it critically for important intellectual content; and (3) approved the final version of the paper before publication.[22] These criteria made it possible to study if authors of original research articles in *Lancet* papers deserved authorship. Although Yank *et al.* used a very conservative definition of guest authors, 44% of the authors did not fulfil these lenient criteria for authorship.[22]

Studies that rely on what people tell you will underestimate the problems because of social desirability bias. Nonetheless, one such study reported 13% ghost authorship of papers published in six major medical journals and 21% guest authorship.[22]

David Healy has described how frank some companies are towards doctors. 'We have had our ghostwriter produce a first draft based on your published work. I attach it here.' When Healy was unhappy with the glowing review of a drug and suggested changes, the company replied that he had missed some 'commercially important' points and published the paper in another academic's name.[23]

When a little light shines on the ghosts, it is usually in the form of 'XX provided editorial assistance', which means 'XX wrote the paper', and when only a trace of light comes through the shadows, we are told that the authors thank XX for help. With what? Cooking coffee while the overburdened clinicians analysed the data? Hardly.

THE MARKETING MACHINE

With an abundance of flawed literature at hand, it is not difficult to let marketing do the final kill, and even without such literature, marketing works. What is likely the most notorious example of this in medical history is related to treatment of stomach ulcers. Fifty years ago, ulcers were often treated by surgery, but James Black from the US company Smith Kline & French invented cimetidine, a drug that reduces stomach acid. It came on the market in 1977 under the name Tagamet,[24] and Black was awarded the Nobel Prize.

The company's success was to be beaten by Paul Girolami, a financial controller who had worked his way to the top as CEO of the UK company Glaxo. Glaxo was mostly known for milk formulas for infants and had no operations in the United States. In 1983, Glaxo marketed a very similar drug, ranitidine (Zantac), with a highly unusual strategy. Instead of offering a lower price than Tagamet, the price was about 50% higher to suggest to people that it was a better drug. It wasn't, but Girolami launched one of the most expensive and aggressive promotional campaigns ever seen. He hired drug salespeople who already worked for Hoffmann-La Roche in the United States and literally exploded the ailment heartburn. Gallup was paid to survey Americans and dutifully came up with the result he wanted, that almost half of Americans suffered heartburn each month, which led to the campaign Heartburn Across America. Glaxo also hired a celebrity, an actress who told the public how Zantac had helped her.

Already 3 years after the launch, Zantac surpassed Tagamet in sales and became the best-selling drug on earth, and Girolami was knighted by Queen Elizabeth.

This looked more like an evil plot concocted by an imaginative novel writer than reality, but unfortunately it was real, and it showed to the world that even research at Nobel Prize level couldn't beat marketing. It changed the drug industry forever after, as they say in fairy tales, and marked the beginning of an era with a terrible waste of taxpayers' money on industry marketing and very little innovation.

Drug companies institutionalised deception,[24] and Pfizer won the race to the ethical bottom. Right from its foundation in 1849, the company has shown a knack for getting people to take more medicine, so it's no surprise that Pfizer became the world's biggest drug company. When its CEO retired in 2000, he said that he recently bought a boat but as he had nowhere to put it, he bought a marina too.[24]

The tight information control goes under the radar of most doctors, but their patients may think otherwise:[25]

'My patient scanned the prescription I had handed her, then idly glanced at the elegant ballpoint pen I had used to sign it. The same brand name appeared on both. She said nothing, but I knew what she was thinking.'

General practitioners rely on the drug industry as their main information source.[11,26,27] In one study, 86% of them reported seeing drug salespeople,[27] and in Australia, 86% of the specialists had seen a drug salesperson within the last year.[28] Free samples of drugs are usually left behind after such visits,[29] and such samples are highly effective in getting doctors to use expensive drugs. This explains why the value of the samples amounted to about one-quarter of the industry's total marketing costs in 2004.[30] It is a nice gesture to give away a pill box for free, but some doctors actually sell them to their patients or bill their government for them.[31,32]

Doctors are surprisingly naïve and don't realise how much they are being manipulated. Most doctors believe the information they get from the industry is helpful for them.[27,33-35] When interviewed, they question the objectivity of the industry, but nevertheless consider the information to be factually accurate and also feel able to separate credible from misleading information.[27] The truth – which has been demonstrated in many research studies – is that doctors are *not* able to separate correct from misleading information.[26,33,35] How could they when they are only presented with misleading information?[35]

Physicians believe that their actions are motivated by how good the drugs are, but studies have shown that their beliefs more closely match marketing claims. A survey of 85 physicians, of which one-third were specialists in internal medicine, showed that 71% believed that impaired cerebral blood flow was a major cause of senile dementia, and one-third had found cerebral vasodilators useful in managing confused geriatric patients.[26] However, dementia isn't caused by impaired blood flow and the drugs didn't work! Half of these doctors also believed that a morphine derivative, propoxyphene, is more effective than aspirin, although it's worse and hardly better than a placebo.

I doubt that these same doctors would privately buy a washing machine that costs 10 times more than other machines, just because the maker has compared it with the cheaper machines and claims that his machine is best. But healthcare is different. Doctors are not held financially accountable for their choices and often prescribe drugs that are 10 times or more expensive than older drugs, although the only information they have comes from the manufacturer.

Because marketing is so effective, industry spends vast amounts of money on it. Already 20 years ago, the industry spent $8000–$15 000 per physician every year in the United States.[36] The current expenditure exceeds $1 billion a year in the United States; there is one salesperson per five office-based physicians, and 12% of a random sample of doctors had received financial incentives to participate in studies. You and I pay for all this through our taxes. We not only pay for the extravagant marketing but also for reimbursement of the drugs because they are so expensive that people cannot afford them.

Meeting with drug salespeople leads to formulary addition requests for the company's drugs, although most of the requested drugs present little or no therapeutic advantage over existing drugs; it leads to higher drug costs and decreased prescribing of generic drugs; and it leads to irrational prescribing in other ways.[33] A study showed that physicians were more likely than other physicians to request these drugs to be added if they had met with salespeople from the companies (odds ratio 13) or had accepted money from them (odds ratio 19).[37]

Sponsored meals lead to formulary addition requests, even when the information spread at lunch rounds about the sponsor's and competitor's drugs is inaccurate.[33] In a study where the salespeople knew their pitches were tape-recorded, 11% of the statements about the sponsor's drug were inaccurate and favoured the drug, whereas none of the statements about competitors' drugs were favourable.[34] There is reason to suspect it's much worse when it's a one-to-one interaction without witnesses.

Whenever research studies have examined dose–response relationships, they existed.[33] Thus, the more exposure to industry people, the worse for the patients and our national economies.

So-called educational events are not any better. The sponsor's drug is always preferentially highlighted and prescribing practice changes in favour of the sponsor's drug.[33]

One of the best things a company can do is to invite doctors to a lavish resort. On an all-expenses-paid trip to the Caribbean, the doctors learned about a new intravenous antibiotic and a new intravenous cardiovascular drug.[38] Only one of 20 doctors admitted that such a trip could possibly influence prescribing decisions; the other 19 denied it. However, usage at the hospitals more than trebled for the first drug and more than doubled for the second, whereas little happened in national usage patterns for the two drugs. Interestingly, the new drugs did not replace the old ones; they simply increased overall drug usage just as we have seen for other areas, e.g. NSAIDs (*see* Chapter 14) and SSRIs (Chapter 17). For some reason, the names of the drugs were not revealed, but hospital owners and tax-payers pay for trips like this many times over what they cost for the companies.

It is not surprising that a major source of income for the drug industry is their me-too drugs. They are rarely any better than old drugs,[2,39] but we are usually left in the dark about this, as the industry generally avoids to perform head-to-head comparisons of similar drugs, and as those that are carried out are often rigged.[2–15,40,41] Publicly funded trials that compare a new drug with an old one commonly reveal that we have wasted vast amounts of money on drugs that were not any better than cheaper alternatives.[40–45]

A study from British Columbia showed that even with a generous definition of what constitutes a therapeutic advance, 80% of the increase in drug expenditure between 1996 and 2003 was explained by new, patented drugs that didn't offer a substantial improvement.[39] If only half of the me-too drugs had been priced to compete with the older alternatives, the state could have saved a quarter of its total expenditure on prescription drugs.

Doctors say they don't take drug ads in medical journals seriously, but they are influenced by them, otherwise they wouldn't be there. A 2003 paper reported on 287 advertisements for anti-hypertensive or lipid-lowering drugs and found 125 promotional claims with references.[46] However, 23 references were unretrievable, as they referred to data on file or inaccessible monographs, and 45 of 102 referenced claims were not supported by the reference provided, which was therefore pure window-dressing to make the ad look 'scientific'.

An analysis of 109 full-page advertisements in 10 leading medical journals showed that in half of cases, they would lead to improper prescribing if the physician had no other information about the drug.[47]

An industry insider who responded to a paper in the *BMJ* where we had compared Cochrane reviews with industry-supported meta-analyses of the same drugs in the same disease[48] gave an amusing account of the issue of the unretrievable references under the heading, 'Pharmaceutical lies':[49]

> We have doctors from all over the world who drop into Australia on a first class all expenses paid junket/trip telling us how great a particular medicine is. If you read the small print on a pharmaceutical company flier you will find most references are 'on file' or have been presented at a midnight session of the Darfur Cardiologists Conference. As a medical director of a pharmaceutical company I learnt how to get articles published in journals with one journal promising publication if we purchased 2000 reprints at $10 each.

Summing all this up, a systematic review of 58 studies showed that the information from the drug industry leads to higher prescribing frequency, higher costs and lower prescribing quality.[50] We should ask our politicians to forbid marketing of drugs, as it is harmful,[33–38,51,52] just like marketing of tobacco is, which is why we have prohibited tobacco advertisements.

Drug companies use the rhetoric of liberalism to defend their right to advertise but liberalism is about the right of people to do what they like as long as it doesn't harm others, not about companies having a right to do immense harm to people and society with impunity.[11]

Actually, most physicians agree that drug salespeople as speakers should be banned,[23] but they are highly inconsistent as most of them meet with salespeople every week.[33] And it gets worse all the time. In 2004, there were 237 000 meetings and talks in the United States sponsored by drug companies featuring doctor salespeople as speakers and 134 000 led by company salespeople; just 6 years earlier, doctors and industry salespeople delivered together only 60 000 talks.[53]

There are also the planted messages. The industry has armies of paid bloggers that distribute pharma material disguised as opinion on the internet, and most major media outlets have pharma ties. For example, James Murdoch, son of Rupert Murdoch, was on the board of GlaxoSmithKline and Time Inc's CEO Laura Lang formerly worked at Pfizer and Bristol-Myers Squibb. This helps explain why we so often see completely uncritical articles in the media that are copy-and-paste versions of company press releases about their wonder drugs. Like the drug industry, the media are immensely powerful, and when the two join forces, falsehoods are at their worst. The industry also tries to get access to making changes in Wikipedia to ensure pharma friendly messages appear there too.

HARD SELL AD NAUSEAM

Drugs against nausea and vomiting tell a story about how the voluntary efforts of 100 000 patients were wasted because of poor research conduct. Ondansetron is a showcase for this. When 108 trial reports were examined more closely, it turned out that 14 of them were not new trials but reports that included some of the same patients reported on before.[54] None of these additional reports had a clear cross-reference to the original reports, although this is required, and some had a completely new set of authors. Some had combined data from two trials, added a new treatment arm, added more data, used a different anaesthetic, used other numbers of patients or reported other patient characteristics than in the original report. One would have thought it impossible to have a new treatment arm and to use a different anaesthetic in the same trial as reported elsewhere.

The trials published more than once were the most positive ones. The NNT to prevent vomiting compared with placebo was 16 for the trials that were not duplicated and only 3 for the duplicated ones. The manipulations, which give the readers a false impression of the drug, were generally not detected, as papers and a textbook cited the same very favourable trial more than once, as if it were separate trials.

Ondansetron was originally marketed by GlaxoWellcome for nausea and vomiting after chemotherapy, but the company wanted to sell it also for postoperative problems. In 1993, an advertisement in the *BMJ* talked about 'Making history of postoperative nausea and vomiting', but all five references were to studies in cancer.[55] In 1994, 18 placebo-controlled trials of ondansetron for postoperative problems had been published, compared to only four trials with an active comparator. Considering that several effective medicines were already available, this wealth of placebo-controlled trials was neither ethical nor helpful for the patients and their doctors, but it was certainly helpful for Glaxo's marketing machine: Although ondansetron was very expensive, it was highly used instead of the much cheaper alternatives.

When ondansetron ran out of patent, its effectiveness evaporated overnight it seemed, as there were now other patented 'setrons' that were much more expensive. One was granisetron. Its effect on the prevention of postoperative nausea was assessed in the largest Cochrane review ever performed.[56] It runs over 785 pages and includes 737 trials (103 237 patients) comparing a drug with placebo or another drug, or doses or timing of administration. This is a colossal waste of resources and abuse for a commercial purpose of the patients' trust in medical research. Much fewer trials and patients would have sufficed to tell us what we need to know. However, these trials inadvertently show us something about fraud and other manipulations with the data. The nausea trials do not show a symmetric pattern as in Figure 9.1, and the bias in trials comparing granisetron with placebo is huge (*see* Figure 9.2). The most dramatic effects were seen in small trials, and it is clear that many small trials with poor effect, or showing that placebo was better than the drug, are missing. The bias was similarly large in trials that had compared granisetron with an old, cheap drug, droperidol. Trials that had been performed by a particularly prolific author, Yoshitaka Fujii, were also heavily biased; he was later found to have fabricated his data in 172 studies of which 126 were randomised trials.[57,58] This is a world record.

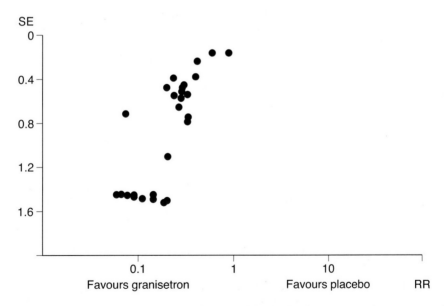

Figure 9.2 Bias in trials comparing granisetron with placebo for postoperative nausea and vomiting. Results are shown for the use of a rescue antiemetic

Despite the huge amount of data, the Cochrane review couldn't conclude anything about the possible differences between the drugs. This must also be some sort of record for research waste; after 737 trials and 100 000 patients no reliable conclusion can be made, although it's so simple to study postoperative nausea and vomiting!

I have been a member of the drug committee at our hospital for 20 years and, in 2012, the clinicians wanted to get permission to use some new antinausea drugs as standard. One was palonosetron, which cost 44 times more than ondansetron and 17 times more than granisetron. We were told that in those trials that had been submitted to the drug agency for obtaining marketing approval, palonosetron had a similar effect to the older setrons when heavy chemotherapy was used, but was slightly better when the chemotherapy caused less nausea and vomiting (81% and 69%, respectively, did not develop nausea). I couldn't participate in the meeting but warned the chairman of the committee against selective publication of the most positive results. I also noted that we needed access to the unpublished trials and their protocols, and that a full Cochrane review was needed if we wanted to know whether the new drugs were any better than the cheap ones.

The minutes from the meeting said that it was agreed to allow the clinicians to use the expensive drugs when heavy chemotherapy was used (where there was no advantage of palonosetron), including a drug that cost 300 times as much as the cheapest one, and that the clinicians should carefully consider when the drugs should be used. Experience has shown that such recommendations rarely prevent people from using expensive drugs, although it's impossible that they can be 300 times more valuable than the cheap ones.

I withdrew my membership of our drug committee after 20 years of uninterrupted disappointment. No matter how shaky or irrational the arguments, or how expensive the new drugs, drug committees almost always please the clinicians. I think it's about not getting into trouble. Heads of departments are powerful and often on industry payroll, and if too many complaints are being made, top managers might not get their tenure renewed. It also takes time to say no, as protests are likely to ensue, and those at the top have far too little time already. I have discussed this with chairmen of drug committees elsewhere and they have also experienced a lack of management support for unpopular decisions.

We don't live up to our values as a profession. Drug salespeople may come to heads of departments and ask whether they will make an application to the drug committee, with the tacit understanding that those who refuse will be out of favour come conference time, and that is also how it works.[59]

The interactions between physicians and the industry were until recently chiefly of interest to medical ethicists.[60] That is not the case any longer, and two previous editors of the *New England Journal of Medicine*, Marcia Angell and Jerome Kassirer, and a previous editor of the *BMJ*, Richard Smith, each wrote a book with a telling title after they had stepped down as editors:

> *The Truth about the Drug Companies: how they deceive us and what to do about it.*[32]

On the Take: how medicine's complicity with big business can endanger your health.[61]

The Trouble with Medical Journals.[62]

HIGHLY EXPENSIVE DRUGS

I have tried to find out just how expensive drugs can be compared to the benefit they offer and yet succeed getting used. Treatment of one patient with biologic agents can cost up to €16 000 a year in Denmark, which is 120 times as much as treatment with conventional drugs.[63] Biologic agents are widely used for rheumatoid arthritis, but a 2010 meta-analysis showed that they are not any better in retarding joint damage than a combination of two cheap disease-modifying antirheumatic drugs (DMARDs).[64] Unfortunately, the meta-analysis came 4 months too late. The European League Against Rheumatism (EULAR) had posted new recommendations stating that biologic agents should be initiated without first trying therapy with a combination of DMARDs in patients whose arthritis was not sufficiently responsive to therapy with a single DMARD.

The EULAR recommendations were based on a review of only a fraction of the published studies, but once an organisation has issued new guidelines, it is extremely difficult to change them, even though, as in this case, billions of Euros could be saved in the EU every year (in Denmark alone, the cost for biologic agents was €130 million in 2011). The authors of the meta-analysis recently conducted a more sophisticated network meta-analysis that confirmed their results (Graudal, personal communication).

In 2010, the *BMJ* reported that a vaccine – not to *prevent* cancer but to treat metastatic prostate cancer – was approved by the FDA.[65] It cost $93 000 for three doses, and who knows whether the doctors would try more doses if they didn't see signs of the expected effect, which is a life extension of merely 4 months.

In 2012, Denmark decided to pay for a drug against metastatic melanoma that cost about $100 000 for one patient and which prolongs life by 3.5 months.[66] The oncologists sold the idea to the public by claiming that 10% of the patients would be cured,[67] although the trials didn't in any way justify this generous interpretation. A member of the working group that decided to pay for the drug couldn't see it was a problem that she received money from the company that stood to benefit from her decision.[68] In 2006, a new drug for head and neck cancer cost about $110 000 a year.[69]

The wooden spoon in futility I have seen so far goes to erlotinib for treatment of pancreatic cancer. Both the FDA and the EMA approved it, although it only prolongs life by 10 days, is toxic and will cost almost $500 000 for 1 year of life gained (10 days for each of 36 patients that aren't even pleasant).[70]

Examples of even more expensive drugs follow in Chapter 20, but here is one about a drug that didn't work. Intravenous alpha-1 antitrypsin is used in some countries for patients with lung disease caused by inherited alpha-1 antitrypsin deficiency. Some lung specialists had successfully lobbied a political majority in the Danish Parliament to agree to reimburse the drug, which may cost up to €116 000 annually per patient and which is to be used in many years, as the deterioration in lung function is slow, and very slow if the patients don't smoke.

Before the decision was made, I was asked to review the trials and I found out that there is no convincing evidence that the drug is effective. It took me only 4 weeks to produce the report, which we later published.[71] It made the politicians decline to reimburse the drug, which saved Danish taxpayers at least €30 million every year.

Something is terribly wrong in the way we prioritise. The most intensive and expensive therapy is often given in the last few days or weeks of life. It would be much better if we used this precious time constructively with our loved ones, instead of being pestered by the toxic effects of chemotherapy in a fight we cannot win.

Such simple ideas have powerful enemies in interest groups. After prominent doctors had declared publicly that they would abstain from life-prolonging chemotherapy if they got lethal cancer,[72] the chairman of the Danish Cancer Society, Frede Olesen, reprimanded them, saying they harmed the trust between patients and doctors.[73] They didn't; they gave very sound advice to the public. Why should the patients not have the same privileges as health professionals? Few oncologists and nurses are willing to accept the chemotherapy their patients endure for minimal benefit.[74] In elderly patients, aggressive treatment is even more misplaced. What is most important to them is to maintain their independence and dignity,[75] not a few extra intolerable weeks.

What is even more remarkable is that the conservative attitude cancer societies don't like may in some cases not only improve the patients' quality of life but also make them live longer. A randomised trial in patients with newly diagnosed metastatic non-small-cell lung cancer showed that those assigned to palliative care early on received less aggressive treatment and lived 3 months longer.[76] Drugs can kill you also when your life is almost over.

EXCESSES IN HYPERTENSION

What we need more than anything else to put a brake on the exploding expenditures on new drugs and their harms is independent drug trials. One such trial, the 2002 ALLHAT trial, shows how strong the counteracting forces of the medico-industrial complex can be. With 33 357 patients, it was the largest hypertension trial ever conducted.[42] It compared four drugs: doxazosin (an alpha-blocker from Pfizer), amlodipine (a calcium channel blocker from Pfizer), lisinopril (an ACE inhibitor) and chlorthalidone (a diuretic). The doxazosin arm was stopped prematurely, as the drug was clearly inferior. However, Pfizer started a damage control campaign, which was very effective, as there was no decline in sales the same year. When the ALLHAT study was presented at a large congress in California, Pfizer invited the doctors on sightseeing to ensure they didn't learn about the results.[77]

In a press release, the American College of Cardiology urged doctors to 'discontinue use' of doxazosin, but this was changed within hours after Pfizer had contacted the College which now said that the doctors should 'reassess' its use.[77] Rather unfortunate advice about a drug that had just been proven inferior, but it might have played a role that donations from Pfizer to the College exceeded

$0.5 million annually. ALLHAT demonstrated that the cheapest of the four tested drugs, the diuretic, was also the best. The chair of the ALLHAT steering committee, Curt Furberg, estimated that the use of the expensive calcium channel blockers and ACE inhibitors cost an excess of $8–10 billion without providing any benefit to patients, and in some instances adding more risk. The use of inferior drugs had caused heart failure in 40 000 patients in the United States at the same time as they had to pay 20 times more for the inferior drugs.[78]

Unsurprisingly, the results generated a huge 'controversy,' with innumerable letters and papers written by seemingly independent whore doctors who were hired guns for the company.

A paper from 2003 reported that Pfizer's other ALLHAT drug, amlodipine, was the most sold antihypertensive drug in Norway, although it was 10 times as expensive as a diuretic, and although the evidence for a preventive effect on heart disease didn't exist.[79] If doctors had used a diuretic rather than amlodipine, $750 million could have been saved annually in Germany, the UK and the United States.[80] In 1996, amlodipine was the most heavily advertised drug in the *New England Journal of Medicine*, while there wasn't a single ad for diuretics.[32] The ALLHAT trial wasn't published in this journal, but in *JAMA*.

An article from 2009 reported that the difference between the cost for the cheapest and the most expensive ACE inhibitor was a factor of 30 and that Denmark could save about €40 million a year by using the cheapest drug.[81] It looked like a no brainer, but no. The chairman of the Danish Society for Hypertension, Hans Ibsen, declared that we needed to be very cautious about changing drugs in patients with a well-regulated blood pressure, whereas another hypertension specialist, Ib Abildgaard Jacobsen, said that he had changed many patients' drugs without problems. Which of the two specialists was on industry payroll? *That's* a no brainer!

A year later, Ibsen shared his thoughts with us. He initially supported the use of losartan, the first angiotensin II receptor antagonist, marketed by Merck, which was one of Ibsen's benefactors.[82] When new similar drugs were introduced, Ibsen recommended those instead, although they were 10–20 times more expensive, with the argument that hypertension research would disappear from Denmark if we didn't use the expensive drugs. In this, Ibsen was supported by the medical director of Novartis, another of his benefactors, who stated that Novartis conducted research to introduce their products on the market so that they would be used and that she saw no great future for trials in Denmark if there wouldn't be subsequent sales. It was rather bold that Novartis – which sold one of the highly expensive new angiotensin II receptor antagonists – didn't try to hide the fact that its 'research' wasn't research but marketing. A colleague who, like me, is a member of Doctors Without Sponsors remarked about the astonishing revelations that when the purpose of research was to teach the doctors to use far too expensive drugs, it might be better that the research was performed elsewhere.[82] We could have saved €67 million in just 1 year if all doctors had used losartan,[83] which is an enormous amount of money for a small country.

I mention this story because I cannot recall any other where people have been so honest about their shady motives. Ibsen once attacked me in our medical journal saying I should be more positive towards the drug industry and acknowledge the important work sincere researchers did in collaboration with sincere drug companies. In reply, I asked what Ibsen meant by a sincere company and noted that he collaborated with Merck, Pfizer, AstraZeneca and Novartis, all of which had received giant fines for fraud, and that tens of thousands of patients had lost their lives because of the misdeeds committed by Merck and Pfizer.[84] Since these patients died from cardiovascular events, which hypertension experts try to avoid, it might have been expected that Ibsen would have refused to collaborate with such companies for the rest of his professional life, rather than calling them sincere. Doctors have a remarkable capacity for denial, whereas the bereaved spouses cannot deny that their loved ones are dead because they took a drug they didn't need.

PATIENT ORGANISATIONS

A chapter on hard sell wouldn't be complete without mentioning patient organisations. They are usually funded by – and speak with the same voice as – big pharma. In 2006, a pan-European cancer campaign, Cancer United, was presented as a pioneering effort by a coalition of doctors, nurses and patients to push for equal access to cancer care across the EU.[85] It was entirely funded by Roche, the world's leading drug pusher (see Chapter 3) and maker of cancer drugs, some of which are exceedingly expensive, e.g. Herceptin for breast cancer and Avastin for bowel cancer. Roche's PR firm was the secretariat and the principal study on which the propaganda was based was funded by Roche. The study report was written by Nils Wilking from the Karolinska Institute in Stockholm and Bengt Jönsson from Stockholm School of Economics. It received a lot of publicity but was seriously flawed, and its conclusions were unsupported by the data.[86] It concluded 'It is clearly in the best interest of cancer patients that new, innovative drug therapies are made available to them as soon as possible. Reduced or delayed access to cancer drugs has a very real impact on patient survival.'

Traditional company speak it was, and the promotional material said that the campaign aimed to collect one million signatures and would press the European Commission for an EU-wide strategy. The chairman of the European Cancer Patients Coalition found herself listed as a member of the campaign's executive board without her agreement. She and members of the European Parliament withdrew from the board. The chair of the executive board, Professor John Smyth, who committed editorial misconduct in his role as editor of the *European Journal of Cancer* in relation to one of our studies on mammography screening,[87] wrote the foreword to the Karolinska report, said the campaign was his idea and expressed a wish that people should stop seeing the industry as the enemy.

NOVOSEVEN FOR BLEEDING SOLDIERS

In 2011, Novo Nordisk agreed to pay $25 million to resolve its civil liability arising from the illegal promotion of its haemophilia drug, NovoSeven.[88] Haemophilia is a very rare disease, but Novo promoted the drug, which contains factor VII, unlawfully to healthcare professionals as a coagulatory agent for trauma patients and similar uses, resulting in false claims to be submitted to government healthcare programmes that were not reimbursable by those programmes. The case involved a whistle-blower lawsuit and an expansive Corporate Integrity Agreement with the Department of Health and Human Services.

The Justice Department suit alleged that Novo improperly paid influential US Army physicians to use and promote NovoSeven and provided illegal incentives also for researchers.[89] The company engaged in a 'fraudulent scheme to use kickbacks and off-label promotion' to boost sales, which trebled in 5 years to $750 million in 2004 and exceeded $1 billion in 2007. The activities involved speaking engagements, positions on advisory boards and unrestricted research grants for people working at the US Army Institute of Surgical Research.

In 2005, a heavily manipulated trial in 301 severely bleeding trauma patients was published in a little-known journal that purported to show that NovoSeven worked.[90] If true, it would have been sensational and we would have expected to see the trial published in the *New England Journal of Medicine* or the *Lancet*, with huge reprint orders. The abstract was highly misleading and described two trials, although it was only one trial. The data analysis was seriously flawed, using a new outcome that wasn't specified in the protocol and an arbitrary cut-off for number of transfusions, and excluding patients from analysis who died within the first 48 hours. The data massage was so clumsily made that it was fairly easy to see that the trial hadn't shown any effect.

The trial was funded by Novo and had a Novo employee and four physicians on Novo payroll among the authors. It was torn into pieces by experts, also in the journal where it was published which spoke of 'information laundering',[91] but Novo's research director, Mads Krogsgaard Thomsen, maintained that it was the physicians who stood for the positive conclusions and that the company had had limited input into the paper.[92] This is hard to believe, as the statistician was also from Novo. A physician from my hospital had acquired access to the protocol, which made it possible for him to see the manipulations. Some people believed in this mockery of science, and Novo embarked on a new trial, which my hospital declined to participate in. We had seen enough already.

In 2006, five FDA physicians reported that 185 thromboembolic events were linked to NovoSeven.[89] In April 2011, two large studies concluded that there was no evidence that the drug prolonged life in any of its off-label uses, and in some studies of strokes and heart surgery, NovoSeven actually increased the risk of stroke and heart attacks.

What galled Sidney Wolfe from Public Citizen the most was how Novo spent years pushing doctors to endorse off-label uses for NovoSeven and then issued a warning stating the drug could cause potentially fatal blood clots if used in patients who don't have haemophilia. Novo promoted NovoSeven for soldiers from 2005 through 2007 with conferences and seminars that bore titles such as 'Stop the bleeding! Bleeding management in military trauma care', 'Damage control resuscitation in Iraq' and 'Blood product effect on survival for patients with combat related injuries'.[93] The company got off easy in terms of the amount of money they paid and no one went to jail.

Novo denied wrongdoing,[89] and in an interview on Danish radio in 2008, Mads Krogsgaard Thomsen stated that the experts knew that the drug worked, even though it could not be documented scientifically, and that this was the explanation for its extensive use.[94] An interesting comment from a research director and a company that created a blockbuster out of hot air. This is how proponents of alternative medicine argue.

REFERENCES

1 Brody H. *Hooked: ethics, the medical profession, and the pharmaceutical industry.* Lanham: Rowman & Littlefield; 2008.

2 Gøtzsche PC. Bias in double-blind trials (thesis). *Dan Med Bull.* 1990; **37**: 329–36.

3 Gøtzsche PC. Methodology and overt and hidden bias in reports of 196 double-blind trials of nonsteroidal, antiinflammatory drugs in rheumatoid arthritis. *Controlled Clin Trials.* 1989; **10**: 31–56 (amendment: 356).

4 Bero LA, Rennie D. Influences on the quality of published drug studies. *Int J Tech Assessm Health Care.* 1996; **12**: 209–37.

5 Safer DJ. Design and reporting modifications in industry-sponsored comparative psychopharmacology trials. *J Nerv Ment Dis.* 2002; **190**: 583–92.

6 Melander H, Ahlqvist-Rastad J, Meijer G, *et al.* Evidence b(i)ased medicine – selective reporting from studies sponsored by pharmaceutical industry: review of studies in new drug applications. *BMJ.* 2003; **326**: 1171–3.

7 McGauran N, Wieseler B, Kreis J, *et al.* Reporting bias in medical research – a narrative review. *Trials.* 2010; **11**: 37.

8 Boutron I, Dutton S, Ravaud P, *et al.* Reporting and interpretation of randomized controlled trials with statistically nonsignificant results for primary outcomes. *JAMA.* 2010; **303**: 2058–64.

9 Gøtzsche PC. Meta-analysis of grip strength: most common, but superfluous variable in comparative NSAID trials. *Dan Med Bull.* 1989; **36**: 493–5.

10 Gøtzsche PC. Patients' preference in indomethacin trials: an overview. *Lancet.* 1989; i: 88–91.

11 Braithwaite J. *Corporate Crime in the Pharmaceutical Industry.* London: Routledge & Kegan Paul; 1984.

12 Bero L, Oostvogel F, Bacchetti P, *et al.* Factors associated with findings of published trials of drug-drug comparisons: why some statins appear more efficacious than others. *PLoS Med.* 2007; **4**: e184.

13 Kelley C, Helfand M, Good C, *et al.* Drug class review. Hydroxymehylglutaryl-coenzyme A reductase inhibitors (statins). 2002 Dec. Available online at: www.pbm.va.gov/reviews/hmgstatins04-09-03.pdf (accessed 11 November 2012).

14 Lundh A, Sismondo S, Lexchin J, *et al.* Industry sponsorship and research outcome. *Cochrane Database Syst Rev.* 2012; **12**: MR000033.

15 Heres S, Davis J, Maino K, *et al.* Why olanzapine beats risperidone, risperidone beats quetiapine, and quetiapine beats olanzapine: an exploratory analysis of head-to-head comparison studies of second-generation antipsychotics. *Am J Psychiatry.* 2006; **163**: 185–94.

16 Moffatt B, Elliott C. Ghost marketing. *Perspect Biol Med.* 2007; **50**: 18–31.

17 Rennie D. When evidence isn't: trials, drug companies and the FDA. *J Law Policy.* 2007 July: 991–1012.

18 Healy D, Cattell D. Interface between authorship, industry and science in the domain of therapeutics. *Br J Psychiatry.* 2003; **183**: 22–7.

19 Sismondo S, Nicholson SH. Publication planning 101: a report. *J Pharm Pharmaceut Sci.* 2009; **12**: 273–9.

20 Gøtzsche PC, Hróbjartsson A, Johansen HK, *et al.* Ghost authorship in industry-initiated randomised trials. *PLoS Med.* 2007; **4**: e19.

21 Yank V, Rennie D. Disclosure of researcher contributions: a study of original research articles in *The Lancet. Ann Intern Med.* 1999; **130**: 661–70.

22 Flanagin A, Carey LA, Fontanarosa PB, *et al.* Prevalence of articles with honorary authors and ghost authors in peer-reviewed medical journals. *JAMA.* 1998; **280**: 222–4.

23 Healy D. Shaping the intimate: influences on the experience of everyday nerves. *Soc Stud Sci.* 2004; **34**: 219–45.

24 Petersen M. *Our Daily Meds*. New York: Sarah Crichton Books; 2008.

25 Zuger A. How tightly do ties between doctor and drug company bind? *New York Times*. 2004 June 27.

26 Avorn J, Chen M, Hartley R. Scientific versus commercial sources of influence on the prescribing behavior of physicians. *Am J Med*. 1982; 73: 4–8.

27 Prosser H, Almond S, Walley T. Influences on GPs' decision to prescribe new drugs – the importance of who says what. *Fam Pract*. 2003; 20: 61–8.

28 Henry D, Doran E, Kerridge I, et al. Ties that bind: multiple relationships between clinical researchers and the pharmaceutical industry. *Arch Intern Med*. 2005; 165: 2493–6.

29 Campbell EG, Gruen RL, Mountford J, et al. A national survey of physician-industry relationships. *N Engl J Med*. 2007; 356: 1742–50.

30 Gagnon M-A, Lexchin J. The cost of pushing pills: a new estimate of pharmaceutical promotion expenditures in the United States. *PLoS Med*. 2008; 5: e1.

31 Harris G. As doctors write prescriptions, drug company writes a check. *New York Times*. 2004 June 27.

32 Angell M. *The Truth about the Drug Companies: how they deceive us and what to do about it*. New York: Random House; 2004.

33 Wazana A. Physicians and the pharmaceutical industry: is a gift ever just a gift? *JAMA*. 2000; 283: 373–80.

34 Ziegler MG, Lew P, Singer BC. The accuracy of drug information from pharmaceutical sales representatives. *JAMA*. 1995; 273: 1296–8.

35 Steinman MA, Harper GM, Chren MM, et al. Characteristics and impact of drug detailing for gabapentin. *PLoS Med*. 2007; 4: e134.

36 Blumenthal D. Doctors and drug companies. *N Engl J Med*. 2004; 351: 1885–90.

37 Chren MM, Landefeld CS. Physicians' behavior and their interactions with drug companies. A controlled study of physicians who requested additions to a hospital drug formulary. *JAMA*. 1994; 271: 684–9.

38 Orlowski JP, Wateska L. The effects of pharmaceutical firm enticements on physician prescribing patterns. There's no such thing as a free lunch. *Chest*. 1992; 102: 270–3.

39 Morgan SG, Bassett KL, Wright JM, et al. 'Breakthrough' drugs and growth in expenditure on prescription drugs in Canada. *BMJ*. 2005; 331: 815–6.

40 Johansen HK, Gøtzsche PC. Problems in the design and reporting of trials of antifungal agents encountered during meta-analysis. *JAMA*. 1999; 282: 1752–9.

41 Jørgensen KJ, Johansen HK, Gøtzsche PC. Flaws in design, analysis and interpretation of Pfizer's antifungal trials of voriconazole and uncritical subsequent quotations. *Trials*. 2006; 7: 3.

42 ALLHAT Officers and Coordinators for the ALLHAT Collaborative Research Group. Major outcomes in high-risk hypertensive patients randomized to angiotensin-converting enzyme inhibitor or calcium channel blocker vs diuretic: The Antihypertensive and Lipid-Lowering Treatment to Prevent Heart Attack Trial (ALLHAT). *JAMA*. 2002; 288: 2981–97.

43 Lieberman JA, Stroup TS, McEvoy, et al. Effectiveness of antipsychotic drugs in patients with chronic schizophrenia. *N Engl J Med*. 2005; 353: 1209–23.

44 Jones PB, Barnes TR, Davies L, et al. Randomized controlled trial of the effect on Quality of Life of second- vs first-generation antipsychotic drugs in schizophrenia: Cost Utility of the Latest Antipsychotic Drugs in Schizophrenia Study (CUtLASS 1). *Arch Gen Psychiatry*. 2006; 63: 1079–87.

45 Woo WWK, Man S-Y, Lam PKW, et al. Randomized double-blind trial comparing oral paracetamol and oral nonsteroidal antiinflammatory drugs for treating pain after musculoskeletal injury. *Ann Emerg Med*. 2005; 46: 352–61.

46 Villanueva P, Peiró S, Librero J, et al. Accuracy of pharmaceutical advertisements in medical journals. *Lancet*. 2003; 361: 27–32.

47 Wilkes MS, Doblin BH, Shapiro MF. Pharmaceutical advertisements in leading medical journals: experts' assessments. *Ann Intern Med*. 1992; 116: 912–19.

48 Jørgensen AW, Hilden J, Gøtzsche PC. Cochrane reviews compared with industry supported meta-analyses and other meta-analyses of the same drugs: systematic review. *BMJ*. 2006; 333: 782–5.

49 Malhotra D. Pharmaceutical lies. *BMJ*. 2006 Oct 28.

50 Spurling GK, Mansfield PR, Montgomery BD, *et al*. Information from pharmaceutical companies and the quality, quantity, and cost of physicians' prescribing: a systematic review. *PLoS Med*. 2010; 7: e1000352.

51 Bowman MA, Pearle DL. Changes in drug prescribing patterns related to commercial company funding of continuing medical education. *J Contin Educ Health Prof*. 1988; 8: 13–20.

52 Bowman MA. The impact of drug company funding on the content of continuing medical education. *Möbius*. 1986; 6: 66–9.

53 Can I buy you a dinner? Pharmaceutical companies increasingly use doctors' talks as sales pitches. 2005 Aug. Available online at: www.worstpills.org (accessed August 2005).

54 Tramèr MR, Reynolds DJ, Moore RA, *et al*. Impact of covert duplicate publication on meta-analysis: a case study. *BMJ*. 1997; 315: 635–40.

55 Aspinall RL, Goodman NW. Denial of effective treatment and poor quality of clinical information in placebo controlled trials of ondansetron for postoperative nausea and vomiting: a review of published trials. *BMJ*. 1995; 311: 844–6.

56 Carlisle J, Stevenson CA. Drugs for preventing postoperative nausea and vomiting. *Cochrane Database Syst Rev*. 2006; 3: CD004125.

57 Carlisle JB. A meta-analysis of prevention of postoperative nausea and vomiting: randomised controlled trials by Fujii *et al*. compared with other authors. *Anaesthesia*. 2012; 67: 1076–90.

58 Does anesthesiology have a problem? Final version of report suggests Fujii will take retraction record, with 172. *Retraction Watch*. 2012 July 3.

59 Boseley S. Junket time in Munich for the medical profession – and it's all on the drug firms. *The Guardian*. 2004 Oct 5.

60 Studdert DM, Mello MM, Brennan TA. Financial conflicts of interest in physicians' relationships with the pharmaceutical industry – self-regulation in the shadow of federal prosecution. *N Engl J Med*. 2004; 351: 1891–900.

61 Kassirer JP. *On the Take: how medicine's complicity with big business can endanger your health*. Oxford: Oxford University Press; 2005.

62 Smith R. *The Trouble with Medical Journals*. London: Royal Society of Medicine; 2006.

63 Heissel A. ['The bomb' has been defused]. *Dagens Medicin*. 2011 Feb 4.

64 Graudal N, Jürgens G. Similar effects of disease-modifying antirheumatic drugs, glucocorticoids, and biologic agents on radiographic progression in rheumatoid arthritis: meta-analysis of 70 randomized placebo-controlled or drug-controlled studies, including 112 comparisons. *Arthritis Rheum*. 2010; 62: 2852–63.

65 Tanne JH. FDA approves prostate cancer 'vaccine' treatment. *BMJ*. 2012; 340: 998.

66 Hodi FS, O'Day SJ, McDermott DF, *et al*. Improved survival with ipilimumab in patients with metastatic melanoma. *N Engl J Med*. 2010; 363: 711–23.

67 Andersen NV. [Drug with trivial effect]. *Politiken*. 2012 Feb 5.

68 Rasmussen LI. ['How can Henrik Dibbern believe that I have interests in the company?'] *Ugeskr Læger*. 2012; 174: 248–9.

69 Cuatrecasas P. Drug discovery in jeopardy. *J Clin Invest*. 2006; 116: 2837–42.

70 Sullivan R, Peppercorn J, Sikora K, *et al*. Delivering affordable cancer care in high-income countries. *Lancet Oncol*. 2011; 12: 933–80.

71 Gøtzsche PC, Johansen HK. Intravenous alpha-1 antitrypsin augmentation therapy for treating patients with alpha-1 antitrypsin deficiency and lung disease. *Cochrane Database Syst Rev*. 2010; 7: CD007851.

72 Jensen JH, Korsgaard P. [We would drop chemotherapy and enjoy life]. *Ekstra Bladet*. 2012 March 16.

73 Dreier J. [Chemotherapy or not?]. *Danish Cancer Society*. 2012 March 19.

74 Slevin ML, Stubbs L, Plant HJ, *et al*. Attitudes to chemotherapy: comparing views of patients with cancer with those of doctors, nurses, and general public. *BMJ*. 1990; 300: 1458–60.

75 Watts G. Why the exclusion of older people from clinical research must stop. *BMJ*. 2012; 344: e3445.

76 Temel JS, Greer JA, Muzikansky A, *et al*. Early palliative care for patients with metastatic non-small-cell lung cancer. *N Engl J Med*. 2010; 363: 733–42.

77 Lenzer J. Spin doctors soft pedal data on antihypertensives. *BMJ*. 2003; 326: 170.

78 Järhult B, Lindahl S-O. [Doxazosin and heart failure: trustworthy information for patients' sake]. *Läkartidningen*. 2003; **48**: 4011–12.

79 Fretheim A, Aaserud M, Oxman AD. The potential savings of using thiazides as the first choice antihypertensive drug: cost-minimisation analysis. *BMC Health Services Research*. 2003; **3**: 18.

80 Drachmann H, Andersen NV. [Millions to spare on drugs]. *Politiken*. 2003 Dec 27.

81 Hagerup A. [Focus: drugs]. *Ugeskr Læger*. 2009; **171**: 203–5.

82 Lindberg M. [Interesting statements by Hans Ibsen and Novartis related to new rules for reimbursement of drugs]. *Ugeskr Læger*. 2010; **172**: 2476.

83 Ebdrup N. [Cheap antihypertensives equally good as expensive ones]. *Videnskab.dk*. 2012 April 13.

84 Gøtzsche PC. Reply. *Ugeskr Læger*. 2011; **173**: 599.

85 Boseley S. Concern over cancer group's link to drug firm. *The Guardian*. 2006 Oct 18.

86 Coleman M. New drugs and survival: does the Karolinska report make sense? *Cancer World*. 2006 Sept–Oct: 26–35.

87 Gøtzsche PC. *Mammography Screening: truth, lies and controversy*. London: Radcliffe Publishing; 2012.

88 US Department of Justice. *Danish pharmaceutical Novo Nordisk to pay $25 million to resolve allegations of off-label promotion of Novoseven*. 2011 June 10.

89 Christenson S, Finley D. Drug firm's wooing made whistleblower suspicious: Fort Sam doctor was early backer of medication to halt bleeding. *San Antonio Express*. 2011 June 26.

90 Boffard KD, Riou B, Warren B, *et al*. Recombinant factor VIIa as adjunctive therapy for bleeding control in severely injured trauma patients: two parallel randomized, placebo-controlled, double-blind clinical trials. *J Trauma*. 2005; **59**: 8–18.

91 Webert KE, Blajchman MA. Randomized trials in patients with blunt and penetrating trauma. *J Trauma*. 2006; **60**: 242–3.

92 Andersen NV, Ellesøe M. [Novo blockbuster buried]. *Mandag Morgen*. 2008; **27**: 9–13.

93 Tedesco J. Military medicine scheme is alleged: S.A. nonprofit tied to alleged scam to influence decisions by doctors. *San Antonio Express*. 2011 July 20.

94 Mogensen T. [Who is guarding the guardian?]. *Ugeskr Læger*. 2008; **170**: 3076.

Impotent drug regulation

> If the American people knew some of the things that went on at the FDA, they'd never take anything but Bayer aspirin.

Len Lutwalk, FDA scientist[1]

We don't have safe drugs. The drug industry more or less controls itself; our politicians have weakened the regulatory demands over the years, as they think more about money than patient safety; there are conflicts of interest at drug agencies; the system builds on trust although we know the industry lies to us; and when problems arise, the agencies use fake fixes although they know they won't work.

I have great respect for the work conscientious scientists do at drug agencies. They have prevented many useless and harmful drugs from being approved and have withdrawn many drugs from the market. However, they work in a system that is fundamentally flawed and where the benefit of doubt protects companies and not patients.

This becomes clear if we compare drugs with cars. My 15-year-old car must be inspected biennially. If I turned up next time without the car but with 10 m of paper and told the inspectors they shouldn't examine my car but the enormous pile of paper where all the results of my careful testing of my car were reported, they would think I was crazy.

Isn't it then crazy that we have accepted a system where this is exactly what the drug industry does? The clinical documentation for just three drugs can take up 70 m of binders (*see* Chapter 11). In my 10 m of paper, I could have hidden somewhere that the brakes were failing without the inspectors ever finding out. Similarly, court cases have revealed that drug companies may hide serious harms in their mountains of documentation that drug agencies will never find. The difference is that if my brakes fail, I might kill myself and perhaps a few others, whereas if a company hides lethal harms of its drug, it might kill tens of thousands of people. We should therefore be much more cautious about drugs than about cars, but we aren't.

Why did we create a system where the industry is its own judge when it so clearly doesn't make sense? Testing drugs should be a public enterprise, but it isn't, and industry money is everywhere; even our drug agencies are paid by industry and therefore compete about being most forthcoming.

Another fundamental problem is that it's a value judgement – not a scientific question – whether a drug is too dangerous compared to its benefits. What should we do about a drug that kills relatively few people while it improves the condition for many? There is no gold standard for such judgements, and regulators are no better than ordinary citizens at deciding where the line should be drawn. Unfortunately, regulators don't consult with the public; they consult with people with vested interests: people from the company that owns the drug and specialists, many of whom have financial conflicts of interest in relation to the drugs they are evaluating. The regulators themselves may also have financial conflicts of interest, and even if they don't, the benefits from a positive decision could be just around the corner in the form of a lucrative position in the company.

CONFLICTS OF INTEREST AT DRUG AGENCIES

There are pervasive financial conflicts of interest in drug regulation,[1,2] and regulators may go back and forth between the industry and drug agencies, the 'revolving door' phenomenon. FDA commissioner Lester Crawford left the agency after the Vioxx scandal (*see* Chapter 13).[3] Crawford approved Vioxx, a Merck drug, and after resigning he became senior council for Merck's PR firm, Policy Directions Inc.[4] Crawford later received a fine of $90 000 for falsely reporting he had sold stock in companies regulated by the FDA while he still owned the shares.[5] These companies included Pepsico, which sells soft drinks and junk food that make people obese, and at the same time, Crawford was head of FDA's obesity working group.[6]

Eyebrows were also raised in Denmark when the drug regulator who helped Nycomed get approval for a slimming pill, Letigen (which means 'light again'), went directly to a senior post in the company that was going to market the drug. Letigen was a bad drug. It contained ephedrine, and was later taken off the market because of its cardiovascular harms.

Members of advisory committees at drug agencies also contribute to the corruption of scientific integrity. Some of them work for both sides and extort the drug companies by commanding unusually high consulting fees from them, which are difficult to decline if the companies want to have their drugs approved.[2] Obviously, people who are paid by the industry to be its voice at committee meetings cannot possibly be advocates also for their patients, which means that their role as 'independent experts' doesn't exist.

Drug agencies don't live up to laws about impartiality in public administration, although this would seem easy to do. In Denmark, for example, an expert isn't allowed to give advice on matters where the expert has a conflict of interest that could influence the advice, if it's possible to get qualified advice from an expert without conflicts. Some years ago, there was uproar in the press when the Danish drug agency had employed psychiatrist Bente Glenthøj in its registration committee, which not only gives advice but make decisions about approval of new drugs.[7] She had many conflicts of interest in relation to drug companies, but couldn't see this was a problem. That's how virtually everyone in the world evaluates their financial conflict of interest: no problem.

The drug agency defended itself by saying it wasn't possible to get the expertise it needed unless it accepted conflicted people. That argument was impossible to swallow. In 2011, there were 1201 registered psychiatrists in Denmark, and only 92 of these (8%) had permission to work for a drug company. The drug agency wanted us to believe that none of the remaining 1109 psychiatrists were qualified.

Nonetheless, the Ministry of Health granted her an exemption from the law provided she didn't participate in cases where doubt could be raised about her impartiality. Now wait a minute. If she couldn't deal with cases where she was an expert, in psychiatry, there was no argument for retaining her at the agency. But of course nothing was done. The fake fix was in place.

The Danish case is typical. What drug agencies do all over the world is not to avoid using conflicted experts but to ask them to declare their conflicts of interest. Excuse me for the comparison, but I think it's relevant: what would your confidence in the police force be if police detectives routinely invited criminals to participate in their work, after the criminals had declared that their conflict of interest was that they hoped the case would never be resolved (because some of their friends had committed the crime)?

Scientists at drug agencies are not only up against a powerful industry, they are also often up against their own superiors and their advisory committees who may have less than ideal motives for their decisions. The bosses often look the other way because they depend on licensing fees and political goodwill, and because questions about harms lead to trouble. A culture develops where many decisions are made that ordinary citizens would not have agreed with if they had been represented in the drug advisory committees.

This is called regulatory capture. The regulators come to work so closely with the industry it regulates that it's inevitable that friendships develop and that they acquire a greater understanding for the industry's problems and positions than those of the patients who are anonymous. The industry is no longer effectively regulated and agencies indulge in protracted and amicable negotiations with the industry instead of acting when there is a public health danger.[1,3] This explains why the culture within the FDA has been described as one of intimidation and fear and as overly industry-friendly.[1,2,8-12] The general public is viewed as a hysterical and irrational mob who should be protected from any suggestion of product hazards.[8] However, it's curious that citizens participate in town planning in a democratic fashion, whereas they are not supposed to know anything about what goes on in drug agencies.

In 2006, the Institute of Medicine wrote a critical report and suggested radical changes,[13] but the response from the FDA was inadequate and demonstrated an almost total lack of understanding of the magnitude of the changes required to create a culture of safety.[14] When FDA scientists find signs of serious harms, they are often overruled and intimidated by their superiors – even to the point of being prevented from presenting their findings of lethal harms of drugs at advisory meetings – or are assigned to another job.[1,8-10,15] It doesn't even stop there. As described in Chapter 3, the FDA has accepted safety data it knew were fraudulent,[12] and – on many occasions – data that clearly showed the drug was *not* safe.[16]

If we look at what happens after approval, it doesn't exactly warrant blind trust in drug agencies either. They are much too slow to react to reports of lethal harms of drugs, if they react at all.[1,9,12,15,17-19] One reason is that, most unfortunately, drug regulation doesn't build on a precautionary principle but on a permissive principle where the benefit of doubt is consistently awarded to the drug industry and not the patients. For example, FDA approved Vioxx because it lacked 'complete certainty' that the drug increased cardiovascular risk,[9] although this was expected based on the drug's mode of action (*see* Chapter 13). Another reason is about saving face. Warnings about a drug, or its withdrawal from the market, suggest that the agency failed when it approved it.[20]

It is really scaring that a survey showed that *70% of FDA scientists are not confident that products approved by the FDA are safe*.[9,21] And that 66% lack confidence in the FDA's safety monitoring of marketed drugs.[22] The citizens have a similar view. In a public poll, 76% worried that the FDA didn't communicate safety issues effectively.[23]

These concerns are supported by facts. No less than 51% of drugs have label changes because of major safety issues discovered after marketing; 20% of drugs get new black box warnings; and more than 1 in 20 are withdrawn from the market.[24–26]

It's actually much worse than this. Post-marketing studies are few and generally of poor quality, and spontaneous reports of harms are a hugely inadequate method to detect even serious harms. There can therefore be no doubt that many of our drugs are dangerous, but the problem is we don't know which ones. Associate Director David Graham, who has spent 40 years working for the FDA's Office of Drug Safety, has illustrated the regulatory impotence with excruciating sharpness:[9]

> 'The way FDA approaches safety is to virtually disregard it. FDA believes there is no risk that cannot be managed in the post-marketing setting ... The case of antidepressants and suicidality is a perfect example. How does the FDA handle this? With labelling changes. FDA knows that labelling changes don't change physician behavior. Yet they act as if they are doing a great public good when they change the warning ... Rather than ensuring with 95 percent certainty that a drug is safe, what FDA says is: We can't be 95 percent certain this drug will kill you, therefore we will assume it doesn't – and they let it on the market ... if we wanted drugs that are safe, we could have it tomorrow. It is easy to design those studies. But FDA is not interested in that.'

People behind desks make decisions that won't work in real life and they know it. I shall say more about this in Chapter 21.

CORRUPTION AT DRUG AGENCIES

It must be very tempting for drug companies to bribe officials at drug agencies, as an enormous amount of money is at stake. The approval of a new drug can be the difference between life and death for a company and a recent case illustrates these issues. I don't suggest any wrongdoing, I just give the information. In 2012, Danish Lundbeck and its Japanese partner Takeda submitted vortioxetine, an SSRI, for regulatory approval in the United States.[27] This doesn't appear too exciting, as we already have lots of antidepressants, but it could be important for Lundbeck, as its blockbuster, escitalopram, will soon run out of patent. A spokesman said the company would receive a $43 million milestone payment from Takeda if the FDA accepted the drug.

We don't know much about corruption at drug agencies, but some of what I describe in this book is difficult to explain unless money is involved in one way or another, which could be a future reward in terms of a well-paid job in the industry or insider trading of drug company stocks (see below). Here is an example.[28] In 2006, the FDA introduced new labelling regulations, but after the 5-year period of comments had expired, the agency quietly added a new section that would make it virtually impossible for patients to file liability claims against the companies when the patients had been harmed by their drugs.

The FDA said that any label it had approved, 'whether it be in the old or new format, pre-empts ... decisions of a court of law for purposes of product liability litigation'. This immunity would apply even if a company failed to warn prescribers or patients adequately about a known risk, unless a patient could prove that the company intentionally committed fraud. This is what was so outrageous. Not only must there be fraud, but it should be intentional. How can a patient know what goes on in a company executive's brain? I have often wondered myself. And how can a patient prove it was fraud?

The data may be in the company's archives, but that doesn't prove it was fraud not to analyse them and tell the world about them. Understandably, several politicians objected vigorously to this provision, as well as to the fact that there was no opportunity to debate it before the regulations were made final. For years, the industry had tried to obtain legislation that immunised them against litigation but Congress had consistently rejected the idea, and suddenly, out of the blue, there it was, produced by the very agency that is supposed to have the American people's interests as their first duty. How can this be explained – all done discreetly, in essence secretly, after the comments period had expired – if there wasn't corruption?

In 2009, nine FDA scientists wrote to President Obama about widespread corruption in the FDA at the highest levels, including several commissioners.[4,29] The scientists were frustrated and outraged and gave many examples of the corruption, which they described as systemic and violating the law. They noted that there was an atmosphere at FDA in which the honest employee fears the dishonest employee, and that senior officials had suppressed or altered scientific or technological findings and conclusions, had abused their power and authority, and had engaged in illegal retaliation against those who spoke out.

In 2012, it was revealed that FDA management had installed spyware on the computers of five scientists who had alerted the FDA to safety problems to no avail and therefore had informed the politicians.[30] This came to light because thousands of confidential documents from the scientists' computers were posted on a public website, apparently by mistake, by a private document-handling contractor that worked for the FDA. The posting of the documents was discovered inadvertently by one of the scientists the FDA had fired who did Google searches to check for negative publicity that might hinder chances of finding work.

There were other revelations in 2012. A former FDA scientist, Ronald Kavanagh, spoke out about crimes and gangster methods at the agency:[31]

While I was at FDA, drug reviewers were clearly told not to question drug companies and that our job was to approve drugs ... If we asked questions that could delay or prevent a drug's approval – which of course was our job as drug reviewers – management would reprimand us, reassign us, hold secret meetings about us, and worse. Obviously in such an environment, people will self-censor ... Human studies are usually too short and the number of subjects in them too small to adequately characterize the most dangerous risks. That's why even a single case has to be taken seriously ... I frequently found companies submitting certain data to one place and other data to another place and safety information elsewhere so it could not all be pulled together and then coming in for a meeting to obtain an agreement and proposing that the safety issue is negligible ... if reviewers say things that companies don't like, they will complain about the reviewer or they will call upper management and have the reviewer removed or overruled. On one occasion, the company even told me they were going to call upper management to get a clear requirement for approval that they did not want to fulfill eliminated, which I then saw happen. On another occasion a company clearly stated in a meeting that they had 'paid for an approval' ... Sometimes we were literally instructed to only read a 100–150 page summary and to accept drug company claims without examining the actual data, which on multiple occasions I found directly contradicted the summary document. Other times I was ordered not to review certain sections of the submission, but invariably that's where the safety issues would be ... FDA's response to most expected risks is to deny them and wait until there is irrefutable evidence postmarketing, and then simply add a watered down warning in the labeling ... When you do raise potential safety issues, the refrain that I heard repeatedly from upper management was, 'where are the dead bodies in the street?' Which I took to mean that we only do something if the press is making an issue of it ... Later, I found that the FDA had internal documents that had the same conclusion [as] my analysis but they had been withheld from the advisory committee ... After FDA management learned I had gone to Congress about certain issues, I found my office had been entered and my computer physically tampered with. I saw strange cursor movements on my computer when I was just sitting at my desk reading that I suspected was evidence of spying ... The threats, however, can be much worse than prison. One manager threatened my children – who had just turned 4 and 7 years old – and in one large staff meeting, I was referred to as a 'saboteur.' Based on other things that happened and were said, I was afraid that I could be killed for talking to Congress and criminal investigators ... I found evidence of insider trading of drug company stocks reflecting knowledge that likely only FDA management would have known. I believe I also have documentation of falsification of documents, fraud, perjury, and widespread racketeering, including witnesses tampering and witness retaliation ... In fact, thanks in part to the Prescription Drug User Fee Act [in which drug companies pay for expedited reviews], thalidomide could not be stopped today.

About 50 years ago, Henry Welch, chief of FDA's antibiotics division, collected more than a quarter of a million dollars in private fees from companies while he was certifying the efficacy and safety of their antibiotics.[32] Welch also edited a journal and shared papers in print with drug companies saying he would make changes they suggested in return for reprint orders and steering advertising revenues his way.[33] There have been other cases of named FDA officials being bribed in return for approval of drugs, which have involved delivery of confidential information from competitors' files at the FDA and prison terms, both for FDA officers and company staff.[34]

When I worked in the industry, a colleague told me that his previous company had paid a clinical pharmacologist what corresponded to about 1 year's salary for browsing a registration application before it was submitted to the drug agency. A pretty handsome payment for a few days of work, and the doctor wasn't likely to reveal the arrangement when she later sat on the other side of the table in the drug agency and contributed to evaluating the same application.

Duilio Poggiolini, general manager of the pharmaceutical department of the Italian Ministry of Health, was arrested in 1993 due to a series of charges related to forgery and bribery favouring the entry of useless drugs.[35] The scandal involved the minister of health who arranged for drug companies to pay bribes in order to get their drugs approved and sold at 'suitable' prices.[36] The corruption network also involved academics who received shares of the bribes in return for expert advice in favour of the drugs, some of which were dangerous and sold at exorbitant prices. It has been estimated that just by taking five of the useless drugs off the market, Italy could have saved $3 billion back in 1993. Poggiolini went to jail while the minister had parliamentary immunity. In 2012, Poggiolini was fined €5 million, a small amount considering that the authorities had initially charged Poggiolini with having accumulated $180 million over 30 years.[37] Crime certainly pays in healthcare.

In 2008, the vice president of the Italian Drug Agency, Pasqualino Rossi, one of Italy's most senior representatives at the EMA, was arrested.[38] Six drug company lobbyists were also arrested, and the case concerned alleged falsification of clinical data in return for cash, revealed by wire tapping and covert cameras. The prosecutor said the corruption had resulted in concealment of life-threatening harms of the drugs. It was a soap opera right from the beginning. The drug agency issued a statement that none of its employees were under investigation, but when the Italian press named the senior officials arrested, the statement was removed and a new one was being prepared. Just like when the drug industry has been caught – it denies everything, even in the face of indisputable evidence.

Internal documents from Pfizer show that UK psychiatrist Stuart Montgomery deliberately avoided to inform the drug regulator for which he worked that he also worked for Pfizer at the same time. He advised Pfizer about how the regulator had reasoned in relation to its application for sertraline (Zoloft) and what the company should do in order to get the drug approved.[39]

The United States is more open about its scandals than other countries, but the little we know confirms US experiences. When a scientist at the German drug agency called for deregistration of a dangerous antibiotic, which had been taken off the market in most other countries, his career came to a stop. The director of the agency, Karl Überla, whom he later described as corrupt, moved him into a post where he was supposed to take care of 'research that didn't exist'.[40] The antibiotic was marketed by the German firm Hoechst, and Überla, who had previously lobbied for the US tobacco industry, accepted favours from Hoechst.

The multitude of regulatory decisions provide many opportunities for buying off regulators. In some Asian countries, drug registration can be secured for small amounts of money.[8]

In Chapter 17, I shall describe how the antidepressant Prozac was approved in Sweden through bribery.

THE UNBEARABLE LIGHTNESS OF POLITICIANS

The drug industry also does what it can to corrupt politicians. In the United States, the drug industry contributes generously to election campaigns and there is more than one lobbyist for each member of Congress, which makes it the strongest lobby in Washington.[41,42] The drug industry also contributes handsomely to political campaigns, and most of the money go to the Republicans.[41] Between 1998 and 2006, the industry spent $1.2 billion on lobbying and political contributions,[43] and in 1994, the Republicans attempted to eliminate the FDA altogether and let the drug industry regulate itself![33]

Lobbying is also strong in Brussels, which until 2010[44] had resulted in extreme secrecy in European drug regulation.[45,46] The lobbying has been so successful that FDA executives now see the industry, and not the American people, as their clients[1,2,15] and even negotiate with industry about performance goals.[22] Politicians have consistently pushed the FDA in this direction, e.g. in the 1990s, President Clinton urged FDA leaders to trust industry as 'partners, not adversaries'.[15]

In 2002, the nomination of a new FDA commissioner, Alastair Wood, was withdrawn in the last minute, and a senator said that Wood put too much emphasis on drug safety.[2,47] Fair enough. It surely must be a mortal sin to be interested in drug safety when offered the highest position in America's drug regulatory agency. Wood was replaced by Mark McClellan who echoed the outrageously false claim from industry that the high drug prices are a consequence of the high development costs (see Chapter 20),[2,48] and he also argued against price controls.[2,49] The title of an article in the Boston Globe didn't leave any doubt about what had happened: 'Drug industry costs doctor top FDA post'.[47] The industry had demonstrated its omnipotence again.

As this example illustrates, political interference with FDA matters contributes to what has been described as the moral decline of the work in the agency. In Europe, politicians in the Danish Parliament and in the EU Parliament have vividly explained to me how they are constantly being haunted by representatives from big pharma. The industry pushes the politicians through lobbying, donations and sometimes outright bribery – which I have also been informed about – into introducing new laws that sacrifice public health for profits. Taxpayers don't write the tax laws, but in considerable measure drug companies write the drug regulations.[8]

In the United States, the politicians have demanded shorter turnaround times, which have resulted in more superficial evaluations of the safety of drugs, also for marketed drugs, as those working with drug safety have become more and more understaffed. The focus is on getting drugs approved quickly, thereby boosting the national economy through exports.[15,25] These influences have caused a marked deterioration in drug regulation. Only 1.6% of drugs approved in 1993–96 were later withdrawn from the market because of serious harms, which increased to 5.3% of drugs approved in 1997–2000.[25,26] Furthermore, drugs approved just before the official deadline – which the politicians had pushed the FDA into accepting although it is way too short for a careful assessment of most drugs – were double as likely to be withdrawn from the market than drugs that, despite the intentions, didn't make it in time and were approved after the deadline.[50,51]

Adverse drug event reporting to the FDA shows the same decline in safety of drugs. From 1998 through 2005, reported serious adverse drug events increased 2.6-fold and fatal adverse drug events increased 2.7-fold, and reported serious events increased 4 times faster than the total number of outpatient prescriptions.[52] There was a disproportionate contribution of pain medications and drugs that modify the immune system, but there was also a substantial increase for other drugs.

Other data confirm the untoward consequences of the FDA's increasing focus on speed rather than on safety.[15] In 1988, only 4% of new drugs introduced into the world market were approved first by the FDA; 10 years later, it was 66%. By the end of the 1990s, the FDA was approving more than 80% of the industry's applications for new products, compared with 60% at the beginning of the decade. The FDA, once the world's unrivalled safety leader, was the last to withdraw several new drugs in the late 1990s that were banned by health authorities in Europe.

In Canada, it's similarly bad.[53] The probability of a new active substance approved between 1995 and 2010 acquiring a serious safety issue after approval was 24%, and for accelerated priority reviews of drugs that were not even major therapeutic advances, the rate was 36%.

This demise of the FDA started in 1992 with the Prescription Drug User Fee Act, after which the companies paid the FDA for its services.[54] For the first 10 years, Congress prohibited the FDA from applying user fees to evaluate drug safety after approval.[55] The FDA demoralised the Office of Drug Safety by pulling scientists from it, shortened review times, approved drugs based solely on their effect on a surrogate outcome (see what the problem with this is below), and broadened its interpretation of potentially life-saving drugs, which were approved under expedited programmes.[14,54] These medicines now included drugs for common chronic conditions, although it is hard to believe that any of the drugs could be life-saving. Further, several of them were later withdrawn for safety reasons, such as troglitazone (Rezulin) for diabetes, dexfenfluramine (Redux), for obesity and rofecoxib (Vioxx) for pain. This looks scandalous to me. I have never heard of slimming pills or pain pills that were life-saving, but I have heard of many that were deadly and I shall say more about these drugs later.

Understandably, the morale of FDA scientists is low, which is very sad. Few jobs are more important than being a scientist at a drug agency. Their responsibility is huge, as a misjudgement can sometimes result in thousands of deaths among rather healthy citizens. They should therefore be exceptionally well paid and effectively protected from any improper influence from their bosses, the politicians, and the drug industry and its patient pressure groups, and they should be allowed the time they need to review the applications carefully and to ask uncomfortable questions. All of this is so far from reality that it seems almost a joke to suggest it, but in 2007 four previous FDA commissioners agreed that the agency should be funded through the Treasury rather than industry payments.[54] Nothing changed, however. Governments argue they cannot find the money, but it's wrong. The user fee system leads to approval of far too many highly expensive drugs that have nothing to offer, which carry a much larger burden on the public purse than if drug agencies were allowed to do a more thorough job without having to please the industry. Furthermore, the money could be provided by a minute tax on prescriptions; as little as 0.5% would suffice.

Politicians interfere directly with FDA decision making although this is equally unacceptable as if politicians interfered with a judge's verdict. A poll showed that 61% of FDA scientists were aware of such political interference.[21] An example was mentioned in a 2009 FDA report that said that four congressmen and the FDA's former commissioner, Andrew von Eschenbach, had unduly influenced the process that led to approval of a malfunctioning patch for injured knees. It occurred despite the fact that the agency's scientific advisers repeatedly and unanimously over many years had deemed the device unsafe because it often failed, forcing the patients to get another operation.[56] The FDA report talked about extreme, unusual and persistent pressure, which started shortly after the congressmen had received campaign contributions by the manufacturer, but as always, the accused said they weren't influenced by the money. An FDA manager said that Eschenbach not only demanded an expedited process but also a favourable outcome. Less than a year after the device was approved, the FDA stated it would revisit its decision.

Patient safety is particularly poor for medical devices. Cardiovascular devices are far more risky than a knee patch and therefore subjected to the most stringent type of assessment. Even so, the requirements are minimal although they should be higher for cardiovascular devices than for drugs, as devices are implanted and cannot be removed as a drug can.[57] A review of 78 applications for cardiovascular devices that received premarket FDA approval showed that only 27% of studies were randomised, 65% of the applications were based on just one study, and in 31%, the control group was retrospective, which is an extremely poor study design that almost always puts the new intervention in a good light.[57] Adding insult to injury, the US Supreme Court has decided that patients harmed by an FDA-approved device cannot sue the company!

Transcatheter aortic valve implantation (TAVI) offered hope to patients too old or too ill for conventional aortic valve replacement operations, and since its introduction, 40 000 implantations have been done.[58] However, it is very costly, and its effect was thrown into doubt by a follow-up study authorised by the FDA, in which more patients died when given TAVI instead of standard therapy. *This trial remains unpublished, and when independent researchers asked for access, they were rebuffed by the FDA and the study sponsor.*

This complete lack of respect for the patients – some of whom died because they were treated with an inferior device – is unbelievable. Unfortunately, there is little hope that the politicians will help us create a better system. After the British House of Commons Health Committee had examined the drug industry in detail in 2004–2005,[17] the members of Parliament felt that the drug agency wasn't competent to undertake its duties as a guardian of public health, but the government declined a public hearing and also a recommendation that a drug should not be launched until full clinical trial data were put on a public register.[59] The excuse for not demanding access to the trial data – that this would require a change in EU regulations – was a red herring. *We can decide not to buy or reimburse new drugs until the clinical data have been made available.* That would save us a lot of money. What is available in the published literature in the years immediately following approval of new molecular entities is a heavily biased selection of all the results that are available at drug agencies.[60]

Also in the EU, industry lobbying leads to curious proposals that are not in the patients' interest. In 2007, the European Commission published a tragicomic document called *Strategy to Better Protect Public Health*.[61] The Commission proposed to delete the clause that marketing authorisation for a drug shall be refused if its therapeutic efficacy is insufficiently substantiated by the applicant! How it might better protect public health to allow ineffective drugs onto the market is hard to explain. Health Action International (HAI) Europe, a large consumer organisation, protested against this and many other harmful proposals, e.g. to bring new medicines to the market faster to provide faster return on investments, which would be obtained by making conditional authorisations the norm rather than awarding them only in exceptional circumstances, when there is an urgent therapeutic need.[62] The EU document is horrific, as it goes on and on, undermining patient safety. For example, the proposal that the companies should be entrusted with the task of gathering and analysing data, issuing warnings and informing of their products' adverse effects after marketing approval is a recipe for public health disasters. The Commission's proposals provided for the industry's intervention at every level of decision making, putting them in the position of both judge and defendant. HAI noted that the companies' pharmacovigilance systems cannot under any circumstances become a substitute for national public pharmacovigilance systems, which unequivocally serve the public interest.

The Commission also proposed that for post-authorisation studies, it should be up to the firms to: 'consider whether the results of the study impact on the product labelling' or 'might influence the risk-benefit balance of the medicinal product'. It's unbelievable that politicians can be so far away from reality and cool facts. My whole book is about patients being harmed tremendously because we allow the industry to be its own judges. HAI Europe strongly condemned the Commission's proposals and called on it to refocus its efforts and defend the public interest, in accordance with its remit to protect European citizens that follows from Article 125 of the Treaty establishing the European Community. It's *so* depressing that a consumer group needs to say the obvious. It cannot be repeated too often that – even without such foolish initiatives – in the United States and Europe, *drugs are the third leading cause of death after heart disease and cancer* (*see* Chapter 21).

Another example of how damaging ignorant and ideologically driven politicians can be for public health is related to the Danish system for handling alleged cases of scientific misconduct. We had one of the oldest and best systems in the world. However, in 2005, the Danish Minister of Science, Helge Sander, who knew nothing about science but introduced professional football in Denmark, decided that the misconduct committee from now on could only handle alleged cases of misconduct for private researchers and companies if these people accepted an investigation, whereas publicly employed researchers could still be investigated whether they liked it or not.[63] There was a storm of protests from all corners of society, even from Novo Nordisk whose spokesperson said that whether research was private or public, it should be done properly. The minister's comment? Research in the Danish drug industry should not be controlled by civil servants. All hell broke loose after this stupid remark. The minister's next comment? No comment.

Novo Nordisk was right, but the Danish Association of the Pharmaceutical Industry used the opportunity for a most shameless response. They said they were tired of doctors who accused its members in the press for skewing their research results.[64] (These 'doctors' were more or less one person: me!) The Association stated that it was completely wrong that its members skewed its results and added that publication of its research was the responsibility of the doctors. The Association was willing to let its members be subjected to investigations provided that the committee would agree to investigate possible scientific misconduct for those doctors who criticised trials that named companies had performed. I have rarely seen anything so shameless and appalling. Companies routinely manipulate the data they publish, so every time a doctor criticised this, whether in the press or in a letter to the editor of the journal where the research was published, the doctor should be referred to the committee for scientific dishonesty for investigation. This is like in the Soviet Union where people criticising those at power were subjected to psychiatric examinations and sometimes incarcerated for life, if they weren't just murdered right away.

It's detrimental to public health that the politicians have allowed direct-to-consumer advertising in the United States. When drugs switch from prescription status to over-the-counter status, the information about their harms and contraindications may disappear.[65] Such a lack of balanced information is harmful for our citizens who are already overdosed, also in countries that don't allow this additional assault on the good health most of us have, after all.

It is nauseating to see US TV commercials, which are delivered in a soft female tone like when stewardesses on an airplane express their hope that you will choose their airline again, or in a deep masculine voice aimed at instilling confidence. These commercials invariably end with something like, 'Ask your doctor whether Lyrica is right for you.' They can also end with, 'You might have a disease you don't know about.' I agree, I surely have cancer, as cancer can be demonstrated in all of us who are above 50, if only we are investigated thoroughly enough.[66,67] But I prefer not to know, as I don't have a 'disease' and treatment of these pseudocancers isn't harmless.

Celebrity advertising is extensively used in the United States, e.g. in TV news and talk shows where the industry sponsorship isn't revealed so that the testimony appears genuine.[41] In Denmark, we don't have this, but in 2004, we nevertheless experienced a curious case of celebrity advertising, imported directly from the highest circles in the United States.[68] Merck was unhappy that its drug against osteoporosis, alendronate (Fosamax), hadn't achieved maximum reimbursement, and it dragged the Danish government into court. It also arranged a meeting between our Minister of Health and the former US Secretary of State, Madeleine Albright, under the pretence that they should discuss the Danish healthcare and reimbursement system. Two days before the meeting, she asked whether she could also bring the director of Merck Denmark, which was accepted. However, during the meeting, which our minister couldn't attend, Albright mentioned the drug she took against osteoporosis. She didn't win many friends on this stunt, which is not how we behave in Denmark, and the embarrassment we felt was exposed in a newspaper: 'Drug giant uses American pressure in Danish drug case.'[68]

Occasionally, we do see a little progress. Until recently, the European Medicines Agency was part of the Directorate General for Enterprise and Industry in the EU,[46] but it has now been moved into the Directorate General for Health & Consumers. And in 2007, new legislation gave the FDA more power to react.[69] However, we also see developments for the worse. In 2012, the US Senate proposed a further expansion of expedited review, with a new category for 'breakthrough drugs'.[70]

DRUG REGULATION BUILDS ON TRUST

Economic theory predicts that firms will invest in corruption of the evidence base wherever its benefits exceed its costs. If detection is costly for regulators, corruption of the evidence base can be expected to be extensive.

Alan Maynard, unpublished manuscript

Drug regulators have told me that the regulatory system builds on trust, which they think is fine, as it would have too serious consequences for the companies if they cheated and it was detected. As Maynard explains, this argument doesn't hold. Furthermore, as we have seen, big pharma means big crime, and where else in society would we trust what criminals tell us? Rats in toxicology studies may never have existed; they may have died more than once; they may be dead, although being described as being in good health in toxicology reports; tissues may be missing; data may have been fabricated; and the animals may have died too early before they developed drug-induced cancers.[8,16]

Drug firms don't trust each other, but drug agencies are supposed to trust the entire industry.[16] The authorities know perfectly well that they cannot trust the industry and the reason they say the opposite is pragmatic. They cannot review more than a tiny fraction of the mountains of documents they receive. As an extreme example, one study report for a Tamiflu trial consisted of 8545 pages, which is a 1000 times greater than its published version.[71] Understandably, most regulators only read summaries most of the time and, to my knowledge, it is only the FDA that routinely does its own statistical analyses on the submitted data, but the EMA now intends to do the same (*see* Chapter 11).

Many of the thousands of pages are pretty useless, and I have no doubt that the industry deliberately drowns the regulators in data, which gives the industry two advantages. First, they reduce the risk that the regulators detect anything that might prevent the drug from being approved, or might hamper sales because of warnings on the label. Second, if problems arise, the industry can claim they didn't conceal anything and that the regulators are therefore to blame. Although this isn't entirely true, it might work out in court.

The regulators are apparently so overloaded that they don't even check that everything is there, which they should. We have found many examples that important appendices have been left out or that pages in the middle of a report were missing. Whole trials can also be missing, e.g. two out of seven negative studies of SSRIs in children,[72] although this is against the law.

It is not surprising that serious harms of new drugs may pass unnoticed, as they may be hidden so well in registration applications and other submissions that it would require time-consuming detective work to unravel them.[1,73,74] An example of this is long-acting beta-agonists for treatment of asthma. In the 1990s, there were concerns that these drugs might increase asthma-related deaths rather than decrease them, and the FDA asked GlaxoSmithKline to carry out a large trial of salmeterol, the SMART trial.[73] Glaxo's handling of the trial was a bit *too* SMART, however, as the company manipulated the results it sent to the FDA.

In 2003, the findings were presented at a meeting for chest physicians where Glaxo claimed that the results were inconclusive, but that was misleading. The Data and Safety Monitoring Board for the study had recommended its termination after 26 000 of the planned 60 000 patients had been enrolled, as there were more asthma-related deaths in the salmeterol arm than in the placebo arm, or alternatively, that 10 000 more patients were recruited.[73]

The trial period was 28 weeks, but the investigators could – if they wanted – report serious adverse events that occurred in an additional 6-month period. The FDA assumed of course that the data they reviewed stemmed from the rigorously controlled randomised double-blind period. Only when the agency specifically queried the company as to which dataset had been provided, did Glaxo reveal that it had included the 6-months follow-up data. That made a huge difference. There was no statistically significant increase in asthma-related deaths when the follow-up data were included, whereas the risk was four times higher when only the trial data were considered, which was statistically significant. Independent researchers concluded that in the absence of the transparency associated with the advisory committee meetings at the FDA, these deceptions would never have come to public attention.[73] Glaxo responded to the revelations by saying it had 'acted responsibly and transparently'.[74]

That wasn't even all. Almost 3 years after the trial was finished, it still hadn't been published. The SMART results confirmed the results of a large trial Glaxo had run and published already in 1993.[75] Glaxo had compared salmeterol with its short-acting drug, salbutamol, and three times as many patients died from asthma when they received the long-acting drug (P = 0.11 for the difference). In

2006, a meta-analysis including the SMART study confirmed that long-acting beta-agonists increase asthma-related deaths.[76] At a superficial glance, the absolute risk of dying seems small, only one per 1000 patients per year of use. However, salmeterol was one of the most prescribed drugs in the world and the increased risk translates into 4000–5000 extra asthma-related deaths every year in the United States alone.[76]

In July 2005, the FDA considered whether long-acting beta-agonists should be removed from the market, but, instead, the agency opted for strong warnings and a recommendation that the drugs should only be used after other asthma drugs had failed.[76] In 2010, the FDA warned again, this time about the increased risk of severe exacerbation of asthma symptoms, leading to hospitalisation and death, and said that these drugs must never be taken alone but should be combined with an inhaled corticosteroid.[77] However, it doesn't solve the problem to add inhaled corticosteroids, e.g. the risk of admission to hospital is still increased two-fold. The FDA also required the manufacturers to conduct additional clinical trials to further evaluate the safety of these drugs when used in combination with inhaled corticosteroids. I find this odd. FDA requirements of additional studies are usually ignored by the companies, and the FDA doesn't enforce them. These drugs are dangerous – likely also when combined with steroids – and we don't need them, so why not take them off the market?

When Glaxo finally published the SMART trial in *Chest*, they mentioned the increase in asthma-related deaths, but the last two sentences in the abstract were interesting:[78]

'Subgroup analyses suggest the risk may be greater in African Americans compared with Caucasian subjects. Whether this risk is due to factors including but not limited to a physiologic treatment effect, genetic factors, or patient behaviours leading to poor outcomes remains unkown.'

Smoke and mirrors and the paper stinks: 'Subpopulations were based on baseline characteristics *such as* [my emphasis] inhaled corticosteroid (ICS) use and study phase. Additionally, outcome events were analyzed separately for white and African-American subjects.'

Such as? Glaxo doesn't even tell us how many times they massaged the data before they found a subgroup result they could use to fool the readers into believing that the drug was only harmful for African Americans. *Even the data massage itself was misleading*. There wasn't a test of interaction, which is what one needs to do before one can say there is a difference between the results in two subgroups. And, in fact, the relative risk for asthma-related deaths was very similar for Caucasians and African Americans. The Discussion section of the paper tells us about only one of the subgroups, which is misleading: '*post hoc* analyses showed no significant differences between treatments … in the Caucasian population'. Glaxo converted a clear harm into no harm. Words fail me, but it says a lot about why *we cannot trust industry-sponsored trials*. Two of the five authors were Glaxo employees and the other three were on Glaxo payroll.

It seems that Glaxo did what it could to protect its drug rather than the patients.[79] In a scathing editorial in the *New England Journal of Medicine*, the editors explained that Glaxo refused to provide a placebo inhaler for an NIH trial of salmeterol. The investigators had to spend $900 000 of taxpayers' money to repackage the active drug and to create a visually identical placebo for use in the trial. The editors furthermore wrote:

> Glaxo's stated goal is 'to improve the quality of human life' but companies are able to develop and sell their treatments only because they can tap into a community resource: Patients who are willing to put themselves at risk as they participate in clinical trials. Companies, for their part, must therefore be willing to put their products at risk by providing them to legitimate third parties for study. Failure to do so is an unacceptable double standard.

Drug companies may not only cheat the authorities in their submissions; they may also lie when questioned directly. In documents prepared for a 2005 FDA hearing, Pfizer denied that its NSAID celecoxib causes heart attacks, based on an analysis of 44 000 patients.[80] But big numbers offered by the industry when it is on the defensive are often deceptive. Pfizer had unpublished evidence to the contrary,[80,81] e.g. a 1999 trial in Alzheimer's disease, and a Pfizer official admitted in an interview that its analysis didn't include outside studies that indicated its drug causes heart problems. One such study, which Pfizer knew about,[82] was conducted by the NIH and had been terminated after finding that high doses of celecoxib more than tripled the incidence of heart attacks and strokes.

Other companies have also deceived the FDA by hiding studies and results showing that their drugs cause lethal harms.[1,8,16,73,83–85]

There is one other reason why we know too little about the harms of drugs. Clinicians are supposed to report serious adverse events to the authorities but a common estimate is that only about 1% of such events get reported.[86] Doctors are busy and may tend to think that an event isn't drug-related and dismiss it, as this is convenient for them. If they report an event, they may learn never to do it again, as they might get harassed by a drug representative who keeps coming back with all sorts of questions about the patient, other drugs the patient was taking, etc. No one is really interested in harms it seems, apart from the victim. When I worked at a department of infectious diseases, I learned why many serious events in industry-funded AIDS trials didn't get reported. The record forms were long and complicated and we didn't have time for endless discussions with the drug company.

INADEQUATE TESTING OF NEW DRUGS

When I lecture doctors in training to become clinical pharmacologists and explain why the regulatory demands for new drugs are inadequate and cannot ensure effective and safe drugs, and how the drug industry often manipulates its research, I'm met with mixed reactions. Some agree heartily and others are quite hostile, as if I had explained to a child that Santa Claus doesn't exist. This worries me, as these are the doctors who are most likely to gets jobs in drug agencies and in the drug industry. I sometimes get the feeling that it's already too late to talk sense to them.

We could easily do far better than we currently do in protecting public health and avoiding wasting our money, and I shall give some examples.

Only two placebo-controlled trials showing an effect isn't enough

Drug agencies consider efficacy to have been demonstrated if two placebo-controlled trials have shown an effect. As explained in Chapter 4, this is fairly easy to do for almost any drug for any condition because drugs have side effects, which will be expected to bias the assessment of a subjective outcome. If the sample size is large enough, any effect will become statistically significant, and the drug will be approved, if not too toxic.

If the company didn't succeed in its first two tries, it can perform more trials until two of them confess. On this background, it's amusing that the Danish Minister of Health, after having consulted with the drug agency, replied to a politician that there is no requirement that a drug needs to be better than an existing drug to become approved, but it must be at least equally good, and under no circumstances worse than existing drugs. However, when only placebo-controlled trials are needed, we have no way of knowing whether new drugs are worse than existing ones.

Companies are obliged by law to submit all trials they have carried out when they ask for drug approval, but the problem with this is that we cannot trust the drug companies. Trials may be missing and if they were conducted in countries with little public oversight, it might be impossible to know they existed.

Cough medicines don't work,[87,88] but the drug industry has nevertheless succeeded getting hordes of medicines approved for cough and the sales are high.[89] No less than 20% of all children up to 4 years are treated with asthma drugs such as terbutaline, which shows that the shady marketing I participated in when I worked for Astra was highly effective (*see* Chapter 2).

In the United States, over-the-counter cough and cold medications were used by 39% of households during 3 years.[90] Many of the drugs came on the market before 1972 when there was little control with medicines, but poison control centres had reported more than 750 000 calls of concern in 7 years related to such products, and the FDA had identified 123 deaths in children under six in its database. Adverse effects of the drugs include cardiac arrhythmias, hallucinations, depressed consciousness and encephalopathy. Manufacturers' advertisements describe the drugs as safe and effective, both of which are untrue.

A petition required the FDA to review the drugs, but the manufacturers claimed that the injuries could be prevented through parent education, which is a horrendous lie. In 2011, the FDA announced that the products shouldn't be used in children below 2 years of age and that the 'FDA strongly supports the actions taken by many pharmaceutical manufacturers to voluntarily withdraw cough and cold medicines that were being sold for use in this age group.'[91] Why didn't the FDA withdraw these useless and potentially dangerous products from the market? And why, after 4 years, was the FDA still reviewing the safety and expected to communicate its recommendations in the near future, as they said? Not even when *useless* drugs kill our children do the regulators act, whereas they have withdrawn many effective products, even though they caused fewer deaths. Drug regulation is not a consistent enterprise.

I once discussed cough remedies with a drug regulator and he alerted me to studies included in a registration application that purported to have shown that the drugs worked. It is one of the weirdest papers I have ever seen (and I have seen a lot). The studies had been carried out in India. A sensitive miniature microphone developed by Procter & Gamble attached to the patient's nose registered every little sound that perhaps was, or could develop into, a cough.[92] All three drugs tested (guaiphenesin, bromhexine and dextromethorphan) had an effect. Surprise, surprise. These recordings were completely irrelevant for the patients. Two of the drugs also increased sputum volume. What are we to make out of that? If they increased sputum production, they would also increase 'expectorant effects' measured as sputum volume, but that would not be a beneficial but a harmful effect. The studies were published in *Pulmonary Pharmacology*, an obscure journal I'd never heard about. It's not the regulators' fault that they have to accept such nonsense; it's the politicians' fault that they have not required outcomes that matter to patients.

Drug trials in countries with widespread corruption

Nowadays, drug trials are outsourced more and more to countries with little oversight and widespread corruption. How are we to know whether the results have been made up when we have no possibility of controlling the trials? Despite considerable opposition from scientists, ethicists and consumer groups, the FDA decided in 2008 that clinical trials performed outside the United States no longer had to conform to the Declaration of Helsinki if used to support applications for registration of products in the US.[93] Pardon me, but have they gone completely mad at the FDA? Has the FDA leadership never heard about the Nürnberg processes? Or about medical experiments on US prisoners where the Declaration of Helsinki wasn't an issue? Or about the Tuskegee affair where researchers in Alabama followed 399 black men infected with syphilis without treating them for 40 years to study the natural course of the disease while preventing them from accessing treatment programmes available to others, and while many died of syphilis, wives contracted the disease and children were born with congenital syphilis?[94] Or that drug companies do research in poor countries for particularly dangerous drugs because peasants don't sue big corporations for injury and because informed consent regulations either don't exist or are weakly enforced?[8] The most well-known example of the use of third world guinea pigs is oral contraceptives, which were first tested in Puerto Rico, later in Haiti and Mexico, and when tested in the United States, poor people were chosen, 90% of whom were either of Mexican or African origin.[8]

In contrast to this indefensible move, the US Court of Appeals ruled shortly afterwards that the Declaration of Helsinki constituted a sufficient customary norm to be considered binding in Pfizer's meningitis trial in Nigeria where the parents didn't know that their children participated in a trial. The court reversed a dismissal by a lower court of a lawsuit by families of children who died or were injured while they received Pfizer's experimental antibiotic, trovafloxacin, although a better drug was freely available through Médecin sans Frontières.[95] Pfizer hired investigators to look for evidence of corruption against the Nigerian attorney general in an effort to persuade him to drop the legal action.[96] It didn't work out and Pfizer had to pay compensation to families whose children died. The drug was never intended for Africa. Pfizer planned to sell it in the United

States and Europe, but its licence was withdrawn in Europe because of concerns over liver toxicity.

An effect on a surrogate outcome isn't enough

One of the most harmful practices in drug regulation is to approve drugs based on their effects on surrogate outcomes. As this mistake has cost the lives of hundreds of thousands, or perhaps even millions, of patients (see below), it's difficult to understand that the regulators don't require proven effects on relevant outcomes.

Here is an example. When I had been a doctor for only 2 years, I diagnosed mild type 2 diabetes in an old man that had been admitted for something else to the department of hepatology where I worked. I wrote in his files that it was common practice to start treatment with tolbutamide, but since the only large trial of tolbutamide ever performed was stopped prematurely because of an excess of cardiovascular deaths, and since those patients who took most of the their daily doses were also those that had the highest event rate, I decided not to institute treatment with tolbutamide.

My superior in the hierarchy blew me up when he saw my notes. 'How dare you not start tolbutamide in violation of the guidelines the endocrinologists have written?' I explained calmly but firmly that I knew more about this drug than the endocrinologists because I had read the trial report carefully, plus the many articles and letters that followed, and also a book that discussed the issues. The study – the University Group Diabetes Project (UGDP) – had been carried out independently of the drug industry, and it had been heavily debated and reanalysed by several other groups than those who conducted the study. I had no doubt about who were right.

Tolbutamide lowers blood glucose but this is a surrogate outcome. We don't treat patients to lower their blood glucose; we treat them to prevent complications to diabetes, in particular cardiovascular ones. I therefore considered it absurd, and still do, that people used this drug when the only trial studying cardiovascular complications was stopped because the drug killed the patients. It was particularly convincing that good compliers with tolbutamide had a greater mortality rate than poor compliers,[97] because patients who do what they are told are generally more healthy than others and therefore have better survival even when the drug is placebo. A trial of a lipid-lowering agent, clofibrate, demonstrated this.[98] There was no difference in mortality between drug and placebo, but among those who took more than 80% of the drug, only 15% died, compared to 25% among the rest (P = 0.0001). This doesn't prove that the drug works of course, and the same difference was seen in the group that received placebo, 15% versus 28% (P = $5 \cdot 10^{-16}$).

Upjohn, the maker of tolbutamide, launched an aggressive campaign to discredit the UGDP study findings by using leading and well-remunerated academics, and the arguments became increasingly ad hominem.[99] Lawsuits were brought by the company to prevent the FDA from mentioning the study's results in the package inserts, and the FDA was even forced to carry out an investigation that concluded that the data in the study hadn't been falsified![97]

The use of tolbutamide should have been stopped by withdrawing the drug from the market, at least temporarily, while those who were sceptical towards the trial's result conducted another trial. But the FDA never required Upjohn to do this and it was never done.

No one seems willing to learn anything – or at least not much – from history when it comes to drug regulation. History repeats itself all the time. For the next 40 years after the UGDP trial, industry simply stopped performing trials that might have revealed that their diabetes drugs increased cardiovascular events, and our drug regulators let them get away with this,[99] which is pretty scandalous. Rosiglitazone is a recent example of a diabetes drug that was approved based on its effect on blood glucose, but as this drug also increased the cardiovascular complications it was supposed to prevent, it was taken off the market in Europe in 2010 after having killed thousands of patients (*see* Chapter 16).

Similar stories can be told from other therapeutic areas.[100] A cardiac arrhythmia suppression trial (CAST) was stopped prematurely because the two active drugs, encainide and flecainide, killed the patients. This trial was originally designed as one-sided, which means that the drug can only be beneficial or neutral, since the cardiologists couldn't imagine that the treatments could be harmful.[101] At the peak of their use in the late 1980s, anti-arrhythmic drugs were likely causing about 50 000 deaths every year in the United States alone, which is of the same order of magnitude as the total number of Americans who died in the Vietnam War.[102] The drugs were widely used because they had an effect on a surrogate outcome, the ECG, and although the FDA had serious safety concerns, they gave in to the pressures of the companies, which – quite predictably – led to the drugs being used in many completely healthy people with benign rhythm disturbances that many of us have.

Tumour shrinkage is another popular but misleading surrogate outcome. Cancer patients' primary interest is to stay alive, but some treatments that reduce the size of the cancer increase mortality, e.g. radiotherapy in women who had their breast cancer diagnosed at screening.[103] This can be said about many, if not most, cancer drugs. High doses may have a better effect on the cancer but may also kill more patients. If the dose is high enough, all cancers will die but so will all patients. This shows how absurd this surrogate outcome is.

In 2008, FDA granted bevacizumab (Avastin) accelerated approval for treatment of metastatic breast cancer, although it didn't increase survival, only progression-free survival.[104] This is not only a surrogate outcome but also one that is prone to bias, as it is pretty subjective to decide whether progression has occurred. The FDA obligated the company to conduct more trials and these didn't show an effect on progression-free survival whereas they showed serious harms, including deaths. Three years later, the drug, which cost the same every year as several new cars, about $88 000, was revoked for breast cancer.[105]

Lack of adequate safety data isn't acceptable

It's a gross failure in drug regulation when drugs with known harms are approved without adequate safety data. The COX-2 inhibitors are a perfect example, as their mechanism of action predicted an increased risk of cardiovascular mortality.

When I discussed this with a drug regulator, he replied that if they were to demand such data, it would delay the introduction of valuable drugs for years.

I don't buy the argument. A drug company could easily perform a large trial of its COX-2 inhibitor that could tell us what the risks are and it's the industry's own fault when it thinks it can get away with cutting corners. If rofecoxib (Vioxx) had been studied in relevant patient populations, its harms would have been detected very quickly, as the number needed to treat for 1 year to cause one extra myocardial infarction is only 70 patients.[19] There is also an overriding ethical issue, which cannot be trumped by petty claims about practicalities and potential loss of income. Unfortunately, the drug agencies give in to the drug companies' unsustainable arguments.

Vioxx was withdrawn in 2004 and valdecoxib (Bextra) in 2005. Before Bextra was pulled off the market, nine of the 10 FDA advisers with industry ties voted to keep it on the market![106]

In 2008, the FDA considered whether, in future, it should require post-marketing studies with relevant outcomes such as cardiovascular morbidity and mortality.[107] However, only one-third of such studies are ever performed,[46] and the FDA is known not to enforce them because it lacks the authority to do so.[22] From 2007, failure to perform a post-marketing study or to make a needed label change can result in fines, but only up to $10 million.[54] As this is peanuts for big pharma, it's window-dressing, or a fake fix. Even when studies *have* been carried out, they might show that a drug has killed thousands of patients, which we could have avoided by requiring relevant trials *before* drug agencies decide whether a drug should be approved. Post-marketing studies are therefore a very bad idea compared to rejecting the application for marketing authorisation. We need relevant data for every new drug in a therapeutic class, as a new drug might kill people even though 10 similar drugs didn't.

An additional problem is that required post-marketing studies are not necessarily randomised trials but may merely be observational studies, which are very poor in detecting signals of harm. Those who are being treated differ in many ways from a control group that is not being treated, and a doubling in the rate of heart attacks in elderly people may simply be because these patients are more prone to get a heart attack than other patients. Patients with rheumatoid arthritis, for example, are more prone to get heart attacks than other people of the same age, which makes it difficult to detect that COX-2 inhibitors kill them.

The spontaneous reporting of serious adverse events to the regulators for marketed drugs is also a weak method for harm detection. In 2010, the FDA warned Pfizer in a 12-page letter for failing to quickly report serious and unexpected potential side effects from its drugs after having conducted a 6-week inspection of Pfizer's headquarters.[108] *Pfizer had misclassified or downgraded reports to non-serious without reasonable justification* and had failed to submit reports on blindness caused by Viagra (sildenafil) and similar medications within the agency's 15-day deadline. Pfizer was also warned in 2009, but the FDA noted that the company's delays in telling the agency about harms had only grown. Pfizer was told that failure to fix the problems could result in legal action without notice and delays in approving the company's pending drugs.

In 2012, Roche was reprimanded by the EMA for failing to report up to

80 000 possible adverse reactions from its drugs, including 15 161 deaths in the United States.[109] Regulators identified additional deficiencies related to the evaluation and reporting to national drug agencies of suspected adverse reactions in 23 000 other patients and 600 participants in clinical trials.

TOO MANY WARNINGS AND TOO MANY DRUGS

All drugs come with a long list of warnings, contraindications and precautions, for example explaining types of patients, conditions or other drugs the patients take that make it risky to use the drug. Have a look at an advertisement in a medical journal and you'll see how overwhelming it is; there can be more than 20 warnings for a single drug. Here is an example.

Statins

Some of my colleagues are obsessed with cholesterol and believe that everyone over 50 should take a statin, no matter what their cholesterol level is, as it will reduce their risk of dying. They also say that statins have no side effects worth mentioning, or even that they have *no* side effects.[110] Let's have a look at an advertisement that appeared on the first pages of *JAMA* on 19 September 2012. It said, 'Try LIVALO® to lower LDL-C and improve other lipid parameters'.

That's not why you might consider taking a statin, is it? You would want it to reduce your risk of dying, not to improve some laboratory values. Can you be sure that a particular statin reduces your risk of dying? No, you cannot, as statins are approved based on their effect on plasma lipids. LIVALO might reduce your risk of dying from heart disease but it might also increase your risk of dying from other causes, so you cannot know what your chances are with and without LIVALO.

Just by reading the first two lines in the ad, I would say no thanks. We shouldn't take 'life-saving drugs' without knowing whether they will decrease or increase our risk of dying.

But let's go on. Page 2 of the ad says, 'Drug therapy should be one component of multiple-risk factor intervention in individuals who require modifications of their lipid profile. Lipid-altering agents should be used in addition to a diet restricted in saturated fat and cholesterol only when the response to diet and other nonpharmacological measures has been inadequate.'

Aha. This is not what my well-meaning colleagues say when they are close to proposing we should get statins with our drinking water. I am not on a diet or on some 'other nonpharmacological measures' (what on earth is that?) and how can anyone decide whether I require a modification of my lipid profile? Can you see how subjective all this is and how woolly the regulatory language is?

Further ahead comes what I wanted to know, but curiously under a subheading called 'Limitations of use':

- Doses of LIVALO greater than 4 mg once daily were associated with an increased risk for severe myopathy in premarketing clinical studies. Do not exceed 4-mg, once-daily dosing of LIVALO.

- The effect of LIVALO on cardiovascular morbidity and mortality has not been determined.

I knew it! We don't have a clue whether LIVALO does what we want it to do. And I would run a risk of severe muscle damage. People absorb and metabolise drugs differently, and some will undoubtedly get severe muscle damage even if they don't exceed 4 mg a day. It could be me. At this point, my free interpretation of the drug's name is LEAVE ME ALONE!

Page 1 of the ad doesn't tell us about the possible benefit of the drug, apart from the headline about the lipids, which isn't useful. The rest of the page is about harms, which are called 'Important safety information'. My scepticism increases:

'Cases of myopathy and rhabdomyolysis with acute renal failure secondary to myoglobinuria have been reported with HMG-CoA reductase inhibitors, including LIVALO.' Such effects increase with dose, with advanced age (>65 years), renal impairment, inadequately treated hypothyroidism, and in combination with fibrates or lipid-modifying doses of niacin (≥1 g/day).

And then it becomes really difficult. 'LIVALO therapy should be discontinued if markedly elevated CK levels occur or myopathy is diagnosed or suspected', and 'Advise patients to promptly report unexplained muscle pain, tenderness, or weakness, particularly if accompanied by malaise or fever, and to discontinue LIVALO if these signs or symptoms appear.'

Good Heavens. CK means creatine kinase, a muscle enzyme. Patients treated with statins often have such symptoms[111] (although the ad wrongly says they are rare), so how would the patients know when to discontinue LIVALO?

We are also told about liver injuries. Liver enzyme tests should be performed before treatment starts and if signs or symptoms of liver injury occur. It seems a bit late to measure liver enzymes if the liver is already injured. 'There have been rare post-marketing reports of fatal and non-fatal hepatic failure in patients taking statins, including pitavastatin.' The drug might kill me.

LIVALO may also increase blood glucose, which will increase my risk of dying from cardiovascular problems, which LIVALO was supposed to protect me against.

I'll stop here, but it's important to realise that drugs are never safe. Life jackets on boats are good to have, as they may save your life. They won't kill you. Drugs are not like that. Taking a statin may reduce your risk of dying from heart disease, but it will also increase your risk of dying from some other causes. Not much, but one of the statins, cerivastatin (Baycol), was taken off the market after patients had died because of muscle damage and renal failure.

Anyone of us will need to consider the pros and cons of taking a drug, and our doctor isn't always the best person to ask, as most doctors have been brainwashed and many have been bribed by the drug industry. What we would like to know is this: how much longer will we live, on average, if we take this drug? The older we are, the smaller the benefit. If we don't die from heart disease, we'll surely die from something else. A male 65-year-old non-smoker with a systolic blood pressure of 140 mm Hg and a cholesterol of 5 mmol/L will be expected to live 3 months longer if he takes a statin for the rest of his life.[112] That's not much, particularly not if the bonus comes when he sits demented and incontinent in a nursing home and would rather have preferred a drug that shortened the length of this misery. We should also ask the patients what their experiences are. A survey of over 10000 people found that muscular side effects were reported in 60% of former users and 25% of current users.[110]

Other lipid-altering drugs are also interesting. It was expected to be beneficial to increase high-density lipoprotein, but a drug that does this had no effect on the progression of coronary atherosclerosis in trials of about 1000 patients.[107] The chemical name of the drug is torcetrapib. Can you pronounce and remember this? One reason why the chemical names, which are invented by the drug companies, are so foolish is that doctors are then forced to use the trade name and therefore less likely to prescribe a cheaper generic when the drug comes off patent. Luckily, the company did a large trial in 15000 patients, and since it showed that the drug kills people, the manufacturer halted the development of the drug.

Another lipid-altering drug, ezetimibe, was approved by the FDA in 2002 because it had lowered low-density cholesterol in the blood by 15%.[107] In 2007, sales of the drug reached $5 billion in the United States, although no one knows whether it's beneficial or harmful.

Warnings are fake fixes

It's impossible for clinicians to know what they need to know about drugs to prescribe them safely, and it's therefore not surprising that doctors make many medical errors. The fundamental problem is that regulators think about drugs one by one and don't care that doctors cannot possibly know all the warnings about the drugs they use. What matters to regulators is: not our fault, we did warn you, didn't we?

Every doctor knows that the anticoagulant warfarin can interact dangerously with other drugs and some food items, but doctors cannot even use this drug safely. In one study, 65% of the patients were given at least one other drug that could increase the risk of bleeding with warfarin, and in another study, about a third of the patients received such drugs.[113]

Cisapride (Propulsid from Johnson & Johnson) was supposed to promote gastric emptying, but it is no longer on the market as it causes cardiac arrhythmias that kill people. In 1998, the FDA warned about the contraindications for the drug through additions to the black box label, and practitioners were furthermore warned through a dear doctor letter sent by the manufacturer. These warnings had barely any effect.[114] In the year prior to regulatory action, cisapride use was contraindicated for 26%, 30% and 60% of users in three study sites, and in the year after regulatory action use was contraindicated for 24%, 28% and 58% of users. Johnson & Johnson sold the drug for more than a billion dollars each year, although it should never have been approved. When the FDA called for a public meeting in 2000, a company executive admitted that they had not even been able to show that the drug worked.[85] Again, regulatory insufficiency resulted in tragedies for real people:[115]

'Vanessa was a healthy girl. She didn't drink or smoke or take drugs – with one exception: over the past year, she had periodically taken cisapride, an acid-reflux drug marketed as Prepulsid. Her doctor, who'd diagnosed her with a minor form of bulimia, prescribed it after she complained of reflux and feeling bloated after meals. Neither their doctor or pharmacist mentioned risks.' On 19 March 2000, her father watched his 15-year-old daughter collapse on the floor at home. 'She was rushed to hospital, where she died a day later. The cause: cardiac arrest.' Five months later, the drug was withdrawn from the market, but it was too late for Vanessa.

Because of the loss of his daughter, her father became active in politics and got elected to the Canadian Parliament, as he wanted to change drug regulation. He expressed incredulity that prescription drugs aren't regulated as stringently as other public safety threats: *'The minister of transportation doesn't "negotiate" with truckers to keep unsafe vehicles off roads,'* he said. By law, doctors must report unfit drivers and are paid to do so. *Fast-tracking drugs to market is like 'air-traffic controllers being told to land planes more quickly'.* Eleven years after his daughter's inquest, none of his major recommendations for reforms had been implemented.

We have thousands of drugs at our disposal, and I wonder why no one ever studied whether the availability of so many drugs does more harm than good. I am sure that's the case. Otherwise, drugs wouldn't be the third leading cause of death.

The doctors cannot know about all the dangers, but the patients can. They can read the package insert carefully and stop taking the drug if they think it's too risky for them. I also hope my book may contribute to making so many citizens angry that they will protest and demonstrate until we force our politicians into introducing some much-needed reforms.

We know very little about polypharmacy

Most patients are in treatment with several drugs, particularly elderly patients. A Swedish study of 762 people living in nursing homes found that 67% were prescribed 10 or more drugs.[116] One-third were in treatment with three or more psychoactive drugs; around half received antidepressants or tranquillisers; and anticholinergic drugs (e.g. for urinary incontinence) were used in one-fifth. All these drugs may create cognitive impairment, confusion and falls, which carry a considerable mortality among the elderly. The symptoms are often misinterpreted by the patients and their carers as signs of old age or impending disease, e.g. dementia or Parkinson's, but when doctors stop the medicines, many of the patients apparently become many years younger, drop the wheeled walking frame, which they got because they couldn't keep the balance, and become active again. A US study found that almost 18% of Medicare patients took drugs that aren't safe for older people.[85]

Just like regulators, doctors see one problem at a time and usually start drug treatment every time. They very often forget about stopping a drug when it's no longer needed. My most important contribution to internal medicine was to stop drugs in newly admitted patients, only to realise that, quite often, the patients arrived doped with the same drugs by their general practitioner next time they were admitted. It is surely an uphill battle.

We know very little about what happens when patients take many drugs, but we know enough to act. Every one of them may affect many bodily functions, apart from the intended one, and they may interact in unpredictable ways. We also know that old people are much overtreated, with harmful consequences. A randomised trial showed that drug reduction lowered both mortality and admission to hospital, and a subsequent study in 70 patients where number of drugs was reduced from 7.7 to 4.4 per patient showed that 88% reported global improvement in health and most had improvement in cognitive functions.[117] Here is a typical story, apart from the fact that few elderly people are that lucky:[118]

> When my father was 88, he was hospitalised for dizziness, which occurred after his medication was increased. In the hospital, he was given more medication which made him confused, frightened, and incoherent. Then his doctor transferred him to a nursing home, where he was dirty, crying, begging people to hold his hand, and listed as DNR (Do Not Resuscitate) – and given still more medication.
>
> I convinced the doctor at the nursing home to discontinue all medication, and I hired a private nurse to give my father an organic diet – rich in fruits, vegetables, grains, beans, nuts, and seeds. In 3 days, my father made such a miraculous recovery that the nurses on the ward didn't recognise him. When I called to speak to my father, he was back to his old self, and told me that he was bored and looking for a card game. My father was discharged the next day, and died several years later, while relaxing peacefully at home.

Here is another story, of a woman who was also 88. She gets admitted to hospital after a bout of diarrhoea and dizziness.[119] Her family was soon shocked by the quick deterioration in her health and the emergence of some strange new symptoms, including delusions, and they couldn't wake her. They found out that she was taking several new drugs, including a painkiller and an antidepressant, but she wasn't depressed, she was rightly grieving for the loss of her former life, because she was now stuck inside a hospital room. At the same time, a psychiatrist diagnosed Alzheimer's and suggested that she take donepezil (Aricept). Her daughter-in-law refused this and took several of the drugs from her, which had dramatic effects. She became herself again. This experience turned her daughter-in-law into a patients' advocate: 'I was looking at all the other people in long term care facilities, where family members were either unaware of the problems or didn't want to rock the boat, and I thought, "Who the hell is going to speak up for these people?"'

Modern medicine doesn't work well for old people. Every clinician has witnessed the medicalised 80-year-old obsessed with arthritis, Alzheimer's disease, and serum cholesterol levels. Contrast this patient with someone else in the same physical condition, who admits that her knees are bad and that she has trouble remembering things. Which patient is better off?[120]

REFERENCES

1 Mundy A. *Dispensing with the Truth*. New York: St. Martin's Press; 2001.

2 Angell M. *The Truth about the Drug Companies: how they deceive us and what to do about it*. New York: Random House; 2004.

3 Day M. Don't blame it all on the bogey. *BMJ*. 2007; **334**: 1250–1.

4 Bailey RS. FDA corruption charges letter verified. *The Los Angeles Post*. 2012 April 8.

5 Tanne JH. Investigators to review conflicts of interest at NIH. *BMJ*. 2007; **334**: 767.

6 Tanne JH. Former FDA head is fined $90 000 for failing to disclose conflicts of interest. *BMJ*. 2007; **334**: 492.

7 Andersen NA, Drachmann H. [Psychiatrist gets millions]. *Politiken*. 2003 Dec 5.

8 Braithwaite J. *Corporate Crime in the Pharmaceutical Industry*. London: Routledge & Kegan Paul; 1984.

9 Blowing the whistle on the FDA: an interview with David Graham. *Multinational Monitor* 2004; **25**(12).

10 Lenzer J. Crisis deepens at the US Food and Drug Administration. *BMJ*. 2004; **329**: 1308.

11 Moynihan R, Cassels A. *Selling Sickness: how the world's biggest pharmaceutical companies are turning us all into patients*. New York: Nation Books; 2005.

12 Ross DB. The FDA and the case of Ketek. *N Engl J Med*. 2007; **356**: 1601–4.

13 Baciu A, Stratton K, Burke SP, eds. *The Future of Drug Safety: promoting and protecting the health of the public*. Washington, DC: National Academies Press; 2006.

14 Smith SW. Sidelining safety – the FDA's inadequate response to the IOM. *N Engl J Med*. 2007; **357**: 960–3.

15 Willman D. How a new policy led to seven deadly drugs. *Los Angeles Times*. 2000 Dec 20.

16 Abraham J. *Science, Politics and the Pharmaceutical Industry*. London: UCL Press; 1995.

17 House of Commons Health Committee. *The Influence of the Pharmaceutical Industry. Fourth Report of Session 2004–05*. Available online at: www.publications.parliament.uk/pa/cm200405/cmselect/cmhealth/42/42.pdf (accessed 26 April 2005).

18 Graham DJ. COX-2 inhibitors, other NSAIDs, and cardiovascular risk: the seduction of common sense. *JAMA*. 2006; **296**: 1653–6.

19 Jüni P, Nartey L, Reichenbach S, *et al*. Risk of cardiovascular events and rofecoxib: cumulative meta-analysis. *Lancet*. 2004; **364**: 2021–9.

20 Garattini S. Confidentiality. *Lancet*. 2003; **362**: 1078–9.

21 Union of Concerned Scientists. *FDA Scientists Pressured to Exclude, Alter Findings; scientists fear retaliation for voicing safety concerns*. 2006 July 20.

22 Psaty BM, Burke SP. Institute of Medicine on drug safety. *N Engl J Med*. 2006; **355**: 1753–5.

23 Anonymous. Institute of Medicine urges reforms at FDA. *Lancet*. 2006; **368**: 1211.

24 Strom BL. How the US drug safety system should be changed. *JAMA*. 2006; **295**: 2072–5.

25 Abramson J. *Overdo$ed America: the broken promise of American medicine*. New York: HarperCollins; 2004.

26 United States General Accounting Office. *Food and Drug Administration: effect of user fees on drug approval times, withdrawals, and other agency activities*. Sept 2002.

27 Reuters. *Danish drugmaker Lundbeck A/S and Japanese partner Takeda Pharmaceutical Co have submitted a new antidepressant for regulatory approval in the United States*. 2012 Oct 2.

28 Avorn J, Shrank W. Highlights and a hidden hazard – the FDA's new labeling regulations. *N Engl J Med*. 2006; **354**: 2409–11.

29 Letter from FDA scientists to President Barrack Obama. 2009 Apr 2. Available online at: http://gaia-health.com/articles201/000201-letter.pdf (accessed 11 Nov 2012).

30 Lichtblau E, Shane S. Vast FDA effort tracked e-mails of its scientists. *New York Times*. 2012 July 14.

31 Rosenberg M. Former FDA reviewer speaks out about intimidation, retaliation and marginalizing of safety. *Truthout*. 2012 July 29.

32 Brynner R, Stephens T. *Dark Remedy: the impact of thalidomide and its revival as a vital medicine*. New York: Perseus Publishing; 2001.

33 Brody H. *Hooked: ethics, the medical profession, and the pharmaceutical industry*. Lanham: Rowman & Littlefield; 2008.

34 Sibbison JB. USA: dirty work in the drug industry. *Lancet*. 1991; **337**: 227.

35 Wikipedia. Duilio Poggiolini. Available online at: http://en.wikipedia.org/wiki/Duilio_Poggiolini (accessed 10 November 2012).

36 Abbott A. Italian health sector in disarray following more scandals. *Nature.* 1993; **364**: 663.

37 Medawar C, Hardon A. *Medicines out of control? Antidepressants and the conspiracy of goodwill.* Netherlands: Aksant Academic Publishers; 2004.

38 Day M. Italian police arrest drug officials over alleged falsification of data. *BMJ.* 2008; **336**: 1208–9.

39 Pfizer memoranda, 24 and 26 April 1989.

40 Grill M. *Kranke Geschäfte: wie die Pharmaindustrie uns manipuliert.* Hamburg: Rowohlt Verlag; 2007.

41 Relman AS, Angell M. America's other drug problem: how the drug industry distorts medicine and politics. *The New Republic.* 2002 Dec 16: 27–41.

42 Ismail M. *Drug Lobby Second to None: how the pharmaceutical industry gets its way in Washington.* The Center for Public Integrity. 2005 July 7.

43 Bass A. *Side Effects – a prosecutor, a whistleblower, and a bestselling antidepressant on trial.* Chapel Hill: Algonquin Books; 2008.

44 Gøtzsche PC, Jørgensen AW. Opening up data at the European Medicines Agency. *BMJ.* 2011; **342**: d2686.

45 Anonymous. FDA more transparent than EMEA. *Prescrire International.* 2002; **11**: 98.

46 Garattini S, Bertele V. How can we regulate medicines better? *BMJ.* 2007; **335**: 803–5.

47 Kranish M. Drug industry costs doctor top FDA post. *Boston Globe.* 2002 May 27.

48 Goozner M. *The $800 Million Pill: the truth behind the cost of new drugs.* Berkeley: University of California Press; 2005.

49 McClellan MB. Speech before First International Colloquium on Generic Medicine. Available online at: www.fda.gov/oc/speeches/2003/genericdrug0925.html (accessed 18 February 2008).

50 Carpenter D, Zucker EJ, Avorn J. Drug-review deadlines and safety problems. *N Engl J Med.* 2008; **358**: 1354–61.

51 Carpenter D. Drug-review deadlines and safety problems (authors' reply). *N Engl J Med.* 2008; **359**: 96–8.

52 Moore TJ, Cohen MR, Furberg CD. Serious adverse drug events reported to the Food and Drug Administration, 1998–2005. *Arch Intern Med.* 2007; **167**: 1752–9.

53 Lexchin J. New drugs and safety: what happened to new active substances approved in Canada between 1995 and 2010? *Arch Intern Med.* 2012 Oct 8: 1–2.

54 Avorn J. Paying for drug approvals – who's using whom? *N Engl J Med.* 2007; **356**: 1697–700.

55 Psaty BM, Korn D. Congress responds to the IOM drug safety report – in full. *JAMA.* 2007; **298**: 2185–7.

56 Harris G, Halbfinger DM. FDA reveals it fell to a push by lawmakers. *New York Times.* 2009 Sept 25.

57 Dhruva SS, Bero LA, Redberg RF. Strength of study evidence examined by the FDA in premarket approval of cardiovascular devices. *JAMA.* 2009; **302**: 2679–85.

58 Van Brabandt H, Neyt M, Hulstaert F. Transcatheter aortic valve implantation (TAVI): risky and costly. *BMJ.* 2012; **345**: e4710.

59 Collier J. Big pharma and the UK government. *Lancet.* 2006; **367**: 97–8.

60 Lee K, Bacchetti P, Sim I. Publication of clinical trials supporting successful new drug applications: a literature analysis. *PLoS Med.* 2008; **5**: e191.

61 European Commission. *Strategy to Better Protect Public Health by Strengthening and Rationalising EU Pharmacovigilance.* 2007 Dec 5.

62 HAI Europe. *Pharmacovigilance in Europe and Patient Safety: no to deregulation.* Press release. 2008 Feb 1.

63 Larsen H, Nyborg S. [The drug industry asks for control]. *Politiken.* 2006 Mar 5.

64 [Committee on Scientific Dishonesty tamed]. *Ugeskr Læger.* 2005; **167**: 3476–7.

65 Greene JA, Choudhry NK, Kesselheim AS, *et al.* Changes in direct-to-consumer pharmaceutical advertising following shifts from prescription-only to over-the-counter status. *JAMA.* 2012; **308**: 973–5.

66 Welch HG. *Should I be Tested for Cancer? Maybe not and here's why.* Berkeley: University of California Press; 2004.

67 Welch HG, Schwartz L, Woloshin S. *Overdiagnosed: making people sick in the pursuit of health.* Boston, MA: Beacon Press; 2011.

68 Andersen NV. [Drug giant uses American pressure in Danish drug case]. *Politiken.* 2004 Aug 31.

69 Amendment to the Federal Food, Drug and Cosmetic Act. Washington, DC: 4 Jan, 2007. Available online at: www.fda.gov/oc/initiatives/HR3580.pdf (accessed 8 July 2008).

70 Moore TJ, Furberg CD. The safety risks of innovation: the FDA's Expedited Drug Development Pathway. *JAMA.* 2012; **308**: 869–70.

71 Jefferson T, Jones MA, Doshi P, *et al.* Neuraminidase inhibitors for preventing and treating influenza in healthy adults and children. *Cochrane Database Syst Rev.* 2012; **1**: CD008965.

72 Meier B. Contracts keep drug research out of reach. *New York Times.* 2004 Nov 29.

73 Lurie P, Wolfe SM. Misleading data analyses in salmeterol (SMART) study. *Lancet.* 2005; **366**: 1261–2.

74 Rickard KA. Misleading data analyses in salmeterol (SMART) study – GlaxoSmithKline's reply. *Lancet.* 2005; **366**: 1262.

75 Castle W, Fuller R, Hall J, *et al.* Serevent nationwide surveillance study: comparison of salmeterol with salbutamol in asthmatic patients who require regular bronchodilator treatment. *BMJ.* 1993; **306**: 1034–7.

76 Salpeter SR, Buckley NS, Ormiston TM, *et al.* Meta-analysis: effect of long-acting beta-agonists on severe asthma exacerbations and asthma-related deaths. *Ann Intern Med.* 2006; **144**: 904–12.

77 *FDA Drug Safety Communication: new safety requirements for long-acting inhaled asthma medications called Long-Acting Beta-Agonists (LABAs).* 2010 Feb 18. Available online at: www.fda.gov/Drugs/DrugSafety/PostmarketDrugSafetyInformationforPatientsandProviders/ucm200776.htm (accessed 8 October 2012).

78 Nelson HS, Weiss ST, Bleecker ER, *et al.* The Salmeterol Multicenter Asthma Research Trial: a comparison of usual pharmacotherapy for asthma or usual pharmacotherapy plus salmeterol. *Chest.* 2006; **129**: 15–26.

79 Curfman GD, Morrissey S, Drazen JM. Products at risk. *N Engl J Med.* 2010; **363**: 1763.

80 Harris G. Pfizer says internal studies show no Celebrex risks. *New York Times.* 2005 Feb 5.

81 Caldwell B, Aldington S, Weatherall M, *et al.* Risk of cardiovascular events and celecoxib: a systematic review and meta-analysis. *J R Soc Med.* 2006; **99**: 132–40.

82 Sherman M, Marchione M. Pfizer: Celebrex raises heart attack risk. *ABC News.* 2004 Dec 17.

83 Avorn J. *Powerful Medicines: the benefits, risks, and costs of prescription drugs.* New York: Vintage Books; 2005.

84 Avorn J. Dangerous deception – hiding the evidence of adverse drug effects. *N Engl J Med.* 2006; **355**: 2169–71.

85 Petersen M. *Our Daily Meds.* New York: Sarah Crichton Books; 2008.

86 Whitaker R. *Anatomy of an Epidemic.* New York: Broadway Paperbacks; 2010.

87 Smith SM, Schroeder K, Fahey T. Over-the-counter (OTC) medications for acute cough in children and adults in ambulatory settings. *Cochrane Database Syst Rev.* 2012; **8**: CD001831.

88 Tomerak AAT, Vyas HHV, Lakhanpaul M, *et al.* Inhaled beta2-agonists for non-specific chronic cough in children. *Cochrane Database Syst Rev.* 2005; **3**: CD005373.

89 Glintborg D. [Cough medicines for acute respiratory infections, what is the evidence?] *Rationel Farmakoterapi.* 2003 Jan 4.

90 Sharfstein JM, North M, Serwint JR. Over the counter but no longer under the radar – pediatric cough and cold medications. *N Engl J Med.* 2007; **357**: 2321–4.

91 *Public Health Advisory: FDA Recommends that Over-the-Counter (OTC) Cough and Cold Products not be used for Infants and Children under 2 Years of Age.* 2011 Feb 23.

92 Parvez L, Vaidya M, Sakhardande A, *et al.* Evaluation of antitussive agents in man. *Pulm Pharmacol.* 1996; **9**: 299–308.

93 Goodyear MD, Lemmens T, Sprumont D, *et al.* Does the FDA have the authority to trump the Declaration of Helsinki? *BMJ.* 2009; **338**: b1559.

94 Wikipedia. Tuskegee syphilis experiment. Available online at: http://en.wikipedia.org/wiki/Tuskegee_syphilis_experiment (accessed 21 January 2010).

95 Boseley S, Smith D. As doctors fought to save lives, Pfizer flew in drug trial team. *The Guardian.* 2010 Dec 9.

96 Smith D. Pfizer pays out to Nigerian families of meningitis drug trial victims. *The Guardian.* 2011 Aug 12.

97 Chalmers TC, Frank CS, Reitman D. Minimizing the three stages of publication bias. *JAMA.* 1990; **263**: 1392–5.

98 The Coronary Drug Project Research Group. Influence of adherence to treatment and response of cholesterol on mortality in the coronary drug project. *N Engl J Med.* 1980; **303**: 1038–41.

99 Nissen SE. Cardiovascular effects of diabetes drugs: emerging from the dark ages. *Ann Intern Med.* 2012; **157**: 671–2.

100 Gøtzsche PC, Liberati A, Luca P, *et al.* Beware of surrogate outcome measures. *Int J Technol Ass Health Care.* 1996; **12**: 238–46.

101 Pocock SJ. When to stop a clinical trial. *BMJ.* 1992; **305**: 235–40.

102 Moore TJ. *Deadly Medicine: why tens of thousands of heart patients died in America's worst drug disaster.* New York: Simon & Schuster; 1995.

103 Gøtzsche PC, Jørgensen KJ. Screening for breast cancer with mammography. *Cochrane Database Syst Rev.* 2013; **6**: CD001877.

104 D'Agostino RB Sr. Changing end points in breast-cancer drug approval – the Avastin story. *N Engl J Med.* 2011; **365**: e2.

105 Pollack A. FDA revokes approval of Avastatin for use as breast cancer drug. *New York Times.* 2011 Nov 18.

106 Lenzer J. FDA is criticised for hinting it may loosen conflict of interest rules. *BMJ.* 2011; **343**: d5070.

107 Psaty BM, Lumley T. Surrogate end points and FDA approval: a tale of 2 lipid-altering drugs. *JAMA.* 2008; **299**: 1474–6.

108 Heavey S. FDA warns Pfizer for not reporting side effects. Reuters. 2010 June 10.

109 Wise J. European drug agency criticises Roche for failing to report adverse reactions and patient deaths. *BMJ.* 2012; **344**: e4344.

110 McCartney M. Statins for all? *BMJ.* 2012; **345**: e6044.

111 Golomb BA, Evans MA, Dimsdale JE, *et al.* Effects of statins on energy and fatigue with exertion: results from a randomized controlled trial. *Arch Intern Med.* 2012; **172**: 1180–2.

112 Støvring H, Harmsen CG, Wisløff T, *et al.* A competing risk approach for the European Heart SCORE model based on cause-specific and all-cause mortality. *Eur J Prev Cardiol.* 2012 Apr 12.

113 Hampton T. Flawed prescribing practices revealed. *JAMA.* 2006; **296**: 2191–2.

114 Smalley W, Shatin D, Wysowski DK, *et al.* Contraindicated use of cisapride: impact of food and drug administration regulatory action. *JAMA.* 2000; **284**: 3036–9.

115 Kingston A. A national embarrassment. *Maclean's Magazine.* 2012 Oct 17.

116 Kragh A. [Two of three people in nursing homes are in treatment with at least ten drugs]. *Läkartidningen.* 2004; **101**: 994–9.

117 Garfinkel D, Mangin D. Feasibility study of a systematic approach for discontinuation of multiple medications in older adults: addressing polypharmacy. *Arch Intern Med.* 2010; **170**: 1648–54.

118 Mann H. Beware of polypharmacy in the elderly. *BMJ.* 2009 March 8. Available online at: www.bmj.com/cgi/eletters/338/mar03_2/b873 (accessed 12 March 2009).

119 Moynihan R. Is your mum on drugs? *BMJ.* 2011; **343**: d5184.

120 Goodwin JS. Geriatrics and the limits of modern medicine. *N Engl J Med.* 1999; **340**: 1283–5.

Public access to data
at drug agencies

If companies wanted to publish negative studies they could, but companies don't like to publish negative studies. It's amusing so many people are making pronouncements about the data – scientists and physicians – without seeing the data.

Russel Katz, director of the neuropharmacology
division at the FDA[1]

If commercial success depends on withholding data that are important to prescribe drugs rationally and safely, there is something fundamentally wrong with our priorities in healthcare. It is of vital importance for public health that doctors and the public can get access to all data generated from all trials in patients and healthy human volunteers and not just a biased sample, as is currently the case.

A good starting point for total access is the data the drug companies have submitted to drug agencies. Chief statistician Hans Melander and his co-workers at the Swedish drug agency have such access and they showed in 2003 that published trial reports of SSRIs were seriously flawed, compared to the study reports submitted in registration applications.[2] In all 42 trials submitted to the agency but one, the companies had performed both an intention-to-treat analysis and a per-protocol analysis (where dropped-out patients are not accounted for). In only two of the publications, however, were both analyses presented, whereas in the remainder, only the more favourable per-protocol analysis was presented. This created a large misconception about how effective the drugs are (Figure 11.1).[3] Moreover, separate trials were sometimes published as if they were the same trial, cross-references to multiple publications of the same trial were missing, and sometimes there were no author names in common in multiple publications of the same trial.

A 2008 study, also of antidepressants, confirmed that the published data are seriously flawed, compared to data submitted to the FDA.[4] The effect in the published trials was 32% larger than in all trials in FDA's possession, and more than double as large as in unpublished trials. Furthermore, there was spin on the results. Six trials that were deemed questionable by the FDA were positive when published, and when 8 of 24 negative trials were published, 5 were positive. Another study, of 164 trials included in 33 new drug applications, also found that what was published didn't reflect what was submitted to the FDA.[5]

Drug regulators have used absurd arguments to deny researchers access to

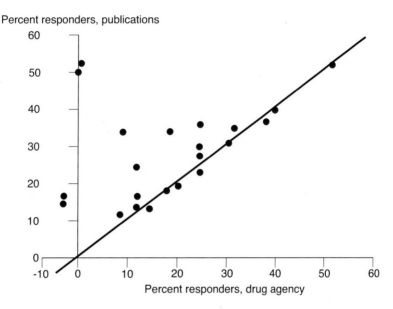

Figure 11.1 Difference in percent responders between an SSRI and placebo as stated in study reports at the Swedish Drug Agency and as stated in publications of the same trials. Points above the line indicate an overestimation of the effect in publications

unpublished trials and data; they have gone so far as regarding suicides occurring while taking a drug that was supposed to *prevent* suicide a trade secret.[6]

The drug industry's arguments have been equally absurd and exploitative of patients. The proposal to register all trials, so that we would know also about the unpublished ones, was rejected in 2000 by drug industry representatives claiming that the very existence of trials was a trade secret![7] Drummond Rennie, deputy editor of *JAMA*, wondered why the FDA had been completely absent from the debate over trial registration and why it didn't correct journal results that directly conflicted with what the FDA knew to be true facts, with the excuse that they have no mandate to inform the public. Wrong. The FDA is supposed to do exactly that: to guard the health of the public.

Iain Chalmers, the founder of the Cochrane Collaboration, considers underreporting of research an equally serious form of scientific misconduct as fabrication of data.[8] I agree. In fact, the consequences for patients are much more devastating, as it is so common. On average, only about half of all studies ever get published,[9] but it can be far worse. A review of dyspepsia caused by five old NSAIDs found 15 published placebo-controlled trials and 11 unpublished trials on the FDA's website.[10] Only one trial was both published and submitted by the companies to the FDA, but the authors of the published paper were completely different from the investigators listed in the FDA report.

Don't you wonder why any type of scientific misconduct flourishes in healthcare, all over the place? If researchers in a single study decided to delete half of their results because they didn't give the result they had hoped for and published the rest, we would call it scientific misconduct. But when whole studies go missing, we accept it as a normal part of life, although it is deeply unethical towards our patients.[7,11] Selective reporting of results is scientific misconduct,[12] which the Danish Association of the Pharmaceutical Industry has acknowledged.[13] But our institutions have generally failed us. Not a single organisation has used its powers, stood up and announced that this must stop, apart from one: the UK Faculty of Pharmaceutical Medicine, a small organisation with about 1400 members.[11]

OUR BREAKTHROUGH AT THE EMA IN 2010

In 2007, PhD student Anders Jørgensen and I decided that the secrecy at drug agencies was so unbearable that we would do everything we could to get access to unpublished studies at the EMA. If we failed, which we expected, we would publish our experiences, particularly the arguments from the regulator, to expose to the world how deeply unethical the secrecy was, and we would then continue our fight from there, till we succeeded.[14]

We chose anti-obesity drugs as our test case because they are so dangerous that most of them have been taken off the market after having caused horrific harms. We asked the EMA for access to the clinical study reports and corresponding trial protocols for rimonabant and orlistat, submitted to the agency.

We outlined the plans for our research and explained that it was essential that the submitted documents became available for independent researchers because of the likely widespread future use of these drugs, the relatively small effect on overweight in published reports and the serious safety concerns that had been raised. In fact, rimonabant was withdrawn from the European market in the middle of the process when independent studies found that adverse effects, including severe depression and increased risk of suicide, were more serious and common than shown by the manufacturer, Sanofi-Aventis, in their clinical studies.[15]

We argued that secrecy isn't in the best interest of the patients because biased reporting of drug trials is common and also noted that we hadn't found any information that could compromise commercial interests in 44 trial protocols of industry-initiated trials we had reviewed previously. Although the EMA's primary aim is to protect the public, the EMA replied – without any comment on our arguments – that the documents could not be released because it would undermine commercial interests.

We appealed to the EMA's executive director, Thomas Lönngren, and asked him to explain why the agency considered that the commercial interests of the drug industry should override the welfare of patients. We argued – with convincing real-life examples – that a likely consequence of EMA's position was that patients would die unnecessarily and would be treated with inferior and potentially harmful drugs because their doctors didn't know what their true benefits and harms were.

Lönngren sent us a similar, cut-and-paste type of letter to the first one, ignoring our request for clarification, and told us we could lodge a complaint with the European ombudsman, P Nikiforos Diamandouros, which we did.[14]

It took 3 years before our case was settled. We described it in the *BMJ*[14] and posted the 27 documents that circulated between the ombudsman, the EMA and us and a comprehensive report of the case on our website (www.cochrane.dk/research/EMA).

To avoid disclosing the documents, the EMA put forward four main arguments: protection of commercial interests, no overriding public interest, the administrative burden involved, and the worthlessness of the data to us after the EMA had redacted them.[14] I'm sure Lönngren felt the armour he had built up was impenetrable, but he had not calculated with the ombudsman, who rejected all his arguments. He stated that commercial interests might be at stake but that the risk of an interest being undermined must be reasonably foreseeable and not purely hypothetical. He could not see that access would specifically and actually undermine commercial interests. After having inspected the relevant reports and protocols at the EMA in London, he concluded that the documents didn't contain commercially confidential information.[14]

The ombudsman indicated that we had established an overriding public interest but noted that this question needed answering only if disclosure undermined commercial interests. He asked the EMA to justify its position that there wasn't an overriding public interest, but Lönngren avoided replying by saying that we had not given evidence of the existence of such an interest. We surely had and, in addition, the argument was irrelevant. A suspect asked for his alibi on the day of the crime doesn't get off the hook by asking for someone else's alibi.[14]

About the administrative burden and the uselessness of the documents after the EMA had redacted them, the ombudsman noted that the requested documents didn't identify patients by name but by their identification and test centre numbers, and he concluded that the only personal data were those identifying the study authors and principal investigators and to redact this information would be quick and easy (when we received the documents, nothing was redacted).

Since the EMA continued to be completely resistant to our arguments and those from the ombudsman – in the most shameless and arrogant fashion – he played his final card, 3 years after our request: he accused the EMA of maladministration in a press release. This had the effect that the agency reversed its stance completely. It now gave the impression that it had favoured disclosure all the time, agreed with the ombudsman's reasoning, and noted that the same principles would be applied for future requests for access. This is how drug companies operate. They fight forcefully against openness, but when there is no escape, they pretend they have been in favour of it all the time. They usually go one step further, as they give the impression that it was their own idea to begin with.

Obviously, it isn't possible to protect the profits of the drug companies and the lives and welfare of the patients at the same time. One has to choose, and our case illustrates beyond a shadow of doubt that the EMA sided with the drug industry and put profits over patients. Moreover, its position wasn't even consistent, which we also pointed out in our letters. It denied access to trial data on adult patients while providing access to data on paediatric trials (which it had to do because of EU legislation).

I felt it was an aggravating fact, which we also pointed out in our letters, that the EMA had helped the drug industry to get away with violating the Declaration of Helsinki, which states that researchers have a duty to make publicly available the results of their research on humans.[16] We also noted that by violating these universal human rights, the EMA was complicit in the exploitation of patients for commercial gains, as the patients are used as a means to an end and treated suboptimally as well, which are both unacceptable.

Furthermore, we drew attention to the declaration's statement 'Medical research involving human subjects must ... be based on a thorough knowledge of the scientific literature' and argued that if the knowledge base is incomplete, patients may suffer and cannot give fully informed consent.[17] Thus, by being secretive, the EMA also acquiesced to unethical research in future. Worst of all, it didn't bother the EMA that it contributed to the unfortunate situation that doctors and patients were unable to select those treatments that provide the best balance between benefits, harms and cost, as they were denied access to the evidence. It didn't bother either that tens of thousands of unnecessary deaths could have been avoided each year, if the public had had access to the unpublished information.[17-24]

Our case was a major breakthrough for public health. In November 2010, the EMA declared it would widen public access to documents, including trial reports and protocols.[25] But it shouldn't have been so difficult to get there, given the fundamental principles on which the European Union is based:[26]

> Any citizen of the Union, and any natural or legal person residing or having its registered office in a Member State, has a right of access to documents of the institutions, subject to the principles, conditions and limits defined in this Regulation.
>
> Openness enables citizens to participate more closely in the decision-making process and guarantees that the administration enjoys greater legitimacy and is more effective and more accountable to the citizen in a democratic system. Openness contributes to strengthening the principles of democracy and respect for fundamental rights as laid down in Article 6 of the EU Treaty and in the Charter of Fundamental Rights of the European Union.

Lönngren made sure my PhD student was unable to do the work we had planned. After his efforts at protecting the industry's commercial interests, he quit the EMA, also in a shameless fashion. Although Lönngren had been told by the EMA that he should not provide product-related advice to drug companies or take managerial, executive or consultative positions in the industry for a period of 2 years, he became director of a new company, Pharma Executive Consulting Ltd, in November 2010 while still employed by the EMA![27]

A year later, the EMA held a workshop at its headquarters that made history.[28] Its new head, Guido Rasi, started by announcing that 'We are not here to decide *if* we will publish clinical-trial data, only *how*.' The industry representatives were stunned. Their usual arguments for secrecy were torn into pieces during the discussions, and the head of the UK drug regulator, Kent Woods, looked like a thing from the past when he tried to argue that there wasn't really a need for the EMA's new openness and transparency. I have never before seen the mighty drug industry lose a public battle so completely as during this afternoon. There is a video in two parts on the EMA's website that takes up 3.5 hours in total, but it is really worth seeing.[28]

There had been another case before ours. Liam Grant, father of a boy who committed suicide while on the acne drug isotretinoin (Roaccutane from Roche), had tried to find out which harms the company had informed the authorities about before marketing approval. The EMA granted access to the reported harms in 2010. In 2002, Danish journalists had also tried to get access to reported adverse events on Roaccutane, the so-called Periodic Safety Update Reports (PSUR), from the Danish medical agency. The agency was willing to give access, but Roche blocked this by arguing it would create a substantial risk for considerable losses for Roche. Roche even threatened to sue the Danish state if disclosure harmed the company's commercial interests![29,30] Sue a state because fewer patients will take a drug after they found out it might kill them? How absurd can healthcare get? This is how gangsters operate: 'If you do anything that will harm our sales of heroin, we'll come after you.' The comparison is appropriate, as Roche built its fortune on massive profits from illegal sales of heroin and morphine (*see* Chapter 3). The fact that Roche regards the harms reported by patients or their relatives as the company's private property demonstrates such an outrageous disrespect for patients and human lives, particularly in this case where the drug had been associated with severe depression and suicide, that I'm speechless.

ACCESS TO DATA AT OTHER DRUG AGENCIES

In 2010, we contacted chief statistician Hans Melander at the Swedish drug agency and asked for access to the placebo-controlled trials and protocols for three SSRIs (citalopram, escitalopram and venlafaxine) submitted to the agency.

We could get everything we wanted, but there was a problem. The reports had been filed in a mountain cave somewhere in Sweden where they took up 70 metres. It would cost about €50 000 to retrieve all this and move it back to the agency in Uppsala, but the agency generously offered to cover this cost. We could then work with the material at the agency, or have it all copied for €0.13 per page, or copy it ourselves at no cost, and take it to Denmark. I estimated that 70 metres in binders was about 500 000 pages, or around €70 000 to get the material copied. In order to work with all this, we needed to scan it, using special software that could also handle tables and convert it to searchable text.

I told Melander to hold the horses and wait while we worked on our pilot study of duloxetine. Over more than a year, we had received documents from the EMA, also on other SSRIs, and they were still coming in. These documents were pdf files, which we converted to searchable text, but even so, it took two of our researchers more than a year before they had extracted the data we needed.

The Dutch regulator was also very forthcoming, but they redacted the adverse effects before they sent us the files, which they were obliged to do according to a court verdict, so the material wasn't very useful.

In 1993, a bill was put before the British Parliament that would lead to greater access to regulatory information about the efficacy and safety of drugs, but it was immediately shot down by the industry aided by its apologists in government, ironically in the same year as the government published its white paper on Open Government.[31]

Contacting the UK regulator to get data on fluoxetine, which the EMA didn't have, was like contacting the MI5. The reply we got was anonymous and we were told that the agency had destroyed the files! The Medicines and Healthcare Products Regulatory Agency (MHRA) destroys the files after 15 years, 'unless there is a legal, regulatory, or business need to keep them, or unless they are considered to be of lasting historic interest'.[32] No legal or historic interest for unpublished drug trials for drugs that are still on the market? Can the irony be deeper than this?

There were also bureaucratic obstacles: 'Each individual document should be requested through a separate request and will be reviewed and assessed in terms of its suitability for release.' We limited our request to very little, which the agency had told us was in their possession, but were then told that 'public authorities are not required to comply with requests that they judge to constitute an excessive use of their resources. The time taken to complete an FOI [Freedom of Information] request should take no longer than 24 working hours, otherwise it is deemed an excessive use of resource. Your request falls into this category ...'.

Undeterred by this, I wrote that members of the European Commission and Parliament had been shocked when I told them that the MHRA destroys its files after 15 years. I suggested that, since the UK was the EU Reference Member State for fluoxetine and only the marketing authorisation holder, Eli Lilly, had the files, the agency should ask Lilly to resubmit the files to the agency, as companies are obliged by law to retain them. Finally, I noted that, based on our collaboration with other drug agencies, what we had requested couldn't come anywhere near 24 hours, and I reminded the MHRA about the basic principles about citizens' access to EU documents and that the UK was in fact a member state in the EU.

New obstacles appeared: 'From my preliminary assessment of your request I will not be able to answer it within the 20 days specified in the Act. It is my initial view that section 43 (commercial interests) of the Act may apply to at least some of the information you have requested.'

Oh boy. This message came a year after the ombudsman's press release accusing the EMA of maladministration and saying there were no commercial interests to protect! In its next letter, the MHRA said it had consulted with Lilly, which had refused to release the documents to us, as such release would harm the company. How could they know? Did they cover up something? Very likely they did (see Chapters 17 and 18).

I changed tactics and asked whether the MHRA had thought about what its attitude might mean for its image. And complained that the MHRA hadn't realised that it needed to update its policies and routines and bring them at par with the recent openness at the EMA.

It worked. After three additional months, and 7 months after our initial request, the MHRA informed us that they would send us the documents. But the MHRA was still the lap dog of big pharma:

'Please bear in mind that the volume of information you have asked for is large, and has taken time to redact and to liaise with the marketing authorisation holder, to ensure that they were fully informed of what we were intending to release to you.'

A good thing was that, in contrast to the files we received from the Dutch agency, adverse effects had not been redacted. Only signatures, names, addresses, investigator CVs, ethics committee information and consent forms were redacted. Why weren't we allowed to see the bits about ethics? Was Lilly afraid we might find out that some of their trials were unethical? We already know that consent forms routinely lie to the patients as they are told they contribute to science when in reality many results are shelved.[11] It doesn't make sense to delete this information, as it isn't commercially confidential information, but it illustrates how arbitrary regulatory decisions are.

The FDA isn't forthcoming.[11] Requests for data need to be very specific, which is difficult when you don't know what is available. And searches on its website to find information may turn up hundreds of documents that are not clearly named, not indexed, don't have a title page, and which exist only as non-searchable scanned images. The documents may not tell you what they are about until you get to page 19.[11] That results in many people giving up, as we did when we tried. Furthermore, data are missing or arbitrarily deleted, e.g. only 16 out of at least 27 trials of celecoxib (Celebrex) were included in the FDA reports requested by researchers according to the Freedom of Information Act.[33] Independent researchers who had access to FDA data nevertheless confirmed the cardiovascular harms of the drug.[34]

For another COX-2 inhibitor, valdecoxib (Bextra, from Searle), 28 consecutive pages had been deleted by the FDA before they were sent to independent researchers, as they contained 'trade secrets and/or confidential information that is not disclosable'.[33] This is totally absurd, as these pages came from an FDA statistical review and evaluation of valdecoxib. There are absolutely *no* trade secrets or confidential information that is not disclosable in such reports.

DEADLY SLIMMING PILLS

The history of the slimming pills is a dire one that confirms that drug regulators aren't willing to learn from history. Phentermine was approved in the United States in 1959 and is still on the market, although it's similar to amphetamine, both chemically and in its effects. In the 1960s, another appetite suppressant with amphetamine effects, aminoxaphen (Aminorex), was very popular in Europe,[35] but it causes pulmonary hypertension and was withdrawn after 7 years when hundreds of patients had died under terrible conditions.

In 1973, fenfluramine (Pondimin), yet another amphetamine-like drug, was introduced on the US market. It increases the neurotransmitter serotonin, which the SSRIs also do (*see* Chapter 17). The drug was withdrawn in 1997, as it causes pulmonary hypertension and a serious form of fibrosis of the heart valves that also kills people. Pondimin was close to never making it to the market, but the FDA scientist who had written a disapproval letter was removed to another job. This led to a congressional investigation of misconduct at the FDA that concluded that a leading FDA officer had misled congress. This officer left the FDA to become an 'expert witness' for drug companies. Of course he did. History surely repeats itself in drug regulation.

In the 1990s, many scientific articles in Europe described Pondimin's detrimental effects, but Wyeth, the maker of the drug, didn't send these reports to the FDA.[35] An obvious reason why Wyeth didn't draw attention to the dangers with Pondimin was that the company was trying to get approval for a similarly deadly drug, dexfenfluramine (Redux), which was simply the *d*-enantiomer of fenfluramine (that consists of two enantiomers, which are mirror images of each other). A researcher who had worked with the drug while being employed by Servier went privately to the FDA with his findings that fenfluramine and dexfenfluramine lead to brain damage in apes and baboons, but he was immediately fired and nothing happened that might have protected the patients.

Everything goes in drug regulation and dexfenfluramine came on the market in Europe. However, its use was severely restricted in 1995 after French researchers had shown that both Pondimin and Redux increase the risk of pulmonary hypertension 10 times. These findings were arrogantly dismissed by the FDA and the industry complained over a critical FDA officer. Nonetheless, the FDA advisory committee rejected the drug because of safety concerns. Wyeth complained and a new meeting was held just 2 months later, which is highly unusual. The committee now included more Redux supporters and the drug was narrowly approved in November 1995 with the votes six to five.[36] When numbers of cases with pulmonary hypertension increased rapidly, FDA doctors tried to convince Wyeth/Interneuron that they should add a black box warning on the label. Instead, they graciously added a notice that Redux could cause hair loss, which had been reported more rarely than pulmonary hypertension![35]

This story of unbelievable crimes towards the patients just continued. Four months after approval of Redux, the damning French results were published in the *New England Journal of Medicine* but with an editorial that praised the drug and said that the risk of pulmonary hypertension was small and outweighed by the benefits of the drug. There wasn't a trace in the editorial that its two authors were paid by the industry, which fact infuriated the editors of the journal when it was revealed by the *Wall Street Journal*. The benefit was a mere 3% weight loss, as stated by the company, e.g. from 100 kg to 97 kg. However, many patients drop out of the trials and the conventional statistical adjustment for this is flawed. Companies use the last recorded weight and carry it forward till the end of the trial. However, much of the weight people lose in the beginning comes back later, and even more important: if people cannot tolerate a drug, they cannot benefit from it. It would therefore be more sensible to carry forward the weight at baseline. In one of our studies, of rimonabant, the last observation carried forward showed a weight loss of 6.4 kg above placebo while baseline carried forward showed a benefit of only 1.5 kg.[37]

While the patients continued to die because of the slimming pills they took, an academic researcher, Mike Weintraub, touted treatment with a combination of *two* amphetamine-like products, fenfluramine (Pondimin) and the old drug phentermine, on TV programmes and elsewhere, although this off-label use had not been approved by the FDA. The combination pill was called Fen-Phen. It became extremely popular even though an article flagged problems with memory loss. In 1996, the total number of prescriptions exceeded 18 million.[38] However, in the summer of 1997, a series of 24 women who had developed valve disease while on Fen-Phen was published in the *New England Journal of Medicine*[38] accompanied by an editorial written by the editor that this time left no doubt that the drugs are dangerous. Based on that paper, the FDA pressed Wyeth/Interneuron to withdraw Redux and Pondimin from the market.[35]

But Wyeth didn't give up. It had plans for 'neutralising' critical doctors and its doubt industry came into gear: hired guns among physicians lent their names to flawed results, and specialist journals lent their pages to the dirty work, above all the *Journal of the American College of Cardiology*, although the cardiologists should have been the most concerned doctors because the patients died from diseases in their specialty. One such cardiologist, Neil Weissman, published a paper in this journal in 1999 and similar papers in other journals purporting there was no problem; he received a total of almost $18 million from Wyeth for his studies. Richard Atkinson, the president of the American Obesity Association, which received money from Wyeth/Interneuron, strongly defended the drugs and aired that the study in the *New England Journal of Medicine* was inadequate. The American College of Cardiology issued a press release declaring that the heart problems disappeared once patients stop taking the pills. This was a blatant lie.

Hired moles asked their colleagues for the medical data that had showed valve disease without revealing they were sent by Wyeth, in one case even indicating they worked for the FDA. The company also launched campaigns trivialising the harms in a hope of getting the drugs back on the market. A famous obesity specialist, George Blackburn, gave many pep talks but filed a sworn affidavit in Boston's court that he had not given talks and had not received any money from the companies. When confronted with his lies and whereabouts, he didn't remember anything.

Wyeth could have warned the public years before independent researchers found out about the harms. Another big company, American Home Products, which marketed Pondimin, behaved similarly badly. It had 160 cases of pulmonary hypertension buried in-house while patients were still being prescribed Pondimin. Starting in April 1996, American Home Products even circulated an internal monthly memo called the Pondimin Monthly Death List. The company obstructed justice by destroying thousands of documents and emails after an order was issued by court *not* to do this. American Home Products denied it had done anything wrong, denied that it had known earlier that its drugs might be dangerous and said that 'We never even promoted Pondimin.'

The only thing that is missing in this soap opera is a denial that the dead patients had ever existed. Perhaps even the company didn't exist but was just a figment of our imagination in line with social constructivism?

When the plaintiffs' lawyers got access to Wyeth's archives, they had close to three million pages copied into computers so that they became searchable. This was an amazing feat. If we stack so many pages, the height of the stack will be about 300 metres! The lawyers found 101 reports of pulmonary hypertension and more than 50 cases of valve disease, which Wyeth had marked as something else. After the FDA had refused to approve Redux at its first meeting, Wyeth sent a document to a different bureau in the FDA, where 52 cases of pulmonary hypertension were well hidden on a little graph in a 40-page document. This Wyeth had the nerve to call 'disclosure'.

An FDA investigation at Wyeth's headquarters uncovered that Wyeth's safety officer had written over the first 13 reports of valve disease the company had received from the Mayo Clinic about Fen-Phen and used the same log numbers for other drugs and less serious adverse effects.[35] However, instead of a criminal investigation the FDA wrote to Wyeth that its reporting system failed to assure that all reports are accurate. This was to put it mildly, but Wyeth's lawyers protested, and a second FDA letter was apologetic about the first letter and politely urged Wyeth to clean up its act. I wonder what kind of society we would have if this was how the police was supposed to address a murderer: 'Dear little thing, we would be *so* happy if you wouldn't do it again. Please accept our profuse apologies that one of our officers accused you of murder and have a nice day.'

There were other revelations. When an FDA officer had threatened Wyeth that if they didn't warn the physicians about neurotoxicity the FDA would, Wyeth went to the top at the FDA and no warning letter was ever sent. It seems that the top of the FDA is capable of almost anything that benefits the drug companies. In 1994, the FDA decided at a meeting that a black box warning was needed for Pondimin telling about 50 cases of pulmonal hypertension, but an addendum to the minutes said that nothing would be done anyhow, without any explanation. An FDA scientist produced a report in 1999 that showed exactly what information the companies had given the FDA about valve disease and when, but FDA lawyers made sure the FDA could not be incriminated by locking it away in a drawer.

As for reports of adverse events, the FDA had left it to the companies to decide themselves whether an event was serious and what to mention first, which had the effect that many cases of reported valve problems were overlooked by the seriously understaffed FDA safety division, as they weren't mentioned on the first page. During court proceedings, 52 cases of *left* valvular disease (which cannot be caused by pulmonary hypertension, as this affects the *right* valves) were discussed, and *none of them had been coded as valvular disease*. The company had also deceived the FDA originally about its animal studies. The valves of the rats' hearts had thickened dramatically and stiffened, but this was hidden under the rather innocent term 'focal fibrosis', which was camouflage for the real thing. What the company told the FDA was only the good news: the rats didn't develop cancer. Marion Finkel, the FDA official who had originally approved Pondimin, but now consulted for drug companies, tried her best to put her client in good light.

Pulmonary hypertension is a terrible disease, and symptoms can start already after a week on the drug. It's uniformly fatal, with a mean survival less than many cancers, and the symptoms feel like strangulation or drowning. The valve disease is similarly devastating. At the time of the mass tort lawsuits, an estimated 45 000 US women were believed to have developed one or both of the two diseases,[35] with an expected death toll of the same size.

These drugs were superseded by sibutramine in 2001, which not only increases serotonin in the brain but also norepinephrine and dopamine. It came as no surprise when it was removed from the market in 2010 because of cardiovascular harms. In 2007, we asked for access to the unpublished trials with this drug at the Danish drug agency, which was granted a year later, but the lawyer of the company, Abbott, blocked the permission for another year by lodging a complaint with the Danish Ministry of Health. Using our Freedom of Information Act we found out that a hired gun, cardiologist Christian Torp-Pedersen, had signed the letter from Abbott to the Ministry, which undoubtedly gave it more credibility. We felt that the cardiologist should have worried more about his patients and the cardiovascular harms of sibutramine than about the company's health.

Why on earth are such drugs still being approved given their history? And why was benfluorex (Mediator from Servier), which is structurally related to fenfluramine and has similar harms, not taken off the European market until 2009 when Pondimin disappeared in 1997? Well, there is nothing new under the sun. There were conflicts of interest among expert advisers and also 'institutionalised cooperation' with the drug industry – the much hyped and lauded public–private partnership.[39,40] Unhealthy ties between the regulator and the industry were also uncovered and there were suspicions that Servier, which is a French company, had obtained far too much political influence. The head of the French drug agency resigned because of the scandal.

Slimming pills are poor drugs that are not liked by the patients. In drug trials, doctors have financial incentives for keeping patients on the drug, but in real life, the situation is very different. A study showed that after just 1 year, less than 10% of the patients still took their drugs (sibutramine or orlistat, a drug that decreases fat absorption) and after 2 years, it was less than 2%.[41]

Recent decisions underline that drug agencies refuse to learn from history. FDA staff explained in 2012 why the FDA had approved two new slimming pills, Belviq (lorcaserin, Arena Pharmaceuticals) and Qsymia (phentermine + topiramate, Vivus).[42] Lorcaserin increases serotonin, increases the incidence of multiple tumours and valvulopathy in rats, and increases valvulopathy by 16% in patients. Topimarate may increase the risk of orofacial cleft if taken during pregnancy, which is a problem the FDA solved with a fake fix we know won't work: tell the women to protect themselves against pregnancy. Both drugs may create psychiatric disturbances and other important adverse effects, and the FDA required a rigorous assessment of long-term cardiovascular safety for the drugs, although it doesn't and cannot enforce such demands, another fake fix. We will surely see new slimming pill scandals.

Obesity specialists have defended the slimming pills all along by saying that the increased risk of dying caused by the drugs is counteracted by the fact that even a minor weight loss in a large population leads to more lives saved than lost. This is a poor argument. First, it hasn't been shown to be true. Second, even if it were true, there is a huge difference between being slowly killed by a drug under terrible suffering and a benefit at population level. It's a fact of life that we may die sooner if we have unhealthy lifestyles. We all know this. If we want to reduce the number of people dying from obesity, we should first and foremost tackle the food industry. Giving people drugs is a fake fix that is very dangerous. A 2008 study of 5743 users of fenfluramines showed that the prevalence of mild aortic regurgitation or moderate mitral regurgitation, or worse, was 20% in women and 12% in men; the risk increased markedly with months of use; and valve surgery was performed in one of 200 patients with drug-induced valvulopathy.[43] And yet the FDA has now approved a similar drug.

REFERENCES

1 Vedantam S. Antidepressant makers withhold data on children. *Washington Post.* 2004 Jan 29.

2 Melander H, Ahlqvist-Rastad J, Meijer G, *et al.* Evidence b(i)ased medicine – selective reporting from studies sponsored by pharmaceutical industry: review of studies in new drug applications. *BMJ.* 2003; **326**: 1171–3.

3 Melander H. [Selective reporting – greater problem than selective publishing?] *Läkartidningen.* 2005; **102**: 224–5.

4 Turner EH, Matthews AM, Linardatos E, *et al.* Selective publication of antidepressant trials and its influence on apparent efficacy. *N Engl J Med.* 2008; **358**: 252–60.

5 Rising K, Bacchetti P, Bero L. Reporting bias in drug trials submitted to the Food and Drug Administration: review of publication and presentation. *PLoS Med.* 2008; **5**: e217.

6 Lenzer J. Drug secrets: what the FDA isn't telling. *Slate.* 2005 Sept 27.

7 Rennie D. When evidence isn't: trials, drug companies and the FDA. *J Law Policy.* 2007 July: 991–1012.

8 Chalmers I. From optimism to disillusion about commitment to transparency in the medico-industrial complex. *J R Soc Med.* 2006; **99**: 337–41.

9 Scherer RW, Langenberg P, von Elm E. Full publication of results initially presented in abstracts. *Cochrane Database Syst Rev.* 2007; **2**: MR000005.

10 MacLean CH, Morton SC, Ofman JJ, *et al.* How useful are unpublished data from the Food and Drug Administration in meta-analysis? *J Clin Epidemiol.* 2003; **56**: 44–51.

11 Goldacre B. *Bad Pharma.* London: Fourth Estate; 2012.

12 Chalmers I. Underreporting research is scientific misconduct. *JAMA.* 1990; **263**: 1405–8.

13 Danish Association of the Pharmaceutical Industry. [Revised collaborative agreement between the Medical Association and the Danish Association of the Pharmaceutical Industry about clinical trials and non-intervention studies]. 2010 June 1.

14 Gøtzsche PC, Jørgensen AW. Opening up data at the European Medicines Agency. *BMJ.* 2011; **342**: d2686.

15 Wikipedia. Rimonabant. Available online at: http://en.wikipedia.org/wiki/Rimonabant (accessed 17 January 2013).

16 World Medical Association. *Declaration of Helsinki – ethical principles for medical research involving human subjects.* 2008.

17 Gøtzsche PC. Why we need easy access to all data from all clinical trials and how to accomplish it. *Trials.* 2011; **12**: 249.

18 Topol EJ. Failing the public health – rofecoxib, Merck, and the FDA. *N Engl J Med.* 2004; **351**: 1707–9.

19 Lenzer J. FDA is incapable of protecting US 'against another Vioxx'. *BMJ.* 2004; **329**: 1253.

20 Anonymous. Institute of Medicine urges reforms at FDA. *Lancet.* 2006; **368**: 1211.

21 Relman AS, Angell M. America's other drug problem: how the drug industry distorts medicine and politics. *The New Republic.* 2002 Dec 16: 27–41.

22 Carpenter D. Drug-review deadlines and safety problems (authors' reply). *N Engl J Med.* 2008; **359**: 96–8.

23 Moore TJ. *Deadly Medicine: why tens of thousands of heart patients died in America's worst drug disaster.* New York: Simon & Schuster; 1995.

24 Cowley AJ, Skene A, Stainer K, *et al.* The effect of lorcainide on arrhythmias and survival in patients with acute myocardial infarction: an example of publication bias. *Int J Cardiol.* 1993; **40**: 161–6.

25 EMA. *European Medicines Agency Widens Public Access to Documents.* Press release. 2010 Nov 30.

26 Regulation (EC) No 1049/2001 of the European Parliament and of the Council of 30 May 2001

regarding public access to European Parliament, Council and Commission documents. *Official Journal of the European Communities*. 2001; L145: 43–8.

27 Hawkes N. Lobby groups call for closure of 'revolving door' between drug regulators and industry. *BMJ*. 2011; **343**: d8335.

28 European Medicines Agency. Access to clinical-trial data and transparency. Workshop report. 2012. Available online at: www.ema.europa.eu/docs/en_GB/document_library/Report/2012/12/WC500135841.pdf (accessed December 2012).

29 Editorial. [Straight talk]. *Information*. 2004 June 30.

30 Alfter B, Teugels M, Bouma J. Media lift lid on secret reports on drug side-effects. *Euobserver*. 2008 Oct 22.

31 Abraham J. *Science, Politics and the Pharmaceutical Industry*. London: UCL Press; 1995.

32 Gøtzsche PC. UK drug regulator destroys all evidence after 15 years. *BMJ*. 2011; **343**: d4203.

33 Jüni P, Reichenbach S, Egger M. COX 2 inhibitors, traditional NSAIDs, and the heart. *BMJ*. 2005; **330**: 1342–3.

34 Caldwell B, Aldington S, Weatherall M, *et al.* Risk of cardiovascular events and celecoxib: a systematic review and meta-analysis. *J R Soc Med*. 2006; **99**: 132–40.

35 Mundy A. *Dispensing with the Truth*. New York: St. Martin's Press; 2001.

36 Avorn J. *Powerful Medicines: the benefits, risks, and costs of prescription drugs*. New York: Vintage Books; 2005.

37 Jørgensen AW. Robustness of results and conclusions in systematic reviews, trials and abstracts [PhD thesis]. Copenhagen: University of Copenhagen; 2011.

38 Connolly HM, Crary JL, McGoon MD, *et al.* Valvular heart disease associated with fenfluramine-phentermine. *N Engl J Med*. 1997; **337**: 581–8.

39 Mullard A. Mediator scandal rocks French medical community. *Lancet*. 2011; **377**: 890–2.

40 Mintzes B. New UK guidance on industry-health professional collaboration. *BMJ*. 2012; **344**: e3952.

41 Padwal R, Kezouh A, Levine M, *et al.* Long-term persistence with orlistat and sibutramine in a population-based cohort. *Int J Obes (Lond)*. 2007; **31**: 1567–70.

42 Colman E, Golden J, Roberts M, *et al.* The FDA's assessment of two drugs for chronic weight management. *N Engl J Med*. 2012; **367**: 1577–9.

43 Dahl CF, Allen MR, Urie PM, *et al.* Valvular regurgitation and surgery associated with fenfluramine use: an analysis of 5743 individuals. *BMC Med*. 2008; **6**: 34.

Neurontin, an epilepsy drug for everything

Several events in 2004 were a wake-up call for those who still believed the drug industry stands for respectable business. Two of the largest US companies had quite different reputations before the scandals broke lose: Pfizer was considered one of the worst whereas Merck (*see* Chapter 13) was known as one of the most ethical drug firms. After 2004, it was hard to tell the difference. The heat was also turned on GlaxoSmithKline in 2004 (*see* Chapter 16).

In 2004, Pfizer agreed to plead guilty to two felonies and pay $430 million to settle charges that it fraudulently promoted the epilepsy drug Neurontin (gabapentin) for unapproved uses.[1] A company whistle-blower would receive $27 million. The fine was small considering that the sales of gabapentin were $2700 million in 2003 alone, and as about 90% of the sales was for off-label use,[1-3] the fine would not be expected to have any deterrent effect.

Warner-Lambert, later bought by Pfizer, paid doctors to allow salespeople to sit with them as they saw patients and to suggest using Neurontin for a wide array of ailments, including bipolar disorder, pain, migraine, attention deficit disorder, restless leg syndrome, and drug and alcohol withdrawal,[1,2] although the drug was only approved for treatment-resistant epilepsy.[2,4,5] A drug index, Drugdex, listed no less than 48 off-label uses for Neurontin, and Medicaid was obliged to pay for the drug if being prescribed for one of these uses.[4] Furthermore, the company that owns Drugdex sells 'medical education', a truly incestuous enterprise.

The common practice of planting salespeople in doctors' offices is euphemistically called 'preceptorship',[4] as if the doctor trained a medical student, but a more appropriate term would be 'predatorship', as it harms patients.[5] The patients are not always aware that the salesperson isn't a medical student, not even when they are examined for breast cancer.[6] A company executive told a salesperson:

'Dinner programs, CME programs, consultantships all work great but don't forget the one-to-one. That's where we need to be, holding their hand and whispering in their ear, Neurontin for pain, Neurontin for monotherapy, Neurontin for bipolar, Neurontin for everything ... I don't want to hear that safety crap.'[7]

Much of the illegal promotion took place at meetings that were supposed to educate doctors. A physician whistle-blower testified that he was trained to distort the scientific evidence,[5] and at some Neurontin meetings, the company paid not only the speakers but also the listeners, treating them to luxury trips to Hawaii, Florida or the 1996 Olympics in Atlanta.[1]

It was very easy to corrupt doctors. Of 40 influential thought leaders identified as potential speakers in north-eastern United States, including 26 current or future department chairs, vice chairs, and directors of academic clinical programmes or divisions, no fewer than 35 participated in company-sponsored activities, and 14 requested or were allocated \$10 250–\$158 250 in honoraria or grants.[6] One doctor received almost \$308 000 to tout Neurontin at conferences.[6]

The speakers were updated on the company's promotional strategies,[6] and Warner-Lambert tracked high-volume prescribers and rewarded them as speakers or consultants, or for recruiting patients in studies. Doctors were also paid to lend their names to ghostwritten articles purporting to show that Neurontin worked for unapproved conditions,[4,6] and a professor requested and received over \$300 000 to write a book on epilepsy.[5,8] It was surely true what was stated in an internal document obtained through US court proceedings: 'Medical education drives this market!'[7]

Other internal documents illustrate the extent to which the company was willing to distort the evidence.[6,9] In relation to the illegal marketing, the company had a publication strategy:

'The results, if positive, will … be published', and 'I think that we can limit the potential downsides of the 224 study by delaying the publication for as long as possible.'

The manipulations also involved selective statistical analyses, selective reporting of outcomes that happened to show a positive effect, inappropriate exclusion or inclusion of patients in the analyses, multiple publication of desirable results, differential citation of Pfizer results, and spin to make negative results appear positive. The bias was already introduced at the design stage, e.g. high doses were used that led to unblinding and biased reporting of subjective outcomes. Pfizer even recognised that unblinding due to adverse events could result in corruption of the study's validity.

The final layer of corruption of the evidence was accomplished by ghostwriters: 'We would need to have "editorial" control'; 'We are using a medical agency to put the paper together which we will show to Dr. Reckless. We are not allowing him to write it up himself' (the doctor's name was actually Reckless); and 'We know Alison wants to make sure that we align publication messages with your global marketing efforts.' A medical writer asked Pfizer: 'How do we make it sound better than it looks on the graphs?'[10]

Kay Dickersin, director of the US Cochrane Center, uncovered all this and summarised what she felt about it: 'Outright deception of the biomedical community, highly unethical, harmful to science, wasteful of public resources, and potentially dangerous to the public's health … As with all the trials I reviewed, selective analyses … could explain any positive findings observed.'[9]

Pfizer was unsure how it should tackle requests from Cochrane researchers about getting access to unpublished data,[9] and a previous case explains Pfizer's dilemma. As explained in Chapter 6, Pfizer got bad publicity in 1999, when my wife and I described in *JAMA* how the company had rigged a series of trials of its antifungal drug, fluconazole, and refused to provide us with the data we needed to sort things out.[11] Even after *JAMA*'s deputy editor had urged the company to reply, Pfizer refused to respond to simple and pertinent questions. The story made front-page news in the *New York Times*. Shortly afterwards, the founder of the Cochrane Collaboration, Iain Chalmers, told me he was visited by a director from Pfizer UK and wanted to show him how easy it is to search in The Cochrane Library. He typed 'Pfizer', which brought him to the Discussion section of our Cochrane review of fluconazole where we wrote:[12]

> We experienced unexpected difficulties in obtaining responses to our requests for additional or clarifying information about the trials ... We did not succeed to get any information from the investigators or Pfizer, the manufacturer of fluconazole, on the most pertinent issues: why oral amphotericin B was used, why the results for this drug were lumped together with those of an ineffective drug ... and whether there was overlap between different trials reports.

Our paper and the media attention gave Pfizer something to think about, which was revealed 2 years later when its vice president for research responded to another Cochrane request by providing a list of references, which was entirely unhelpful. The internal deliberations were interesting:[9]

'I would not send unpublished data to anyone outside Pfizer ... The decision is ultimately yours ... the risk is that in the Cochrane review there is a statement saying Pfizer declined to provide the information requested! which does not look good for the company.'

Three years later, the Cochrane group again reminded Pfizer of its request but in vain. The Cochrane protocol was eventually withdrawn and the review was never completed. In relation to another Cochrane review, Pfizer stated: 'We definitely will not supply any internal data, we all agree on that.'

It is indisputable that the illegal and fraudulent promotion, which was approved by some of the company's top executives, led to harm.[2,6] An internal memorandum showed that doctors who attended dinners given by the company to discuss unapproved uses of Neurontin wrote 70% more prescriptions for the drug than those who didn't attend.[2] The company even insisted on pressing doctors to use much higher doses of Neurontin than those that had been approved, which means higher income for more harm.

A seeding trial, the STEPS study, which had no control group, had the marketing objective to increase the dose of Neurontin and its market share, and it involved 772 physicians who only treated four patients each, on average.[13] Physicians with little or no experience in trials were recruited and the data were very dirty, which the two published papers said nothing about. Drug salespeople collected data and were directly involved in suggesting to the doctors which patients to enrol while being present in the doctors' offices. The trial was deeply unethical, as the patients were not informed about the true marketing purpose of the study, and as the doctors were the actual study subjects without knowing this, as the effect of their participation on sales was closely monitored.

Off-label promotion exposes patients to harms with no assurance of benefit. This criminal activity has increased and its victims have died, suffered heart attacks and strokes, had permanent nerve damage or lost their eyesight.[14] In 2010, a jury found that Pfizer violated the federal Racketeer Influenced and Corrupt Organizations Act (RICO) and the company was to pay $142 million in damages.[15] The jury found Pfizer engaged in a racketeering conspiracy over a 10-year period. Pfizer never told doctors or patients that its studies had shown that Neurontin was no more effective than a placebo for some of its off-label uses.

REFERENCES

1 Tansey B. Huge penalty in drug fraud: Pfizer settles felony case in Neurontin off-label promotion. *San Francisco Chronicle*. 2004 May 14.
2 Harris G. Pfizer to pay $430 million over promoting drug to doctors. *New York Times*. 2004 May 14.
3 Lenzer J. Pfizer pleads guilty, but drug sales continue to soar. *BMJ*. 2004; **328**: 1217.
4 Angell M. *The Truth about the Drug Companies: how they deceive us and what to do about it*. New York: Random House; 2004.
5 Petersen M. *Our Daily Meds*. New York: Sarah Crichton Books; 2008.
6 Petersen M. Suit says company promoted drug in exam rooms. *New York Times*. 2002 May 15.
7 Landefeld CS, Steinman MA. The Neurontin legacy – marketing through misinformation and manipulation. *N Engl J Med*. 2009; **360**: 103–6.
8 Petersen M. Court papers suggest scale of drug's use. *New York Times*. 2003 May 30.
9 Dickersin K. *Reporting and other biases in studies of Neurontin for migraine, psychiatric/bipolar disorders, nociceptive pain, and neuropathic pain*. Available online at: www.pharmalot.com/wp-content/uploads/2008/10/neurontin-dickersin-2.pdf (accessed 10 December 2008).
10 Saul S. Experts conclude Pfizer manipulated studies. *New York Times*. 2008 Oct 8.
11 Johansen HK, Gøtzsche PC. Problems in the design and reporting of trials of antifungal agents encountered during meta-analysis. *JAMA*. 1999; **282**: 1752–9.
12 Johansen HK, Gøtzsche PC. Amphotericin B vs fluconazole for controlling fungal infections in neutropenic cancer patients (Cochrane Review). In: *The Cochrane Library*, Issue 1. Oxford: Update Software; 2000.
13 Krumholz SD, Egilman DS, Ross JS. Study of Neurontin: titrate to effect, profile of safety (STEPS) trial: a narrative account of a gabapentin seeding trial. *Arch Intern Med*. 2011; **171**: 1100–7.
14 Adams C, Young A. Off-label prescription case reflects federal concern over unsafe uses. *Knight Ridder Newspapers*. 2004 May 14.
15 Voris B, Lawrence J. *Pfizer Told to Pay $142.1 million for Neurontin Fraud*. Bloomberg. 2010 March 25.

Merck, where the patients die first

On 30 September 2004, Merck withdrew its COX-2 inhibitor, the anti-arthritis drug Vioxx (rofecoxib) from the market. I was in Canada and browsed the TV stations to induce natural sleep when I learned about it on Fox News. What was more surprising to me than the withdrawal of the drug was that the president of the US Arthritis Foundation lamented for about 10 minutes about what a great loss it was for the patients that Vioxx was no longer available. If I hadn't known who was speaking, I would have guessed it was the CEO of Merck. Company talk all over. For a full 10 minutes. I usually get 30 seconds when I'm on the news.

This speaks volumes about the extent to which patient organisations collude with big pharma. I checked the website for the Arthritis Foundation, and it had Pfizer's logo on its opening page. In contrast to the Foundation's hype about the drug, the jury in a court case stated that Merck showed 'malicious, oppressive, and outrageous' conduct and found it guilty of four counts of fraud in marketing rofecoxib.[1]

It was known right from the start that COX-2 inhibitors, via their mechanism of action, must increase the risk of thrombosis. In 1996, Merck scientists discussed the heart attack risk,[2] and investigators sponsored by Merck found that Vioxx reduced urinary metabolites of prostacyclin in healthy volunteers by about half,[3] which indicates that Vioxx causes thrombosis. However, Merck convinced the authors to change what they had written into a meaningless sentence: 'Cox-2 may play a role in the systemic biosynthesis of prostacyclin.' Also in 1997, a Merck scientist said that if they didn't allow patients to use aspirin in their trials (which decreases the risk of a heart attack), patients on Vioxx might have more heart attacks and that would 'kill the drug'.[4] Merck surely concealed how dangerous Vioxx was. A senior Merck scientist proposed to leave out people with a high risk of cardiovascular problems in the company's planned VIGOR study so that the difference in heart complications between Vioxx and other NSAIDs 'would not be evident'.[5] None of the trials in the FDA submission were designed to evaluate the cardiovascular risk.[3]

As mentioned in Chapter 10, FDA also had serious concerns about the drug. When the FDA approved rofecoxib for marketing in May 1999[4] despite disconcerting evidence in the application, it stated that it lacked 'complete certainty' that the drug increased cardiovascular risk.[4,7]

I find this extraordinary. Imagine how absurd it would be if a doctor said to a patient: 'I'm not completely sure that this drug might kill you, so please take it.'

If there had been patient representatives in the advisory committee, they would probably have rejected the application and demanded of Merck that it tested its drug more carefully, as it was clear that the drug *must* cause thrombosis. Further, as there were many other NSAIDs on the market, the drug wasn't needed.

The scandal of the COX-2 inhibitors is really monumental. The drugs were approved based on small, short-term trials that didn't look for cardiovascular harms, in patients with a low risk for such events, although nearly half of real world patients with arthritis have coexisting cardiovascular disease.[8,9] Merck did conduct two trials, however, trial 090[10-12] and VIGOR[13] that both showed that rofecoxib increased cardiovascular events. Trial 090 ended in 1999 but wasn't published until 2006,[12] 2 years after Vioxx had been withdrawn when the publication couldn't harm the sales.

The other trial, with the catchy name VIGOR, was published in the *New England Journal of Medicine* in 2000.[13] It compared Vioxx with naproxen. A year later, pharmacist Jennifer Hrachovec called a radio show on which the journal's editor, Jeffrey Drazen, appeared and begged him to correct the paper because there were three more heart attacks on rofecoxib on the FDA's website than in the journal article, but Drazen responded evasively.[14] Two months earlier, Hrachovec had sent a letter to the journal, but it was rejected, officially because of 'lack of space', which is an excuse respectable journals cannot hide behind when scientific misconduct relevant for patient safety is suspected.

The VIGOR trial would have looked very different if the three extra heart attacks had not been deliberately omitted from the trial report. Their inclusion would also have undermined the assertion in the article that only those who were already at high risk of a heart attack showed an increased risk after taking Vioxx, as the omitted heart attacks were all in the low-risk group.[14]

There were other editorial blunders. The editors didn't ensure that thromboses were appropriately described and discussed. There were two full tables of gastrointestinal adverse effects in the article, but no table of thromboses; they were only mentioned in a few lines in the text, and only as percentages, which made it impossible to calculate the true number of events, *as not all of them were included!* Based on the percentages, I calculated 32 versus 17 thrombotic events on Vioxx and naproxen, respectively, but there were actually another 15 versus 3 events.[15] That wasn't even all. The FDA reviewer found a death from a heart attack on Vioxx that was coded as something else and, conversely, two deaths too many on naproxen.[11] Thus, the coding of the events favoured Vioxx and many more events disappeared on Vioxx than on naproxen in the published report. This looks like fraud to me.

The editors allowed Merck to say that the reason Vioxx caused more thromboses than naproxen was that naproxen was protective rather than Vioxx being harmful. This interpretation was wholly speculative and later refuted, and it was irrelevant for the patients. As there were more serious events overall with Vioxx, there could be no doubt that naproxen was the better drug.[11]

The editors noted that forensic IT work on the submitted disc revealed that the three cases of myocardial infarction had been omitted from the manuscript 2 days before it was submitted to the journal.[16] They also found out that Merck had selected an earlier cut-off date shortly before the trial ended for the thrombotic events than the cut-off date for the gastrointestinal events, which they were not informed about and which is deceitful.[15] They blamed Merck and the clinical investigators but forgot to mention their own role in allowing the obviously flawed paper to appear in print. After 5 years of silence, when the drug had been withdrawn and the journal ran a risk of getting accused in court cases, the editors finally reacted by publishing an 'expression of concern'.[16] If they had acted earlier, it might have killed the sales of Vioxx instead of killing the patients, as the journal is so influential, and it would also have blunted the impact of the reprint sales.[14] The *New England Journal of Medicine* sold 929 400 reprints of the article – more than one for every doctor in the country – and they brought in between $697 000 and $836 000.[14] The journal won't disclose its revenue, but its owner, Massachusetts Medical Society, listed $88 million in total publishing revenue for the year ending 31 May 2005.

In 2001, independent researchers using FDA data documented that Vioxx doubled the risk of serious cardiovascular events significantly in the VIGOR trial (8076 patients),[17] and in 2004, a meta-analysis performed by independent researchers showed that a clear relationship between Vioxx and increased risk of myocardial infarction existed already by the end of 2000.[6] When this meta-analysis was published, the French drug agency felt it could be interpreted as an accusation of their own incompetence.[18] They therefore wrote a letter to the editor to defend themselves, which, ironically, demonstrated their incompetence. They claimed there was no evidence of an increased risk before 2005 and put forward Merck's false explanation that the reason Vioxx caused more thromboses than naproxen was that naproxen was protective rather than Vioxx being harmful. Sometimes it's better to keep quiet with one's ignorance. The rest of the world, including the FDA, had known since 1999 that Vioxx could cause thrombosis.[7,13,17]

Two other meta-analyses, from 2001 and 2002, one with 28 465 patients and the other with 5435 patients, didn't find an increase in cardiovascular risk with Vioxx compared with placebo, which is highly surprising given the huge number of patients, but not given that all the authors were employees or paid consultants for Merck.[19,20] It is telling that the two meta-analyses performed by independent researchers were published in *JAMA* and the *Lancet*, whereas those performed by Merck were published in specialist journals, *Circulation* and the *American Journal of Cardiology*.[19,20] *Circulation* is owned by the American Heart Association, which accepts drug company sponsorship;[21] over a 10-year period, the association funded more than one billion dollars in research grants.[22] This amount is surreal for a non-American. The website of the *American Journal of Cardiology* advertises many free CME programmes and, like *Circulation*, it also publishes supplements to the journal. The first supplement I came across was a paper that under Acknowledgments said that 'Funding for publication and medical writing assistance were provided by Novo Nordisk Inc.'.[23] Even in 2012, we are told about 'medical writing assistance', which means that the paper wasn't written by its eight authors but by a ghost.

Internal company documents[24] showed that Merck in 2003 got away with publishing a huge seeding trial, the ADVANTAGE trial, which involved 600 sites and 5557 patients, in a prestigious journal, *Annals of Internal Medicine*.[25] It compared Vioxx with naproxen and, as in the VIGOR trial, scientific misconduct was involved.[26] Eight patients suffered heart attacks or sudden cardiac death on Vioxx compared with only one on naproxen, but in the publication, three of the Vioxx cases had disappeared so that the difference was no longer statistically significant. As an example, one of Merck's scientists who had judged that a woman died from a heart attack was overruled by his boss, 'so that we don't raise concerns'. The cause of death was now called unknown, also in Merck's report to the FDA. Merck's top scientist, Edward Scolnick, noted in emails that he would personally pressure senior officials at the FDA if it took action against Vioxx.[26]

The first author on the trial report said that Merck came to him after the study was completed and asked him to help with the editing. He was paid, which is highly unusual for a first author of a trial report, and the report was already written up by Merck; a Merck employee was thanked for 'assistance with manuscript preparation'.[25]

It confirms that we cannot trust drug companies that an independent meta-analysis of Vioxx studies found that those with an external endpoint committee reported four times more heart attacks with Vioxx than with the comparator, whereas trials without an external endpoint committee reported *fewer* heart attacks with Vioxx.[6] Although the members of data and safety-monitoring boards in drug trials are supposed to be independent, even according to Merck's own policy, the head of the VIGOR board was awarded a 2-year consulting contract with Merck 2 weeks before the VIGOR trial ended, and he disclosed family ownership of Merck shares worth $70 000.[3] Before VIGOR was published in 2000, chief scientist Edward Scolnick admitted internally that Vioxx causes thromboses.

Internal company documents show that Merck used guest and ghost authors for many of its papers.[27] To investigate to which extent the medical literature is flawed and misleads the clinicians, we studied 397 abstracts on Vioxx.[28] It was expected from the beginning that the drug would be a double-edged sword compared to older NSAIDs, i.e. causing less gastrointestinal bleeding and more thrombosis. From the patients' point of view, both effects are important and should be investigated, emphasised and reported similarly. However, before the withdrawal of Vioxx, 3.4 times as many abstracts commented on gastrointestinal bleeding as those that commented on thrombotic effects, whereas after withdrawal, 1.8 times as many abstracts commented on thrombotic effects. Thus, the harms of Vioxx came into focus too late when the drug had been withdrawn.

Merck also misled the readers by publishing a fake journal, the *Australasian Journal of Bone and Joint Medicine*, which looked like a peer-reviewed medical journal but was a marketing tool.[29] Most of its articles presented data favourable to Merck products, including Vioxx, without disclosing the sponsorship.[29]

Like Merck, the FDA failed badly in its duty towards the patients. A five times increase in heart attacks in the millions of people taking the drug wasn't a public health emergency in the FDA's eyes.[7,30,31] Life-saving revisions of the Vioxx label took nearly 2 years to complete, as 'We were trying to work out exactly what was acceptable to both sides.'[7,30] I wonder what the thousands of grief-stricken spouses who lost their loved ones during these 2 years will say about this tempo in drug regulation. Many of the tens of thousands of patients who were killed by Vioxx[4] shouldn't have been treated with an NSAID, as paracetamol (acetaminophen) would have given the same effect, or as they could have done well without treatment.

In February 2001, the FDA discussed the VIGOR study with Merck because of the five-fold increase in myocardial infarction with rofecoxib in comparison with naproxen, and the FDA asked Merck to make the doctors aware of these results.[4,32] However, the next day, Merck instructed its sales force of more than 3000 people:

'DO NOT INITIATE DISCUSSIONS ON THE FDA ARTHRITIS ADVISORY COMMITTEE ... OR THE RESULTS OF THE ... VIGOR STUDY.'

If a physician inquired about VIGOR, the salesperson should indicate that the study showed a gastrointestinal benefit and then say, 'I cannot discuss the study with you.'

Merck also produced a pamphlet to its sales force indicating that rofecoxib was associated with one-eighth the mortality from cardiovascular causes of that found with other NSAIDs.[32] The pamphlet presented a misleading analysis of short-term studies and didn't include any data from the large VIGOR study. The card's two references included 'data on file' at Merck and a brief research abstract.[33]

The corruption of the truth was total. In May 2001, Merck produced the press release 'Merck reconfirms favorable cardiovascular safety of Vioxx'.[4] Drug salespeople were only allowed to discuss approved results with the doctors, which were studies that provided 'solid evidence as to why [doctors] should prescribe Merck products'. Distributing studies that raised safety questions about Merck's drugs was 'a clear violation of Company Policy'.[32]

A Merck spokesperson, Kenneth C Frazier, lied when presented with Senator Henry A Waxman's unequivocal account of all these issues.[32] He said that 'Our representatives were instructed to present a balanced description of the risks and benefits of Vioxx', and that the data from the randomised trials (involving more than 28 000 patients) didn't show an increased risk with Vioxx.[34] Waxman replied that it was telling that the company relied on its 28 000 patients meta-analysis, as the FDA already in 2001 found it to have serious methodological limitations.[35]

Eric Topol from Cleveland wrote about the issues 3 weeks after the withdrawal of Vioxx,[4] and two Merck employees misinformed the readers in response.[36] They claimed that the increase in cardiovascular risk began after 18 months of therapy. This marketing trick was widely believed at the time, even by clinical pharmacologists who should have known better. I told them that when you take the first dose of a drug that is thrombogenic, you might get a thrombosis. Merck's misleading claim came from a trial in colorectal adenomas, and they propagated it – surprise, surprise – in the abstract in the *New England Journal of Medicine*.[37] Merck had not used a correct statistical test, and they had excluded all events that occurred more than 2 weeks after stopping treatment, although some of these patients would be expected to have, and actually had,[38] thrombotic events. It took 15 months before Merck was forced to retract its claim from the journal.[39] Topol wrote that the harms were visible early on,[40] and he also showed that two deaths, four heart attacks and three strokes with Vioxx were missing in the VIGOR publication compared with the data the FDA had access to, whereas the total number of such events was the same for the comparator drug, naproxen, in the two datasets. More fraud, it seems.

Trials in Alzheimer's disease were similarly revealing.[41] Internal Merck analyses in April 2001 showed that Vioxx increased total mortality significantly by a factor of three, but these analyses were not submitted to the FDA until 2 years later and they were not made public. Merck continued to recruit patients in one of the trials for an additional 2 years after it knew that Vioxx was deadly. Despite the deaths, the two published papers stated that Vioxx was 'well tolerated'. That must be the most obscene interpretation that exists of a drug being 'well tolerated', but I accept that dead patients cannot complain about lack of tolerance. What Merck did was to discard all deaths that occurred more than 2 weeks after the patients got off the drug, e.g. because of adverse effects, in violation of Merck's own protocol that stated that such deaths should be included in the results.[42] In fact, the risk of thrombosis may be increased a whole year after patients come off the drug. Merck spokespeople lied to the FDA and Congress about what and when the company knew that Vioxx is deadly.

There were lies all over the place. Two months after the withdrawal of Vioxx, the medical director of Merck in Sweden wrote in the *Swedish Medical Journal* that none of the trials before one on adenomas from 2005 had shown an increased risk of Vioxx compared with placebo.[43]

The same year Merck pulled rofecoxib off the market, its CEO received performance-based bonuses worth over $36 million in addition to his base salary[44] and he was never indicted. Merck pleaded guilty in 2012 to a criminal violation of federal law related to its promotion and marketing of Vioxx and was to pay nearly a billion dollars in a criminal fine and civil damages.[45] In 2007, the company announced a settlement worth $4.85 billion.[46] At that time, the company had already spent more than $1.2 billion on legal fees.[47] The crimes involved off-label marketing of Vioxx and false statements about the drug's cardiovascular safety. In relation to our study of Vioxx abstracts, we registered the conditions (apart from arthritis) that rofecoxib was proposed for, in 852 abstracts. Although almost half of the abstracts were published after the withdrawal of rofecoxib, where there was no longer any interest in suggesting new indications for the drug, the number and variety of conditions for which an effect of rofecoxib was proposed was astounding, no less than 30.[28] It was as if the drug – like Neurontin – could be used for everything, e.g. schizophrenia, sclerosis, eight different cancers and premenstrual acne (*see* Table 13.1), and yet we only studied abstracts. There were likely more conditions mentioned in the main text of the papers.

How many patients did Merck kill with Vioxx because of thrombosis? In its trial of colorectal adenomas, Merck assessed thrombotic events and there were 1.5 more cases of myocardial infarction, sudden cardiac death or stroke on rofecoxib than on placebo per 100 patients treated.[37] More than 80 million patients have been treated with rofecoxib,[4] and since about 10% of such events

Table 13.1 Conditions for which an effect of rofecoxib was mentioned in 852 abstracts

Neurological disorders

Hemicrania continua

Schizophrenia

Sclerosis

Alzheimer's dementia

Migraine

Premenstrual migraine

Surgery

Prevention of urethral strictures after TURP

Pre-medication for tonsillectomy

Pre-medication for uterine curettage

Hernia operations

Post CABG

Pre-medication for ear-nose-throat surgery in general

Minor dental surgery (e.g. removal of molars)

Minor orthopaedic surgery

Cancer

Treatment for glioblastoma multiforme

Protection against colorectal neoplasia in familiar polyposis

Treatment of malignant melanoma and sarcomas

Treatment of prostate cancer

Treatment of bone cancer

Treatment of breast cancer

Treatment of lung cancer

Other

Reduction of atherosclerosis among ACS-patients post-infarction

Congenial nephrogenous diabetes insipidus

Menstrual pain

Endometriosis

Non-bacterial prostatitis

Haemophilic arthropathy

Premenstrual acne

Prevention of ectopic ossification in arthroplasty

are fatal, a crude estimate is that rofecoxib has killed about 120 000 people. The patients were treated for 2.4 years, on average, and as many patients in clinical practice are treated for shorter periods, this could be an overestimate. However, other factors tend to lead to underestimation: only events that occurred within 2 weeks after the patients stopped their drug were recorded and the patients were only 59 years of age, on average, and at low risk for thrombotic events.[37] This is a general problem with Merck's trials. Merck only included patients that had an unusually *low* risk of thrombosis, e.g. Medicare patients in Tennessee treated with rofecoxib in clinical practice had a baseline risk of getting a myocardial infarction that was eight times higher than that for the patients in the trials.[6] I therefore believe, also considering that patients with arthritis are usually treated for years with NSAIDs, that my estimate of 120 000 deaths because of thrombosis is realistic. In addition, Vioxx has killed many thousands of patients because of ulcer complications.

In 2006, I saw a TV commercial in the United States on CNN that ended with a very deep voice saying, 'Merck, where the patients come first.' I couldn't help thinking, 'Merck, where the patients die first.'

REFERENCES

1 Tanne JH. Merck appeals rofecoxib verdict. *BMJ.* 2007; **334**: 607.

2 Lenzer J. FDA is incapable of protecting US 'against another Vioxx'. *BMJ.* 2004; **329**: 1253.

3 Krumholz HM, Ross JS, Presler AH, *et al.* What have we learned from Vioxx? *BMJ.* 2007; **334**: 120–3.

4 Topol EJ. Failing the public health – rofecoxib, Merck, and the FDA. *N Engl J Med.* 2004; **351**: 1707–9.

5 Petersen M. *Our Daily Meds.* New York: Sarah Crichton Books; 2008.

6 Jüni P, Nartey L, Reichenbach S, *et al.* Risk of cardiovascular events and rofecoxib: cumulative meta-analysis. *Lancet.* 2004; **364**: 2021–9.

7 Graham DJ. COX-2 inhibitors, other NSAIDs, and cardiovascular risk: the seduction of common sense. *JAMA.* 2006; **296**: 1653–6.

8 Topol E. Arthritis medicines and cardiovascular events – 'house of coxibs'. *JAMA.* 2005; **293**: 366–8.

9 Psaty BM, Furberg CD. COX-2 inhibitors – lessons in drug safety. *N Engl J Med.* 2005; **352**: 1133–5.

10 US Senate Finance Committee. Testimony of David J Graham, MD, MPH. 2004 Nov 18. Available online at: www.finance.senate.gov/imo/media/doc/111804dgtest.pdf (accessed 21 February 2013).

11 US Food and Drug Administration. Memorandum. 2001. Available online at: www.fda.gov/ohrms/dockets/ac/01/briefing/3677b2_06_cardio.pdf (accessed 23 June 2009).

12 Weaver AL, Messner RP, Storms WW, *et al.* Treatment of patients with osteoarthritis with rofecoxib compared with nabumetone. *J Clin Rheumatol.* 2006; **12**: 17–25.

13 Bombardier C, Laine L, Reicin A, *et al.* Comparison of upper gastrointestinal toxicity of rofecoxib and naproxen in patients with rheumatoid arthritis. *N Engl J Med.* 2000; **343**: 1520–8.

14 Armstrong D. *The New England Journal missed Vioxx warning signs.* 2006 May 15. Available online at: www.post-gazette.com/pg/06135/690336-114.stm (accessed 27 November 2012).

15 Curfman GD, Morrissey S, Drazen JM. Expression of concern reaffirmed. *N Engl J Med.* 2006. 10.1056/NEJMe068054. Accessed 23 Feb 2006.

16 Curfman GD, Morrissey S, Drazen JM. Expression of concern: Bombardier et al., 'Comparison of upper gastrointestinal toxicity of rofecoxib and naproxen in patients with rheumatoid arthritis,' N Engl J Med 2000;343:1520–8. *N Engl J Med.* 2005; **353**: 2813–14.

17 Mukherjee D, Nissen SE, Topol EJ. Risk of cardiovascular events associated with selective COX-2 inhibitors. *JAMA.* 2001; **286**: 954–9.

18 Liévre M, Abadie E, on behalf of the French Marketing Authorization Committee. Discontinuation of Vioxx. *Lancet.* 2005; **365**: 23–4.

19 Konstam MA, Weir MR, Reicin A. Cardiovascular thrombotic events in controlled, clinical trials of rofecoxib. *Circulation.* 2001; **104**: 2280–8.

20 Reicin AS, Shapiro D, Sperling RS, *et al*. Comparison of cardiovascular thrombotic events in patients with osteoarthritis treated with rofecoxib versus nonselective nonsteroidal anti-inflammatory drugs (ibuprofen, diclofenac, and nabumetone). *Am J Cardiol*. 2002; **89**: 204–9.

21 Corporate sponsorship. American Heart Association. Updated 2012 Oct 25. Available online at: www.heart.org/HEARTORG/Giving/ForCompanies/SponsorshipOpportunities/Corporate-Sponsorship_UCM_321431_Article.jsp (accessed 31 October 2012).

22 Kassirer JP. *On the Take: how medicine's complicity with big business can endanger your health*. Oxford: Oxford University Press; 2005.

23 Sanon S, Patel R, Eshelbrenner C, *et al*. Acute coronary syndrome in patients with diabetes mellitus: perspectives of an interventional cardiologist. *Am J Cardiol*. 2012; **110** supplement: 13B–23B.

24 Hill KP, Ross JS, Egilman DS, *et al*. The ADVANTAGE seeding trial: a review of internal documents. *Ann Intern Med*. 2008; **149**: 251–8.

25 Lisse JR, Perlman M, Johansson G, *et al*. Gastrointestinal tolerability and effectiveness of rofecoxib versus naproxen in the treatment of osteoarthritis: a randomized, controlled trial. *Ann Intern Med*. 2003; **139**: 539–46.

26 Berenson A. Evidence in Vioxx suits shows intervention by Merck officials. *New York Times*. 2005 Apr 24.

27 Ross JS, Hill KP, Egilman DS, *et al*. Guest authorship and ghostwriting in publications related to rofecoxib: a case study of industry documents from rofecoxib litigation. *JAMA*. 2008; **299**: 1800–2.

28 Jørgensen AW, Jørgensen KJ, Gøtzsche PC. Unbalanced reporting of benefits and harms in abstracts on rofecoxib. *Eur J Clin Pharmacol*. 2010; **66**: 341–7.

29 Grant B. Merck published fake journal. *The Scientist*. 2009. Available online at: www.the-scientist.com/blog/display/55671 (accessed 23 June 2009).

30 Day M. Don't blame it all on the bogey. *BMJ*. 2007; **334**: 1250–1.

31 Psaty BM, Furberg CD. COX-2 inhibitors – lessons in drug safety. *N Engl J Med*. 2005; **352**: 1133–5.

32 Waxman HA. The lessons of Vioxx – drug safety and sales. *N Engl J Med*. 2005; **352**: 2576–8.

33 Waxman HA. *The marketing of Vioxx to physicians. Memorandum*. Congress of the United States. 2005 May 5.

34 Frazier KC. The lessons of Vioxx. *N Engl J Med*. 2005; **353**: 1420.

35 Waxman HA. The lessons of Vioxx. *N Engl J Med*. 2005; **353**: 1420–1.

36 Kim PS, Reicin AS. Rofecoxib, Merck, and the FDA. *N Engl J Med*. 2004; **351**: 2875–6.

37 Bresalier RS, Sandler RS, Quan H, *et al*. Cardiovascular events associated with rofecoxib in a colorectal adenoma chemoprevention trial. *N Engl J Med*. 2005; **352**: 1092–102.

38 Nissen SE. Adverse cardiovascular effects of rofecoxib. *N Engl J Med*. 2006; **355**: 203–4.

39 Correction. *N Engl J Med*. 2006; **355**: 221.

40 Topol E. Rofecoxib, Merck, and the FDA. *N Engl J Med*. 2004; **351**: 2877–8.

41 Psaty BM, Kronmal RA. Reporting mortality findings in trials of rofecoxib for Alzheimer disease or cognitive impairment: a case study based on documents from rofecoxib litigation. *JAMA*. 2008; **299**: 1813–17.

42 Madigan D, Sigelman DW, Mayer JW, *et al*. Under-reporting of cardiovascular events in the rofecoxib Alzheimer disease studies. *Am Heart J*. 2012; **164**: 186–93.

43 Juhlin R. [MSD about Vioxx]. *Läkartidningen*. 2004; **46**: 3720–1.

44 Whelton RS. Effects of excessive CEO pay on U.S. society. Available online at: www.svsu.edu/emplibrary/Whelton%20article.pdf (accessed 6 November 2007).

45 Department of Justice. *U.S. pharmaceutical company Merck Sharp & Dohme sentenced in connection with unlawful promotion of Vioxx*. 2012 April 19.

46 Charatan F. 94% of patients suing Merck over rofecoxib agree to terms. *BMJ*. 2008; **336**: 580–1.

47 Berenson A. Merck agrees to settle Vioxx suits for $4.85 billion. *New York Times*. 2007 Nov 9.

Fraudulent celecoxib trial and other lies

> Companies cannot be expected to play the role of judge and jury, and there is a real risk of fraud.
>
> Prescrire International, about the CLASS study[1]

Pharmacia, later bought by Pfizer, published a large trial, the CLASS trial,[2] of celecoxib (Celebrex) in *JAMA* in 2000, which was fraudulent. All study authors were employees or paid consultants to the company, and eight US medical schools had contributed authors.[3]

According to the paper, celecoxib resulted in fewer stomach ulcers than the two comparators, diclofenac and ibuprofen, and two clinical experts wrote a favourable editorial in *JAMA*.[4] One of the editorialists was furious when he learned later – because of his membership of an FDA advisory committee – that it was not one trial but two trials bundled together to look like one, and that the trials ran for 12 and 15 months, not for 6 months as stated in *JAMA*.

The protocols for the two trials differed markedly from the published paper in design, outcomes, duration of follow-up and analysis, and the advantage of celecoxib disappeared when the protocol-specified analyses were performed by independent researchers.[5]

People in the company knew perfectly well what they were doing. In one email, an associate medical director at Pharmacia disparaged the way the study was being presented as 'data massage', for 'no other reason than it happens to look better'.[6] In another email, a medical director at Pfizer described it as 'cherrypicking the data' even as officials were publicly boasting of the study's success. Internal documents show a game plan on how the company might present unwelcome findings: 'Worse case: we have to attack the trial design if we do not see the results we want … If other endpoints do not deliver, we will also need to strategize on how we provide the data.' A slide proposed explaining poor results through 'statistical glitches'.

The FDA's advisory committee concluded that, based on the full data, celecoxib exhibited no advantage in reducing ulcer complications over the two old, much cheaper drugs. The FDA's statistical reviewer explained why the company's arguments for the 6-month analysis were obviously invalid.[7] A committee meeting in 2005 was also illuminating. All 32 participants considered that celecoxib, rofecoxib and valdecoxib increase the risk of cardiovascular events.[8]

However, the drug agencies continued to drag their feet and downplay the facts. For example, the Danish drug agency changed its product information for etoricoxib (Arcoxia, a Merck product) a week after the FDA meeting, so that it now said that 'Clinical studies suggest that the group of selective COX-2 inhibitors may be associated with a risk of thromboembolic events.' No way! The terms *suggest*, *may be*, and *associated with* document just how difficult it is for drug agencies to acknowledge the harms of drugs they have approved. Here is an honest version: clinical studies have *shown* that the group of selective COX-2 inhibitors *increase* thromboembolic events. Note that I left out *a risk of*. When a harm has been shown to occur in randomised trials, it is not a risk of harm, it is a real harm. We don't talk about the chance of benefit, we talk about benefit and therefore also need to talk about harms. It is so typical for regulators and industry to use different language when they see what they like to see from what they use when they prefer to close their eyes.

Merck Denmark must have welcomed this wool-in-mouth statement, as its letter to Danish doctors 5 days later said that 'selective COX-2 inhibitors can possibly be associated with a risk of thromboembolic events'. Oh dear. Merck had just killed more than one hundred thousand patients with Vioxx but didn't even on this occasion admit the proven cause–effect relationship but said that such drugs are *possibly associated with a risk*. Downgrading the unwelcome facts three times in just five words is something of an achievement.

In 2002, a Pfizer sponsored meta-analysis was published in the *BMJ*,[9] which shows how risky it is to collaborate with the industry, even for a skilled statistician who has done a lot of good work for the Cochrane Collaboration. The paper surprised many of his Cochrane colleagues when it came out. It claimed that celecoxib leads to fewer serious gastrointestinal events, and the abstract only mentioned relative benefit, not absolute benefit, which was far more modest. The authors only included the misleading 6 months data for the CLASS trial, which was by far the biggest one. What was most strange, however, was that, although the gastrointestinal events were described in detail over several pages, including many graphs, there were *no data on thromboses*, which makes the review completely worthless.

The authors, one of which was from Pfizer, explained that the review was limited to assessing only upper gastrointestinal safety, with the excuse that the trials did not report on thromboses. This excuse is pathetic. It is irresponsible not to report the number of thromboses, given that it is the most important harm of COX-2 inhibitors. Furthermore, the clinicians are obliged to report all serious adverse events immediately to the company, which means that the company must have had data on thromboses, whether or not they preferred to forget about them. In fact, thromboses *were* reported in the CLASS trial, and even using only the misleading 6 months data, there were 4.3% serious adverse events with celecoxib and 4.2% with the other two drugs, i.e. no advantage at all for celecoxib.[2]

The manipulations paid off, as they always do. About 30 000 reprints were bought from the publisher and less than 2 years after its publication, the CLASS trial had already been cited 169 times, and sales increased from $2.6 billion to $3.1 billion in just 1 year.[5] The fraud in *JAMA*, which has been propagated in many meta-analyses, must have been worth billions of dollars for the company.

The decision to report only data for the first 6 months was taken post hoc while the trial was running. The company might therefore have known beforehand that it would benefit the drug not to report the full data. In reply to the criticisms, the authors wrote that their decision 'was made before the trial analysis was completed'.[10] This explanation stinks. I'm sure that if Pharmacia/ Pfizer (the other two authors of the meta-analysis weren't involved with the trial, although they say 'we' in their reply) had made this decision earlier, during the trial's execution, the company would have told us. And if they had made the decision without looking at the data, they would have told us, as it would have strengthened their credibility. Another problem was that, in the CLASS trial, adverse events were only recorded if they occurred within 48 hours of stopping the drug in case a patient dropped out because of harms. This appallingly bad trial conduct means the company might have missed many cases of myocardial infarction and other thromboses on celecoxib.

The lies continued. A vice president for clinical research at Pharmacia in the United States claimed in 2002 that the analyses and outcomes were prespecified and that CLASS was a single study.[11] The lies were forcefully rejected by independent researchers, who noted that also in Pharmacia's successor study to CLASS, the SUCCESS-1 study, the company had pooled results from different protocols with different comparator drugs.[12] Pharmacia's statements were also rejected by the FDA's statistical reviewer, who remarked that *the company had conducted at least 34 subgroup analyses that were not prespecified* in violation of the trial protocol that stated that the primary outcome should show a statistically significant difference before any subgroup analyses would be undertaken.[7,13] As with Vioxx, trials purporting not to have found a risk of thromboses found their way to cardiology journals, e.g. *American Journal of Cardiology*.[14]

Even as late as in 2009, Pfizer played games denying the problems with its drug. It funded a trial in general practice, comparing celecoxib with other NSAIDs, but the funding was concealed in the invitation for an investigators' meeting, which said the University of Dundee sponsored the trial.[15] There was a 2-week run-in phase before the randomisation where all patients would receive celecoxib, which invalidates the trial because those who cannot tolerate the drug don't get randomised. The information to the patients stated that the evidence wasn't conclusive as to whether celecoxib increased heart disease and strokes. This lie should have caused the research ethics committee to reject the trial. I have a product summary from February 2005 that mentions the cardiovascular problems and a letter from Pfizer to doctors that acknowledges that the drug causes them and says that celecoxib should not be used in patients with ischaemic heart disease or with cerebrovascular disease.

Furthermore, in 2005, the US National Cancer Institute published a trial of celecoxib for prevention of colorectal adenoma in the *New England Journal of Medicine*, which was terminated prematurely for safety reasons, as celecoxib increased significantly cardiovascular events.[16] And a meta-analysis conducted by independent researchers using FDA data showed in 2006 that celecoxib doubles the number of heart attacks compared with placebo.[17] The authors contacted Pfizer for details about its trials, but Pfizer didn't provide any.

This illustrates that the responsibility of doing trials should be taken away from the drug companies. We let them get away with their frauds and lies far too easily. When Merck withdrew Vioxx from the market in 2004, Pfizer grabbed the opportunity immediately. The next day, the company wrote to Danish doctors that celecoxib had been used in more than 50 million people worldwide and that the company had reviewed clinical trials in more than 400 000 patients (that's what they wrote; I suppose they meant 40 000), and that this had not yielded any signs that celecoxib increased the risk of cardiovascular side effects. The fine for this ruthless misinformation was $2000.[18]

Fifty million people. How many deaths because of thrombosis is this? Using the same calculation as for rofecoxib (see p. 160–1), we get 75 000 deaths. In addition, celecoxib has killed many thousands of patients because of ulcer complications. And that's only up till 2004; the drug is still on the market.

This is similar to the estimated number of deaths caused by Vioxx. I wonder why our drug agencies haven't withdrawn celecoxib and similarly dangerous NSAIDs? The Danish drug agency did react, however. It withdrew the reimbursement of celecoxib and similar drugs 1 month after Vioxx was withdrawn, which saved many lives. Compared to 2003, the use of celecoxib in 2005 was only 10% and in 2007 it was 4%.

Pfizer continued to protect its drug rather than the patients' lives. Four days before the reimbursement disappeared, the company wrote to all Danish doctors complaining it created a dilemma for the doctors and was a step backwards for the patients who were denied access to new medicines. Pfizer's letter contained a form the doctors could use to apply for reimbursement for individual patients, and the company established a separate phone line where doctors could be advised what they should do. The company also put ads in the *Journal of the Danish Medical Association* showing an elderly lady dancing on the table with the text: 'Life is too long to have pain.' I reproduced the ad in a paper I published in the same journal and added: 'and too short to die of myocardial infarction.'[19]

Apart from withdrawing a drug from the market, withdrawal of reimbursement is the most powerful tool the authorities have. The committee that deals with these decisions has received remarkably similar letters of complaint from doctors in the whole country, orchestrated by the company. Another example of drug whores.

Pfizer was very worried that its fraud could lead to many legal proceedings and its lawyers harassed not only *JAMA* but several other prominent journals.[20,21] More than 3000 lawsuits had been raised against Pfizer alleging the company marketed celecoxib and valdecoxib as being without the adverse effects of the old NSAIDs.[20] Pfizer issued subpoenas to get access to all peer reviews, rejected manuscripts and editorial decisions about papers submitted to *JAMA* on the two drugs. Obviously, these unpublished materials couldn't have played any role in Pfizer's appalling marketing conduct, and the judge appropriately quashed Pfizer's subpoenas. Although peer reviewers are guaranteed anonymity, Pfizer asked for their identity. I wonder what the idea was. To sue the peer reviewers, or harass them in other ways, e.g. via their superiors (see Chapter 19)?

The habitual lying took a new turn in 2012 when investors' lawyers accused

Pfizer of having destroyed documents about the development of celecoxib and valdecoxib in bad faith and compounded their initial misconduct by making false statements about the existence of centralised databases.[22] Pfizer denied the existence of electronic databases containing millions of files about the drugs and argued that the existence of the 'e-Rooms were a figment of plaintiffs' imagination'. However, Pfizer officials later acknowledged the rooms existed and turned over documents stored electronically. The lawyers also complained that Pfizer's technical staff undertook 'two dismantling projects while this case was pending'. In response, Pfizer's lawyer filed a new lie saying, 'At no time did Pfizer ever mislead plaintiffs concerning the existence of databases.'

MARKETING IS HARMFUL

A Canadian study showed that the bombardment of doctors with sales pitches about COX-2 inhibitors claiming that the drugs have fewer gastrointestinal adverse effects than the old NSAIDs aggravated the problem. The total sales of NSAIDs (including celecoxib and rofecoxib) increased, and as more patients were now treated, a declining trend in hospital admissions for gastrointestinal haemorrhage changed to an *increase*.[23]

The COX-2 inhibitors are a prime example that fraudulent research and fraudulent marketing are very harmful for patients and very lucrative for the companies and that our most prestigious journals lend their pages to the deceptions. A 2001 review article in the *New England Journal of Medicine* about the coxibs was utterly flawed.[24] The two authors had financial ties to the makers of Vioxx and Celebrex and their paper was a shameful advertisement for the drugs to the point of even mentioning the non-existing advantage of Celebrex that the FDA had forbidden the company to make.[25] The serious harms of the two drugs were dismissed in a most unacademic fashion. I wonder how many millions of dollars the journal made on selling reprints of this totally misleading review. The same year, both drugs were among the top 10 selling drugs in the United States.[25]

Were it not for the power of marketing, the popularity of new drugs would be difficult to understand. The risk of taking a new drug is greater than the risk of using an old one, as it takes time before the harms of new drugs become known. As an example, the COX-2 inhibitor lumiracoxib (Prexige from Novartis) was approved by the EMA in 2006 and withdrawn a year later because of serious liver problems, including deaths. It was never approved by the FDA.

NSAIDs are very dangerous. Even before the COX-2 inhibitors, we caused deaths on a terrible scale with NSAIDs. It has been estimated that 3700 deaths occur each year in the United Kingdom due to peptic ulcer complications in NSAID users,[26] corresponding to about 20 000 deaths each year in the United States. In agreement with this, it was estimated in 1999 that more than 16 000 Americans died from stomach ulcers caused by NSAIDs, roughly the same number as those who died from AIDS.[27] This makes NSAIDs one of the most deadly drug groups (*see* Chapter 21 about drug deaths). The tragedy is that many of these people could have had a good life without NSAIDs, but marketing has lured doctors into using NSAIDs for virtually every kind of pain, assisted by prostituted rheumatologists. A journalist writing about Vioxx and Celebrex called a national society of US rheumatologists in 2000 to speak to an expert who wasn't being paid by either company. She was told there was none.[27]

People who tell the truth get punished (see also Chapters 13 and 19). In 2002, an independent Spanish drug bulletin wrote that the so-called advantages of celecoxib and rofecoxib were scientific fraud.[28] Merck sued while Pfizer did not, perhaps because taking action would lead to a worse outcome for the company. Merck misrepresented the court's verdict, which was that the Spanish article was accurate, that it reflected the debate on the ethics of publications in medical research and echoed the FDA's warnings to Merck regarding misleading information on the cardiovascular adverse effects of rofecoxib in promotional materials.[29]

Merck stated only 6 months before it withdrew Vioxx that '*MSD is fully committed to the highest standards of scientific integrity, ethics, and protection of patient's wellbeing in our research. We have a tradition of partnership with leaders in the academic research community.*'[30] Great. Let's have some more of such ethical partnerships. They often kill our patients while everyone else prospers.

Perhaps Hells Angels should consider something similar in their PR: *We are fully committed to the highest standards of integrity, ethics and protection of citizens' well-being when we push narcotic drugs. We have a tradition of partnership with leaders in the police force.*

REFERENCES

1 Celecoxib and the CLASS trial: data massaging by industry. *Prescrire International.* 2002; **11**: 190–1.

2 Silverstein FE, Faich G, Goldstein JL, *et al.* Gastrointestinal toxicity with celecoxib vs nonsteroidal anti-inflammatory drugs for osteoarthritis and rheumatoid arthritis: the CLASS study: A randomized controlled trial. Celecoxib Long-term Arthritis Safety Study. *JAMA.* 2000; **284**: 1247–55.

3 Okie S. Missing data on Celebrex. *Washington Post.* 2001 Aug 5.

4 Lichtenstein DR, Wolfe MM. COX-2-Selective NSAIDs: new and improved? *JAMA.* 2000; **284**: 1297–9.

5 Jüni P, Rutjes AW, Dieppe PA. Are selective COX 2 inhibitors superior to traditional non steroidal anti-inflammatory drugs? *BMJ.* 2002; **324**: 1287–8.

6 Thomas K. In documents on pain drug Celebrex, signs of doubt and deception. *New York Times.* 2012 June 24.

7 Lu HL. *Statistical Reviewer Briefing Document for the Advisory Committee.* FDA. 2000; NDA20-998.

8 FDA. Summary minutes, AAC & DSaRM. 2005 Feb 16–18. Available online at: www.fda.gov/ohrms/dockets/ac/05/minutes/2005-4090M1: Final.htm (accessed February 2005).

9 Deeks JJ, Smith LA, Bradley MD. Efficacy, tolerability, and upper gastrointestinal safety of celecoxib for treatment of osteoarthritis and rheumatoid arthritis: systematic review of randomised controlled trials. *BMJ.* 2002; **325**: 619.

10 Deeks JJ, Smith LA, Bradley MD. Systematic review of celecoxib for osteoarthritis and rheumatoid arthritis. *BMJ.* 2003; **326**: 335–6.

11 Geis GS. Pharmacia's response to editorial. *BMJ.* 2002; **325**: 161–2.

12 Jüni P, Rutjes AWS, Dieppe P. Authors' reply. *BMJ.* 2002; **325**: 163–4.

13 Hrachovec JB, Mora M. Reporting of 6-month vs 12-month data in a clinical trial of celecoxib. *JAMA.* 2001; **286**: 2398.

14 White WB, Faich G, Whelton A, *et al.* Comparison of thromboembolic events in patients treated with celecoxib, a cyclooxygenase-2 specific inhibitor, versus ibuprofen or diclofenac. *Am J Cardiol.* 2002; **89**: 425–30.

15 Andrade M. In clear sight. *BMJ*. 2009; **339**: 538–40.

16 Solomon SD, McMurray JJ, Pfeffer MA, *et al*. Cardiovascular risk associated with celecoxib in a clinical trial for colorectal adenoma prevention. *N Engl J Med*. 2005; **352**: 1071–80.

17 Caldwell B, Aldington S, Weatherall M, *et al*. Risk of cardiovascular events and celecoxib: a systematic review and meta-analysis. *J R Soc Med*. 2006; **99**: 132–40.

18 Crone M. [Pfizer gets additional fine for illegal marketing]. *Berlingske*. 2004 Nov 16.

19 Gøtzsche PC. [COX-2 inhibitors and other nonsteroidal, anti-inflammatory drugs – what future?] *Ugeskr Læger*. 2006; **168**: 1972–3.

20 DeAngelis CD, Thornton JP. Preserving confidentiality in the peer review process. *JAMA*. 2008; **299**: 1956.

21 Dyer C. Pfizer asks journal for comments made by peer reviewers. *BMJ*. 2008; **336**: 575.

22 Feeley J, Van Voris B. Pfizer destroyed arthritis drugs' files, investors claim. Bloomberg. 2012 Nov 21. Available online at: www.bloomberg.com/news/2012-11-21/pfizer-destroyed-arthritis-drugs-files-investors-claim.html (accessed 10 July 2013).

23 Mamdani M, Juurlink DN, Kopp A, *et al*. Gastrointestinal bleeding after the introduction of COX 2 inhibitors: ecological study. *BMJ*. 2004; **328**: 1415–6.

24 FitzGerald GA, Patrono C. The coxibs, selective inhibitors of cyclooxygenase-2. *N Engl J Med*. 2001; **345**: 433–42.

25 Abramson J. *Overdo$ed America*. New York: HarperCollins; 2004.

26 Blower AL, Brooks A, Fenn GC, *et al*. Emergency admissions for upper gastrointestinal disease and their relation to NSAID use. *Aliment Pharmacol Ther*. 1997; **11**: 283–91.

27 Petersen M. *Our Daily Meds*. New York: Sarah Crichton Books; 2008.

28 Gibson L. Drug company sues Spanish bulletin over fraud claim. *BMJ*. 2004; **328**: 188.

29 Laporte J-R. Merck Sharpe and Dohme versus Laporte. *Lancet*. 2004; **364**: 416.

30 Honig P. Merck Sharp and Dohme versus Laporte. *Lancet*. 2004; **363**: 1079–80.

Switching cheap drugs to expensive ones in the same patients

Seeding trials lure doctors into prescribing new expensive drugs instead of old cheap ones that are equally good or better (*see* Chapters 8 and 9). The worst of them are designed to persuade prescribers to switch patients who are already well treated with the old drug. As doctors are paid for each patient they switch, this kickback clouds clinical judgement.

NOVO NORDISK SWITCHES PATIENTS TO EXPENSIVE INSULIN

Switch campaigns are sometimes carried out without the faintest guise of research. Insulin was obtained from animal pancreas until the 1980s when bio-synthetic human insulin began to replace animal insulins, with important supply implications but no clinical advantage.[1] To overcome this marketing problem, the first worldwide insulin switch campaigns were launched. In 2006, Novo Nordisk paid doctor's assistants and a pharmacy chain to switch diabetic patients to the company's high-priced new insulin products. Novo's district manager wrote to the salespeople:[2]

> 'Our goal is 50 or more scripts per week for each territory ... If you are not achieving this goal, ask yourself if those doctors that you have such great relationships with are being fair to you. Hold them accountable for all of the time, samples, lunches, dinners, programs and past preceptorships that you have provided or paid for and get the business!! You can do it!!'

Such actions are unlawful, as federal anti-kickback statutes prohibit drug companies from offering financial incentives to doctors or pharmacists to encourage or reward the prescribing of particular drugs, but the crimes are highly successful. While Novo's insulin sales rose 364%, Eli Lilly's sales rose only 13%. Health professionals warned that switches to newer, more rapidly acting insulin types could be dangerous and even lethal if the patients have not been thoroughly informed. This wasn't always the case. Some patients first became aware of the switches when they picked up the new medicines at a pharmacy.[2]

Another switch campaign began when human insulin was replaced by genetically engineered insulin analogues at several times the cost.[1] Company reports for 2010 show that insulin glargine, the most successful analogue, helped to give

Sanofi-Aventis insulin sales of around $5.1 billion, compared with $4.7 billion for Novo and $3.1 billion for Eli Lilly. However, the insulin analogues offer little benefit to most people with type 2 diabetes, except those who experience troublesome hypoglycaemia.[1]

In 2012, a paper in the *BMJ* described that Novo had recruited nearly 360 000 patients for questionable 'studies'.[3] Most studies were performed in middle or low income countries, even though the patients may have difficulty affording the more expensive insulin. In India, the new insulin was nine times more expensive than the cheapest human insulin. One of the studies lacked a control arm and a well-defined question, and its results were highly implausible, as almost no one reported hypoglycaemia. Clearly, if one wants to know something about the new insulin, hundreds of thousands of patients aren't needed, but we would need a comparator group that received the old insulin. Some of Novo's 'results' were published, but with selected subanalyses with positive outcomes, and with co-authors or writing support from the company.[1] The doctors were paid, which might constitute kickbacks. Everyone prospers while the poorest patients pay the bill, hardly an example of the 'ethical partnerships' between industry and doctors we hear so much about.

ASTRAZENECA SWITCHES PATIENTS TO EXPENSIVE ME-AGAIN OMEPRAZOLE

The power of money in corrupting doctors' judgements is perhaps best illustrated by the stereoisomers. Usually, only one of the two halves, which are mirror images of each other, is active, but when the patent runs out, the company may patent the active half, a trick called evergreening, or 'me-again'. Our patent laws are really weird since they allow this, which merely benefits the company for no societal gain.

The proton-pump inhibitor omeprazole (Losec, Prilosec), used for stomach ulcers and related conditions, was the world's best-selling drug in the late 1990s. When the patent ran out in 2001, AstraZeneca had extracted the most active half, which has its own chemical name, esomeprazole (Nexium). Generic versions of omeprazole were ready to enter the market at a much lower price than Losec and, in a rational world, all patients would now be treated with a cheap version of omeprazole. This didn't happen. AstraZeneca used illegal methods to keep competitors away.[4] It abused its dominant market position; lied to patent lawyers, patent offices and courts in several countries about the date at which omeprazole had originally been given marketing authorisation; replaced a capsule formulation of the drug with tablets and withdrew the capsule authorisation, which made it impossible for manufacturers of generic drugs to market the capsules.

AstraZeneca produced flawed trials that purported to demonstrate that Nexium was slightly better than Losec. Instead of comparing equivalent doses, AstraZeneca compared 40 mg Nexium with 20 mg Losec, which is a much higher dose.[5] It is ludicrous to 'prove' that something is better than itself. If I drink four beers instead of one, my mental capacity will deteriorate more, but this doesn't mean that a beer is stronger than a beer. AstraZeneca did a meta-analysis of three such trials showing that more patients with reflux oesophagitis were healed on the high dose than on the low dose after 4 weeks.[5] The result was shown as a relative risk of 1.14, which isn't informative. I therefore redid the meta-analysis and found a risk difference of only 0.08. Thus, by treating 13 patients (= 1/0.08) with the high dose, one more patient would get an effect, at a cost that was about 30 times higher.

Thirty times! It would seem impossible to get any doctor to use such a drug, but doctors are willing to do almost anything, no matter how stupid it is, while they say that the information they get from the drug industry is valuable for them (*see* Chapter 9). AstraZeneca's violent attack on common sense worked, aided by a series of shady marketing techniques at extremely high cost; the company used $500 million in the United States for its campaign in just 1 year.[6] *Five hundred million dollars for selling a drug that was 30 times more expensive than a drug that contained the same active substance.* What a waste.

In Germany, AstraZeneca launched seeding trials, and one-quarter of all general practitioners participated in the hoax and were paid for starting patients on Nexium and making a note of how it went.[7]

Seeding trials increased the German drug budget with €1 billion in 2008.[8] Companies pay doctors as much as €1000 per patient; the patients don't give informed consent; and the health insurance companies pay for the drugs. This looks like paying kickbacks, but bribery of doctors is legal in Germany if they work in private practice.[9] Self-employed physicians (about one-third of all doctors) that accept up to €10 000 from drug companies in cash – or gifts such as computers, equipment or even holidays – will not face corruption charges. Germany's Supreme Court ruled in 2012 that drug companies cannot be penalised either when paying German freelance physicians to prescribe their drugs. The case leading to the verdict involved a drug salesperson who paid cash to doctors, amounting to a 5% kickback on each product they prescribed. The company's official explanation was that the money was remuneration for delivering academic presentations, but these seminars never took place. Even more astonishingly, the head of the German Medical Association, Frank Ulrich Montgomery, shared the court's view that the rights of doctors to operate in an independent professional capacity should be protected. He added that the media coverage of the case was part of a wider behind-the-scenes agenda to tarnish the reputation of doctors. I doubt the media are better at tarnishing the reputation of doctors than the doctors themselves.

AstraZeneca was also 'creative' in Denmark, selling Losec to the hospitals for only 1% of the price, whereas the patients had to pay the full price when they left the hospital. The company used the same trick with Nexium, which was sold for 2% of the price. Because of such tricks, hospitals are now obliged to use the same drug as would be preferred outside hospital.

A couple of years ago, I discussed ulcer drugs with a chief gastroenterologist at a meeting. He firmly believed that Nexium was a better drug than Losec and therefore used Nexium. I fail to understand this. Are my colleagues dumb or corrupt? I cannot see other possibilities. Roughly half of those in treatment with proton-pump inhibitors have no appropriate indication,[10] and expenditure on these drugs was €10 billion globally in 2006. It is difficult for patients to stop, as the use of the drugs disturbs the hormonal homeostasis. This builds up an excessive production of counteracting hormones, which may cause severe gastric symptoms if treatment is stopped abruptly.[11]

The rebound phenomenon is a problem with many of our drugs and it is often misinterpreted to mean that the patients need to increase the dose or to take the drug forever, although a much better option would have been to taper off the drug slowly or to take the drug only intermittently, e.g. if you have heartburn. The rebound phenomenon is the reason why we have an epidemic of happy pills (*see* Chapter 17).

Pfizer has provided a most bizarre example of me-again. Aricept (donepezil) was the biggest player in the lucrative market for Alzheimer's disease with over $2 billion in annual sales in the United States alone.[12] Four months before the expiry of the patent, the FDA approved a new dose, donepezil 23 mg, which would be patent protected for three more years, whereas the old doses of 5 and 10 mg were not. The advertising was directed towards patients and contained untrue statements, but the scam worked.

One would have hoped people were clever enough to take either 20 or 25 mg of the drug to save money, but no. And the FDA failed us badly again. Its own medical reviewers and statisticians recommended against approval, as the 23 mg dose didn't produce a clinically meaningful benefit whereas it caused significantly more adverse events, particularly protracted vomiting. The reviewers added that the adverse events could lead to pneumonia, massive gastrointestinal bleeding, oesophageal rupture and death.[13] This didn't impress the director of the FDA's neurology division, Russel Katz, who overruled his scientists.

I must use strong language now. What the hell is going on? We know that big pharma is evil,[14] but what about our drug agencies? Why do they side with evil and deceitful drug companies?

REFERENCES

1 Gale EAM. Post-marketing studies of new insulins: sales or science? *BMJ*. 2012; **344**: e3974.
2 Harris G, Pear R. Drug maker's efforts to compete in lucrative insulin market are under scrutiny. *New York Times*. 2006 Jan 28.
3 Yudkin JS. Post-marketing observational trials and catastrophic health expenditure. *BMJ*. 2012; **344**: e3987.
4 Hawkes N. AstraZeneca must pay €52.5m fine for anticompetitive tactics, rules European court. *BMJ*. 2012; **345**: e8396.
5 Edwards SJ, Lind T, Lundell L. Systematic review of proton pump inhibitors for the acute treatment of reflux oesophagitis. *Aliment Pharmacol Ther*. 2001; **15**: 1729–36.
6 Relman AS, Angell M. America's other drug problem: how the drug industry distorts medicine and politics. *The New Republic*. 2002 Dec 16: 27–41.
7 Grill M. *Kranke Geschäfte: wie die Pharmaindustrie uns manipuliert*. Hamburg: Rowohlt Verlag 2007.
8 Tuffs A. Germany sees rise in post-marketing studies. *BMJ*. 2009; **339**: b4199.
9 Hyde R. German doctors free to take cash from drug firms. *Lancet*. 2012; **380**: 551.
10 Forgacs I, Loganayagam A. Overprescribing proton pump inhibitors. *BMJ*. 2008; **336**: 2–3.
11 McKay AB. Overprescribing PPIs. *BMJ*. 2008; **336**: 109.
12 Schwartz LM, Woloshin S. How the FDA forgot the evidence: the case of donepezil 23 mg. *BMJ*. 2012; **344**: e1086.

13 Lenzer J. FDA is criticised for licensing high dose donepezil. *BMJ*. 2011; **342**: d3270.
14 Goldacre B. *Bad Pharma*. London: Fourth Estate; 2012.

Blood glucose was fine but the patients died

The story of rosiglitazone is one of death, greed, and corruption ... The trust between doctor and patient, researcher and participant, or author and editor is undermined when the foundations on which evidence is built are treated with such casual contempt.

Editorial, *The Lancet*[1]

The FDA approved rosiglitazone (Avandia) in 1999 although there were more thrombotic heart events with the drug than with placebo or active comparators (relative risk 1.8, 95% confidence interval 0.9 to 3.6).[2]

The FDA reviewer had adjusted for time on drug, which brought the relative risk down to 1.1. However, as stated in the package insert, the drug increased LDL cholesterol by 19%, which explains its harmful effect on the heart. The cholesterol-lowering drug ezetimibe was approved in 2002 based on a 15%–18% reduction in LDL cholesterol, which was presumed to confer cardiovascular benefits. Thus, a lowering of LDL cholesterol by 15%–18% *without* evidence of clinical benefit led to drug approval in one case, whereas an increase by the same amount *with* clinical evidence of harm didn't lead the FDA to reject rosiglitazone. This illustrates again the failure at drug agencies in protecting public health.

In Europe, the EMA was so concerned that it rejected the drug, only to approve it a year later despite there being no new evidence. It isn't clear why, but Silvio Garattini was on EMA's committee and has described how the companies bring forward paid opinion leaders who give favourable presentations at committee meetings.[3]

A member of the committee told the *BMJ* that he had been contacted by respected members of the diabetes community who urged him to approve the 'wonder' drug. Garattini's view was that there was no need for the drug, as there already were so many that were more or less the same.[3] He explained that long-term trials required after marketing approval are highly beneficial for the companies, which have every reason in the world to be so slow with the trials that the drug was off-patent when the bad results came in. An even better strategy was to ignore the demands, and in fact, only about a third of FDA requests for post-marketing studies are ever carried out.[3]

In 1999, the company, then known as SmithKline Beecham, completed a trial that found more cardiac problems with rosiglitazone than with pioglitazone, but according to an internal email, 'These data should not see the light of day to anyone outside of GSK.'[3,4] Instead of publishing the results, the company spent the next 11 years trying to cover them up.[4] Mary Anne Rhyne, a GlaxoSmithKline spokeswoman, said that the company had not provided the results of its study because they 'did not contribute any significant new information'.[4] Apparently it did, also for Glaxo, as the results made the company decide against further comparisons!

In 2004, the WHO sent Glaxo an alert about cardiac events and the company performed a meta-analysis that confirmed this, which it sent to the FDA and the EMA in 2006. However, none of the agencies made the findings public because of the proprietary nature of companies' trial results.[3] This absurd interpretation of ownership of data and results is not only deeply unethical, it is also wrong, as it violates the fundamental principles on which the European Union is founded (see Chapter 11).[5] But as long as we allow regulators to believe in their own nonsense and putting profits before the survival of patients, it allows the companies to 'push the drug aggressively and hope they can make a billion dollars before someone finds out', as former editor of the New England Journal of Medicine, Jerome Kassirer, expressed it.[6] Rosiglitazone was Glaxo's second-best-selling drug, at about $3 billion a year,[3] and Glaxo behaved like drug pushers in the street, as they could have informed the public about the dangers with its drug but didn't.

In 2006, Glaxo sent an updated analysis to the FDA with five more trials confirming the harm, but, yet again, the FDA failed to warn the patients and the physicians.[2] Perhaps the FDA was duped by an observational study Glaxo had also submitted, performed by a commercial vendor, which showed no increase in risk? However, Glaxo had carefully avoided to report to the FDA what this study had shown when rosiglitazone was compared with pioglitazone. This comparison showed that rosiglitazone led to more admissions to hospital with myocardial infarction than pioglitazone.[2] I believe the omission is scientific misconduct, given that Glaxo already knew that pioglitazone is a better drug.

Rosiglitazone was now the most sold diabetes drug in the world, but in 2007, all hell broke loose for Glaxo. As part of a legal settlement in relation to the company's fraud with paroxetine (see Chapter 18),[3,7] Glaxo was required to post the results of its clinical trials on a website. This enabled independent researchers Steven Nissen and Kathy Wolski to have a closer look at rosiglitazone. Their 2007 meta-analysis of 42 trials, 27 of which were unpublished, showed that the drug causes myocardial infarction and cardiovascular death.[5,8,9]

Diabetes drugs are supposed to lower cardiovascular mortality, not increase it, but, as just noted, the shocking news was not news for Glaxo.[10] The company had known about this for 8 years but failed to warn the regulatory authorities and the public. Three years later, the US Senate Finance Committee released a 334-page investigation of rosiglitazone and Glaxo, which mentioned internal company emails and documents that give us a rare insight into the conduct of a major drug company.[9]

Nissen and Wolski submitted their meta-analysis to the New England Journal of Medicine on 1 May 2007. The manuscript was sent for peer review and only 2 days after submission, an academic peer reviewer broke the rules and faxed the manuscript to Glaxo.[9] Despite its confidential nature, Glaxo circulated the manuscript to more than 40 scientists and executives at the highest levels in the company.[11] On 8 May, Glaxo's head of research admitted internally that the FDA and Glaxo itself had come to similar conclusions about the increased risk with rosiglitazone as the submitted meta-analysis did.[11] Yet the next day Glaxo had its key lies ready, which they called 'key messages', and which were that the meta-analysis was based on incomplete evidence and that the company strongly disagreed with its conclusions.

Already on 10 May, four Glaxo scientists and executives met with Steven Nissen after having asked for a meeting.[9] As Glaxo had previously threatened John Buse (*see* Chapter 19), Nissen secretly taped the meeting. Because of Nissen's meta-analysis, Glaxo had decided to unblind the collected data on its ongoing RECORD trial, which the EMA had required the company to carry out because of cardiovascular safety concerns when it approved the drug in 2000.[3] An internal email suggested that if the independent academic steering committee for the trial wouldn't agree to publish interim results, the company would pursue the line that 'a decision has been made – live with it'.[11] Glaxo convinced the steering committee that an interim analysis should be published, but the committee didn't know that Glaxo had already unblinded the results 2 weeks earlier. The committee apparently believed it was their decision to unblind the study and publish.

At the meeting with Nissen, an executive said, 'Let's suppose RECORD was done tomorrow and the hazard ratio was 1.12.'[9] This comment was made 4 days before the company claimed it unblinded the trial and 14 days before the steering committee was asked to approve unblinding. The hazard ratio that was published was about the same, 1.11.

Funded by Glaxo, Philip Home *et al.* published what they called 'an unplanned interim analysis' electronically in the *New England Journal of Medicine* only 2 weeks after Nissen and Wolski published their meta-analysis in the same journal on 14 June. Glaxo succeeded to publish a large trial reporting on 4447 patients followed for 4 years, only 7 weeks after they heard about a meta-analysis that threatened the survival of their product. In contrast, it can take companies 5 or 10 years to publish results they don't like, if they publish them at all. Companies are surely able to act fast in the case of a drug emergency.

What made the *New England Journal of Medicine* decide to publish an unplanned interim analysis of an ongoing trial, to publish it so quickly and to accept it despite its poor design (e.g. the trial drugs weren't even blinded)? An FDA scientist, Thomas Marciniak, said that the FDA would have found the trial's design unacceptable.[3] My take on this is that the journal has far lower standards for industry trials than for other types of research and that it has allowed its integrity to be corrupted by big pharma for financial gains (*see also* Chapters 5, 6, 13 and 14).

There were eight authors. One was from Glaxo and the other seven were 'consultants' on company payroll.[11] They talked about 'exceptional circumstances' (but didn't specify that these were that one of their comrades had stolen Nissen's manuscript) motivating them to report unplanned interim findings and they regarded their findings as 'inconclusive'.[12] It's unbelievable and scandalous that the *New England Journal of Medicine* let them get away with this. Nowhere is the reader told what the 'exceptional circumstances' were and the editors didn't ensure the authors explained it in the paper. When the final results were published in the *Lancet* 2 years later,[13] they appeared to be false.[9] The event rate for heart attacks was less than one-third of that observed in a similar trial with pioglitazone, and the paper claimed that rosiglitazone was administered during 88% of the follow-up, which was mathematically implausible, given other information about the trial.[9]

Since the 1950s, the FDA has required drug companies to turn over all individual patient case reports from their studies. This permits reanalysis of how each case was coded[3] and enabled Marciniak to scrutinise the RECORD trial data.[3] The EMA had accepted the company's findings that the risk of complications was the same, 14.5% for rosiglitazone and 14.4% for the comparator.[3] However, when Marciniak studied 549 case reports he found many missing cases of cardiac problems that favoured rosiglitazone four to one.[3,14] For one patient, there were 1438 pages, and for most of the other 4500 patients there were several hundred pages, making a review of all case reports a huge task.[3] Marciniak concluded that the case report forms are essential for understanding a study and he found that rosiglitazone increased cardiovascular risk also in the RECORD trial,[3] in contrast to Glaxo's manipulated results.

Very importantly, Marciniak stated that 'even with blinded adjudication, biased referral for adjudication of cases and data by unblinded investigators and site monitors may lead to biases in event rates'.[14]

> *The importance of this statement cannot be overestimated. The sponsor has access to the data and knows who received which drug, and biased selection of 'unclear cases' for review by an independent committee is an important reason why industry trials should be distrusted.* (see also Chapter 5, p. 54)

Grave suspicions were raised earlier. The editorial that accompanied the interim publication of the RECORD trial mentioned that the trial had found an exceptionally low event rate in a high-risk population of patients with diabetes and noted that the most likely explanation was incomplete ascertainment of events.[15] The editorialists also noted that rosiglitazone increased the risk of a heart attack to the same degree as lipid-lowering statins lower the risk.

However, as always the FDA wanted it otherwise. According to the documents released by the Senate, a top official at the FDA, John Jenkins, director of the agency's office of new drugs, preferred to continue to put patients at risk. He argued internally that rosiglitazone should remain on the market and briefed the company extensively on the agency's internal debate. According to a sealed deposition, a top company official wrote after he spoke with Jenkins that 'It is clear the office of new drugs is trying to find minimal language that will satisfy the office of drug safety'. In the deposition, Rosemary Johann-Liang, a former supervisor in the drug safety office who left the FDA after she was disciplined for recommending that rosiglitazone's heart warnings be strengthened, said of Jenkins' conversations with GlaxoSmithKline that 'This should not happen', and she suggested that 'People have to make a determination about the leadership at the FDA'.

Rosiglitazone was suspended in Europe in September 2010 whereas the process at the FDA continued to be fishy. In July 2010, the FDA held a new advisory committee meeting to decide if the drug should remain on the market. This was 5 months after the damning Senate report, but that didn't deter the higher-ups in the agency from more wrongdoing. In an unprecedented move, the FDA invited additional people to its meeting who had been involved in a similar 2007 meeting but were no longer active members of either committee.[16] Most of these people had voted for keeping the drug on the market in 2007, and their addition to the 2010 meeting tipped the scale from voting for a withdrawal to voting for keeping it on the market, which was what the FDA decided.

The scandal rambled on. In 2009, Glaxo started the TIDE trial, scheduled to end in 2015.[10] It is unethical, as it compares the cardiovascular safety of rosiglitazone and pioglitazone, although the company knew that rosiglitazone increases the risk of myocardial infarction compared to pioglitazone.[10] Furthermore, the information given to patients being asked to volunteer for the trial was seriously misleading and therefore also unethical.[17] Because US and European physicians were not willing to enrol patients, Glaxo exploited developing countries,[2] but in 2010 India's drug controller stopped the trial. Two FDA safety officers also suggested to stop the trial, as it was unethical and exploitative, and to take rosiglitazone off the market, as it causes 500 heart attacks and 300 cases of heart failure every month in the United States.[11] Nothing was done initially, but later the FDA halted the trial.[17]

The same year, Glaxo had the nerve to say in a statement to the *BMJ* that the RECORD trial had shown its drug performed similarly as the comparators.[3] Glaxo also said that a head-to-head trial would prove that rosiglitazone doesn't increase the risk of myocardial infarction and that the evidence suggesting that it does was 'not scientific'.[18] Glaxo's lies are not of this world.

In 2010, Steven Nissen published 'The rise and fall of rosiglitazone', an online editorial in the *European Heart Journal*. Glaxo's head of research and development, Moncef Slaoui, wrote to the journal that Nissen's editorial was 'rife with inaccurate representations and speculation that fall well outside the realm of accepted scientific debate. We strongly disagree with several key points within the editorial, most importantly those which imply misconduct on the part of GSK.'[19] Slaoui asked the journal to withdraw the editorial from its website and not to print it in the journal's hardcopy edition 'until the journal has investigated these inaccuracies and unsubstantiated allegations'. When the journal didn't give in but published the editorial in print, Slaoui said that there was 'absolutely no attempt to suppress' the editorial. Glaxo called Nissen's meta-analysis a hypothesis that had not been confirmed by more recent and considerably more robust evidence from prospective, long-term cardiovascular outcomes studies.[20] *Absolute bullshit.* A meta-analysis of the randomised trials is the most reliable evidence we have and it is not a hypothesis; it provides definitive proof. Glaxo also remarked that 'The American Heart Association and the American College of Cardiology Foundation had said that "insufficient data exist to support the choice of pioglitazone over rosiglitazone".' If that is true, it only shows how corrupt these organisations are. They should be the most concerned when a drug causes heart attacks.

So what *did* the FDA do when it didn't want to lower the number of deaths among diabetes patients by taking the drug off the market as in Europe? It issued meaningless warnings, the standard fake fix.[21] It stated that rosiglitazone should only be used in patients already being treated with the drug, and in those patients whose blood sugar cannot be controlled with other drugs and who, after consulting with their healthcare professional, do not wish to use pioglitazone.

Can you see what's wrong with this advice? At least four things. First, why on earth should a patient continue with a harmful drug only because the patient is already on the drug? I think the patients would prefer a less harmful drug, as you never know when a myocardial infarction strikes.

Second, we don't use drugs to control blood sugar but to lower the risk of complications to diabetes such as cardiovascular events. So, do get off the drug immediately, no matter what the FDA says!

Third, as the endocrinologists thought it was a wonder drug, it might not be a good idea for the patient to consult 'their healthcare professional'. In fact, it has been shown that doctors who take money from manufacturers of rosiglitazone were substantially more prone to recommend the drug than other doctors, even after the FDA had warned about its cardiovascular harms.[22]

Fourth, what plausible reason could there be that a patient would *not* want to use pioglitazone when that drug seems to be safer (see below)?

The FDA's stubbornness is a considerable threat to public health. By 2009, even the heavily industry-supported endocrinologists (*see* Chapter 8) had woken up and a consensus group of the US and the European diabetes associations unanimously advised against using rosiglitazone.[2]

These events are so bizarre that they raise uncomfortable questions. Did someone higher up in the FDA hierarchy receive a load of money from Glaxo at some secret bank account or in a suitcase that left no trails? Considering the enormous sales of rosiglitazone, even $100 million in bribes would be peanuts. I am not saying this happened, but if not, what could then be the explanation for this series of implausible events? Future rewards?

The oddities don't even stop there. The risk of myocardial infarction with rosiglitazone seems to be increased by about 80%, and in 2010, the FDA decided that trials of diabetes drugs should show that the risk of cardiovascular events is clearly less than 80%.[23] To allow this degree of permitted risk is incredible, particularly since we use diabetes drugs to *decrease* the cardiovascular risk, certainly not to allow a certain *increase*.

The asymmetry and lack of consistency in regulatory decision making is dangerous for the patients. In 2007, there was almost unanimous agreement in the FDA advisory committee that rosiglitazone increases cardiovascular risk, but the committee nevertheless recommended the drug should stay on the market. If there had been almost unanimous agreement about the harms when the drug was first submitted for marketing approval, it would hardly have been approved.[24]

Assertions that a drug agency considers that a drug's benefits outweigh its harms, which we hear all the time when troubles accumulate, also for rosiglitazone in 2007,[24] are unhelpful. It's not easy to compare benefits and harms, as they aren't measured on the same scale, and it's never made explicit how agencies arrive at gracious conclusions, which – more than anything else – seem to be convenience statements aimed at getting the agency off the hook and avoid disturbing their industry friends and their powerful allies among the politicians.

The FDA's meaningless warnings about rosiglitazone are typical. If you analyse the text in package inserts, you'll see how illogical and other-worldly it often is. For many years, I joked about the general warning that a drug should be used with caution in pregnancy. How should this be done? Either you use a drug or you don't. I have kept a 1998 Janssen-Cilag package insert from the time when my children suffered repeatedly from pinworms and the whole family needed treatment. It says that the use of mebendazole (Vermox) during pregnancy and breast feeding should always occur in consultation with the doctor because there is no experience with the use of the drug under these conditions. Great advice. What exactly is the doctor supposed to do? In this case, the doctor was me or my wife, as we are both doctors. She wasn't pregnant but if she had been, we would have preferred to live with anal itching rather than running an unknown risk of giving birth to a malformed baby.

Pioglitazone causes heart failure but is still on the market, as it is believed to be safer than rosiglitazone.[11] However, serious questions about trial conduct have been raised also for this drug. A large trial, the PROactive study of 5238 patients comparing pioglitazone with placebo, failed to find a significant benefit ($P = 0.10$) for its primary outcome, which was a composite endpoint of various adverse cardiovascular events.[25] This was the true result. The drug didn't work. The trial protocol had been published and it stated that this outcome was chosen because the aim of the study was to evaluate the overall effects on macrovascular disease.[26] However, when the trial was published in the *Lancet*, there was an additional composite outcome, which consisted of patients who died or had a non-fatal heart attack or stroke, and for which P was 0.03. *This was called the main secondary endpoint, although it didn't exist in the protocol.*

Several observers commented on the discrepancy, and the authors, which included two people from the sponsors, Eli Lilly and Takeda, defended themselves by saying that the new composite outcome was introduced in the final statistical analysis plan, which was released in May 2005 and sent to the FDA.[27] They also said that it's legitimate to change outcomes during a study's conduct provided it's agreed 'before any knowledge of unblinded data by the trialists'. Finally, they stated that 'The PROactive Executive Committee was not aware of any results of the study before the official unblinding of the study on May 25, 2005.'

It is important to be the devil's advocate here, as we know we cannot trust drug companies. The final visits for all patients were completed in January 2005, 4 months before the analysis plan was changed and a new outcome was invented. Both companies were represented at the steering committee and its executive committee. Furthermore, the statements in the authors' defence were carefully worded, as if they had been cleared with lawyers. Could a company statistician have peeped at the data behind the academic investigators' back before the final analysis plan was 'suggested' to them?

Such a scenario isn't speculative. As noted in Chapter 5, we analysed 44 protocols for industry-sponsored trials and found it was stated explicitly in 16 cases that the sponsor had access to accumulating data while a trial was running.[28]

Who knows in how many other cases the sponsor had access to the data but was smart enough not to write this in the protocol? It reflects poor trial conduct and isn't something the companies want to tell the world about, as it was only mentioned in one of the 44 publications.

If that were the case for the PROactive study, all of the statements in the *Lancet* letter might nonetheless have been technically correct. The trialists *might not* have been unblinded and the executive committee *might not* have known about the results. But the company statistician likely knew about the results because the trial had a Data and Safety Monitoring Board, whose job it is to warn about excessive harms that might emerge while the trial is running.

For obvious reasons, we should be deeply sceptical towards companies finalising statistical analysis plans after a lot of data have arrived. The incentive to cheat is huge and, as noted earlier, the difference between an honest data analysis and a less honest data analysis can be worth billions on the world market. It shouldn't surprise anybody that cheating is exceedingly common, but until recently, it was difficult to prove, as trial protocols were regarded as confidential. We succeeded to get access to a cohort of protocols submitted to a research ethics committee in Copenhagen that allowed us to study the extent of cheating with the predeclared outcomes.[29] We identified 102 protocols, which included both industry-funded (about three-quarters) and non-industry-funded trials that had all been published. To our great surprise, at least one protocol-defined *primary outcome* had been changed in 63% of the trials. And in 33% of the trials, a new primary outcome was introduced in the published report that didn't exist in the protocol. Here comes the worst part:

> Not a single publication acknowledged that primary outcomes had been changed!

The reason this is so devastating for the trustworthiness of trials is that there are often many outcomes, which may be further divided or combined, creating even more chances of hitting the bull's eye. Imagine you fire a gun towards many targets that are partly overlapping. Even if you are a poor shot, there is a good chance you'll hit near the centre of one of the targets. If you want to cheat, you'll say that the target you hit was also the one you aimed at. Even better, you may wipe out some or all of the other targets before you invite the audience in to see how good a shot you are. Wiping out other targets corresponds to not mentioning outcomes stated in your protocol, another common practice in clinical trials. We found that 71% of the trials had at least one unreported outcome, and in these trials, a median of four efficacy and three harms outcomes were missing in the publications.[29]

We have published other revealing papers based on our cohort of trial protocols. For example, we found unacknowledged discrepancies between protocols and publications for sample size calculations (18/34 trials), methods of handling protocol deviations (19/43), missing data (39/49), primary outcome analyses (25/42), subgroup analyses (25/25) and adjusted analyses (23/28).[30] Interim analyses were described in 13 protocols but mentioned in only five corresponding publications.

It is clear that trial reports cannot be trusted and that we need to have access to the full protocols and the raw data. The EMA agrees. The rosiglitazone scandal made the EMA's new director Guido Rasi say in 2012 that the agency needs to analyse the raw data rather than accepting aggregated information submitted by drug companies seeking approval.[31]

Speaking of statistics, there is another issue with the PROactive trial that smells. The trial report mentions 14 cases of bladder cancer on drug and 6 on placebo. This difference wasn't statistically significant (P = 0.07) and could therefore be explained away by the company's salespeople.[32] However, 4 years later it was revealed that one of the cases in the placebo group was benign, and 14 versus 5 is statistically significant (P = 0.04). The reason this smells is that such 'errors' always favour the company that controls data analysis and the writing of the report.

A final point that the glitazones illustrate so nicely is that we cannot rely on surrogate outcomes. Rosiglitazone and pioglitazone reduce glucose to the same degree and both increase the risk of heart failure. However, while rosiglitazone definitely increases cardiovascular events, the overall effect of pioglitazone is more uncertain.[24,25,33] In 2011, four members of the EMA committee dealing with an application for generic pioglitazone gave a divergent statement: 'It appears impossible to define a subpopulation of diabetic patients where the benefits of pioglitazone would outweigh its risks.'[33]

Sometimes, researchers declare they have validated a surrogate marker. Don't believe them, as it cannot be done. All drugs have many effects, and we cannot pick just one of them and say that this effect will tell us what we need to know. For example, both rosiglitazone and pioglitazone increase body weight and fractures, and rosiglitazone has an adverse effect on LDL cholesterol, none of which are related to their effect on glucose.[15,25] In the PROactive study, pioglitazone increased body weight by 4 kg compared to placebo, which isn't a beneficial effect for patients with diabetes.[25] It was also worrying that for every 62 patients treated with pioglitazone, one additional patient was admitted to hospital with heart failure, which is a serious condition. In 2011, the FDA warned that pioglitazone 'may be associated with an increased risk of bladder cancer'.[34] There it is again: *may be associated with an increased risk*. Three wool-in-mouth terms in just seven words. Drug agencies just *won't* acknowledge the harms of drugs they have approved. Pioglitazone more than doubles the incidence of bladder cancer and was withdrawn for this reason in France in 2001.[35] When I drink whiskey or have sex, I cannot say it *may be associated with an increased chance* of well-being. It feels good.

Troglitazone (Rezulin) was withdrawn in the UK in 1997 and in the United States in 2000 because it *may be associated with an increased risk* of liver failure; sorry, I meant it *causes* liver failure.[3] It was approved despite doubts about both efficacy and safety,[36] but the experienced FDA medical officer who had reviewed the drug was removed at the request of the company, Parke-Davis, before the advisory committee vote.[37] (I fully understand if you have become angry after having seen so much fraud and abuse of power that harm and kill patients, but that's exactly why I wrote this book: to wake people up to what is happening. The worst is still to come, in the next two chapters about psychiatric drugs.) Parke-Davis cheated the advisory committee by saying that the risk of liver toxicity was comparable to placebo and that additional data from other studies confirmed that the rate of liver damage was 'very, very similar'.[38] When the company provided these additional data a week after approval, they showed a substantially greater risk with the drug than with placebo. As usual, the FDA responded by a fake fix. It advised monthly liver function tests, but they were rarely performed, e.g. in only 1% of patients after four months.[39] What is more serious is that it's a fatally incorrect assumption that liver tests prevent liver failure.[37]

Outright fraud was also an issue. When cases of serious liver damage accumulated, Parke-Davis tightened the criterion for 'abnormal' for those treated with its drug but not for those treated with placebo, whereby they obscured the true risk for the FDA.[38] When a new advisory committee reviewed the drug again in March 1999, the committee voted 11 to 1 to keep it on the market, but *nine of the 10 physicians who reported on safety were paid consultants to the company.*[37] Is there anything the FDA *doesn't* allow?

In Europe, Glaxo Wellcome took Rezulin off the UK market after only 3 months because of rapidly increasing reports of liver damage, and Glaxo and the Japanese company that had developed the product withdrew applications for marketing in 26 additional countries.[38]

At the FDA, however, the story rolled on, as depressing as always: intimidation of scientists that warned about the drug and protection of the drug by higher-ups.[39] David Graham reported that the drug increased the risk of liver failure by a factor of 1200, whereas the company, assisted by nine prominent diabetes experts who were later shown to be on company payroll, claimed the incidence was only one in 100 000. I greatly admire people like Graham who against all odds stay at the FDA and do what they can to protect patients, when most people with their heart in the right place would have run screamingly away from an institution like that.

Parke-Davis continued lying. It wrote to US doctors that Glaxo Wellcome had temporarily suspended marketing and that it only had experience with 5000 patients, although Glaxo's decision was based on cases of liver failure worldwide including those in the United States.[38] The company also reassured the doctors that the new reports had not indicated a greater potential for serious harm than previously estimated.

At the same time, the NIH conducted a trial to see if troglitazone could prevent healthy people becoming diabetic. The director of its diabetes division, Richard Eastman, wrote to the doctors who had enrolled patients that Glaxo's decision was apparently a marketing decision and that the NIH was comfortable with continuing with troglitazone. Eastman had received over $78 000 from the company as a consultant to Parke-Davis, but when this was revealed in a newspaper, neither his boss nor the university-based chairman of the study saw any problems with it.[38] Six months after Eastman's reassuring letter, a healthy teacher died of rapidly progressing liver failure and there was no way the regular liver tests could have prevented this from happening. At this point, the NIH discontinued the troglitazone arm in their study, but the drug remained on the US market for almost another 2 years. Why? Why 3 years more in the United States than in the United Kingdom?

Independent researchers saved the FDA from yet another diabetes scandal. Muraglitazar has a similar mechanism of action to the glitazones, and an FDA advisory committee recommended approval of the drug. However, independent researchers who analysed the trial data submitted to the FDA found that Bristol-Myers Squibb and Merck had produced flawed analyses and that the drug was harmful.[40,41] The companies' presentations to the advisory committee concluded that no significant excess risk of deaths or cardiovascular events occurred with muraglitazar. However, there was a two-fold increased risk in the composite outcome of death, heart attack or stroke and a seven-fold increase in heart failure (albeit with a wide confidence interval). The drug also increased weight and oedema, like the glitazones do. The Freedom of Information Act made the independent analysis possible, and it saved many lives. Although the FDA had already prepared an approval letter, it refused to approve the drug after this analysis.

I have no doubt about what I would do if I should get type 2 diabetes. I would eat less and exercise more. These are highly effective interventions, the best we have, considering also that they won't kill us. However, when the non-profit American Diabetes Association on its website announced that diabetes management involves more than blood sugar control, namely blood pressure and cholesterol control, there was nothing about the best interventions, weight loss and exercise.[42] Perhaps because the so-called non-profit organisations leading this initiative had many corporate sponsors: AstraZeneca, Aventis, Bristol-Myers Squibb, Eli Lilly, GlaxoSmithKline, Merck/Schering-Plough, Monarch, Novartis, Pfizer and Wyeth.

If I decided to take a drug, it would be metformin, which is old and very cheap, and which – in contrast to the other drugs – actually *reduces* cardiovascular morbidity and all-cause mortality, and even reduces body weight slightly. It is clearly the best drug,[43] and was introduced to the United Kingdom already in 1958, in Canada in 1972, but not in the United States until 1995.[44] Perhaps it tells us something about unrestrained capitalism and US healthcare that the FDA has been so quick to approve expensive and harmful drugs while the best and cheapest drug was introduced so late (*see also* Chapter 21).

The extent to which the diabetes area has been corrupted is sickening. The Endocrine Society in the United States is supposed to be an academic society for diabetes doctors, but it invites companies to 'get complete access to the endocrine marketplace by partnering with the Endocrine Society', which offers 'the full range of endocrinologists you want to reach ... to fit your needs'.[37] I could vomit. The Society's first practice guideline recommended testosterone to be measured in all men above 50 years of age and also that treatment might be warranted even if the level wasn't low when the symptoms suggested hormone deficiency.[37] I could vomit again. A horrendously dangerous guideline, as testosterone increases the risk of prostate cancer and as no screening trials have ever been performed that might tell us whether this advice does more harm than good. Such a trial is actually not needed. I am pretty sure it would show that screening for 'low testosterone' – whatever that is supposed to mean – is harmful. I don't understand why my colleagues have sold out of their common sense; money isn't that important, particularly not for people who are already very wealthy. It's greed.

NOVO NORDISK INTERFERES WITH AN ACADEMIC PUBLICATION

In 2011, academic researchers published a paper in *Gastroenterology* that reported an increased risk of pancreatitis and pancreatic cancer in patients with diabetes treated with two glucagon-like peptide-1 drugs. They had used the FDA's database of reported adverse events of drugs and an elegant design. Their results were convincing, and they also agreed with animal experiments and an analysis performed by the Drug Commission of the German Medical Association that found 11 reports of pancreatic cancer with one of the drugs, which was an unusually high number compared with other diabetes drugs.[45]

The study was published on the journal's website in February 2011, which said it was an unedited manuscript that had been accepted for publication, and that the manuscript would undergo copyediting, typesetting and review of the resulting proof before it was published in its final form.

Novo Nordisk has a glucagon-like peptide-1 drug on the market, liraglutide (Victoza), and its research director, Mads Krogsgaard Thomsen, wrote a six-page letter to the editor, 'Potentially damaging controversial analysis to be published in Gastroenterology'. The letter ended by saying: 'On behalf of Novo Nordisk, in order to ensure the most optimal guidance to patients and public reaction, we would urge Gastroenterology to withhold the publication of Elashoff *et al.* until it has been confirmed by an independent statistical analysis.'

There was no threat of litigation, but every editor knows that when a company's sales are threatened and it shows its muscle, this is always a possibility. The editor retracted the article, which was republished in the print journal in July 2011, after the authors had looked at their data again, with the same findings.[46]

It's appalling that a drug company interferes with academic publication. Publication on a journal's website is publication and according to the International Committee of Medical Journal Editors, a journal should in no instance remove an article from its website.[47] People can have their say in letters to the editor and corrections can be posted if needed. It was wrong of the editor to withdraw the paper, and it's essential that we oppose gangster methods and do our utmost to protect our academic freedom, without which the progress of science will wither. We shouldn't be afraid of threats of litigation when we have done honest science; we must stand by it. Elephants often threaten; they rarely attack.

Novo's actions become particularly absurd when we consider the facts. When Novo sought approval of the drug, grave concerns about liraglutide were raised at the FDA by two reviewing pharmacologists and a clinical safety reviewer.[48] The safety reviewer said in her statement that she didn't recommend approval because 'In the United States, there are already 11 classes of drugs approved for glycemic control in type 2 diabetes ... The need for new therapies for type 2 diabetes is not so urgent that one must tolerate a significant degree of uncertainty regarding serious risk concerns.'

Victoza was approved in January 2010 against the advice of the FDA's own reviewers. The director of the FDA's Office of Drug Evaluation II, Curtis Rosebraugh, swept aside their criticisms and explained that while 'many sponsors may responsibly introduce a drug into marketing, theirs is a profit-based business and the pressures to generate revenue are strong. Also, with most classes of drugs, there are similar drugs in development from competitors which places even more pressure to generate profit before there is more competition'. Sydney Wolfe from Public Citizen said about this remark that it was the kind of comment one would expect from the drug's sponsor or from Wall Street, not from a high-ranking FDA official.

In June 2011, Novo had warned all US doctors about the adverse effects of Victoza. The FDA had demanded this after a study had shown the doctors had far too little focus on the harms of the drug.[49] The FDA warned that the drug may cause thyroid tumours and pancreatitis, which is a risk factor for pancreatic cancer. It also stated that it shouldn't be used as initial treatment until additional studies had been completed, and required studies of cardiovascular safety and establishment of a cancer registry to study the occurrence of thyroid and other cancers.[50]

In April 2012, Public Citizen sent a petition to the FDA asking the agency to ban Victoza.[51] Experiments had shown that mice that were genetically predisposed to pancreatic cancer developed pancreatic cancer more quickly than usual in response to one of the glucagon-like peptide-1 drugs.

I believe the academic researchers were right and that we shall see a withdrawal of Victoza because of its harms. Just like so many other diabetes drugs and those that should have been withdrawn but never were, like tolbutamide (*see* Chapter 10) and rosiglitazone in the United States.

REFERENCES

1 Strengthening the credibility of clinical research. *Lancet.* 2010; **375**: 1225.
2 Nissen S. Slides presented at the FDA advisory meeting about rosiglitazone. 2010 July 13.
3 Cohen D. Rosiglitazone: what went wrong? *BMJ.* 2010; **341**: 530–4.
4 Harris G. Diabetes drug maker hid test data. *New York Times.* 2010 July 13.
5 Gøtzsche PC. Why we need easy access to all data from all clinical trials and how to accomplish it. *Trials.* 2011; **12**: 249.
6 Khan H, Thomas P. Drug giant AstraZeneca to pay $520 million to settle fraud case. ABC News. 2010 April 27.
7 Bass A. *Side Effects – a prosecutor, a whistleblower, and a bestselling antidepressant on trial.* Chapel Hill: Algonquin Books; 2008.
8 Nissen SE, Wolski K. Effect of rosiglitazone on the risk of myocardial infarction and death from cardiovascular causes. *N Engl J Med.* 2007; **356**: 2457–71.
9 Nissen SE. Setting the RECORD straight. *JAMA.* 2010; **303**: 1194–5.
10 Mitka M. Critics press FDA to act on evidence of rosiglitazone's cardiac safety issues. *JAMA.* 2010; **303**: 2341–2.
11 Moynihan R. Rosiglitazone, marketing, and medical science. *BMJ.* 2010; **340**: c1848.
12 Home PD, Pocock SJ, Beck-Nielsen H, *et al.* Rosiglitazone evaluated for cardiovascular outcomes – an interim analysis. *N Engl J Med.* 2007; **357**: 28–38.
13 Home PD, Pocock SJ, Beck-Nielsen H, *et al.* Rosiglitazone evaluated for cardiovascular outcomes in oral agent combination therapy for type 2 diabetes (RECORD): a multicentre, randomised, open-label trial. *Lancet.* 2009; **373**: 2125–35.
14 Psaty BM, Prentice RL. Minimizing bias in randomized trials: the importance of blinding. *JAMA.* 2010; **304**: 793–4.
15 Psaty BM, Furberg CD. The record on rosiglitazone and the risk of myocardial infarction. *N Engl J Med.* 2007; **357**: 67–9.
16 Graham D, Gelperin K. More on advisory committee decision. *BMJ.* 2010; **341**: 519.
17 Mello MM, Goodman SN, Faden RR. Ethical considerations in studying drug safety – the Institute of Medicine report. *N Engl J Med.* 2012; **367**: 959–64.

18 Cohen D. FDA puts rosiglitazone post-marketing trial on hold. *BMJ*. 2010; **341**: c4017.

19 Tanne JH. GSK is accused of trying to suppress editorial on rosiglitazone. *BMJ*. 2010; **340**: c2654.

20 Slaoui M. The rise and fall of rosiglitazone: reply. *Eur Heart J*. 2010; **31**: 1282–4.

21 FDA Drug Safety Communication. *Avandia (Rosiglitazone) Labels now Contain Updated Information about Cardiovascular Risks and Use in Certain Patients*. 2011 Mar 3.

22 Wang AT, McCoy CP, Murad MH, *et al*. Association between industry affiliation and position on cardiovascular risk with rosiglitazone: cross sectional systematic review. *BMJ*. 2010; **340**: c1344.

23 Lehman R, Yudkin JS, Krumholz HM. Licensing drugs for diabetes. *BMJ*. 2010; **341**: 513–14.

24 Solomon DH, Winkelmayer WC. Cardiovascular risk and the thiazolidinediones: déjà vu all over again? *JAMA*. 2007; **298**: 1216–18.

25 Dormandy JA, Charbonnel B, Eckland DJ, *et al*. Secondary prevention of macrovascular events in patients with type 2 diabetes in the PROactive Study (PROspective pioglitAzone Clinical Trial In macroVascular Events): a randomised controlled trial. *Lancet*. 2005; **366**: 1279–89.

26 Charbonnel B, Dormandy J, Erdmann E, *et al*. The prospective pioglitazone clinical trial in macrovascular events (PROactive): can pioglitazone reduce cardiovascular events in diabetes? Study design and baseline characteristics of 5238 patients. *Diabetes Care*. 2004; **27**: 1647–53.

27 PROactive Study Executive Committee and Data and Safety Monitoring Committee. PROactive study. *Lancet*. 2006; **367**: 982.

28 Gøtzsche PC, Hróbjartsson A, Johansen HK, *et al*. Constraints on publication rights in industry-initiated clinical trials. *JAMA*. 2006; **295**: 1645–6.

29 Chan A-W, Hróbjartsson A, Haahr MT, *et al*. Empirical evidence for selective reporting of outcomes in randomized trials: comparison of protocols to published articles. *JAMA*. 2004; **291**: 2457–65.

30 Chan A-W, Hróbjartsson A, Jørgensen KJ, *et al*. Discrepancies in sample size calculations and data analyses reported in randomised trials: comparison of publications with protocols. *BMJ*. 2008; **337**: a2299.

31 Jack A. European drugs watchdog to step up scrutiny. *Financial Times*. 2012 March 6.

32 Hillaire-Buys D, Faillie JL, Montastruc JL. Pioglitazone and bladder cancer. *Lancet*. 2011; **378**: 1543–4.

33 European Medicines Agency. *Assessment report, Pioglitazone ratio*. EMA/391408/2012. 2012 May 24.

34 Ray WA, Stein CM. Reform of drug regulation – beyond an independent drug-safety board. *N Engl J Med*. 2006; **354**: 194–201.

35 Hillaire-Buys D, Faillie JL. Pioglitazone and the risk of bladder cancer. *BMJ*. 2012; **344**: e3500.

36 FDA Drug Safety Communication. *Update to Ongoing Safety Review of Actos (pioglitazone) and Increased Risk of Bladder Cancer*. 2011 June 6.

37 Kassirer JP. *On the Take: how medicine's complicity with big business can endanger your health*. Oxford: Oxford University Press; 2005.

38 Avorn J. *Powerful Medicines: the benefits, risks, and costs of prescription drugs*. New York: Vintage Books; 2005.

39 Brody H. *Hooked: ethics, the medical profession, and the pharmaceutical industry*. Lanham: Rowman & Littlefield; 2008.

40 Nissen SE, Wolski K, Topol EJ. Effect of muraglitazar on death and major adverse cardiovascular events in patients with type 2 diabetes mellitus. *JAMA*. 2005; **294**: 2581–6.

41 Brophy JM. Selling safety – lessons from muraglitazar. *JAMA*. 2005; **294**: 2633–5.

42 Abramson J. *Overdo$ed America*. New York: HarperCollins; 2004.

43 Saenz A, Fernandez-Esteban I, Mataix A, *et al*. Metformin monotherapy for type 2 diabetes mellitus. *Cochrane Database Syst Rev*. 2005; **3**: CD002966.

44 Wikipedia. Metformin. Available online at: http://en.wikipedia.org/wiki/Metformin (accessed 12 October 2012).

45 Spranger J, Gundert-Remy U, Stammschulte T. GLP-1-based therapies: the dilemma of uncertainty. *Gastroenterology*. 2011; **141**: 20–3.

46 Elashoff M, Matveyenko AV, Gier B, *et al*. Pancreatitis, pancreatic, and thyroid cancer with glucagon-like peptide-1-based therapies. *Gastroenterology*. 2011; **141**: 150–6.

47 Gøtzsche PC, Mæhlen J, Zahl PH. What is publication? *Lancet*. 2006; **368**: 1854–6.

48 Public citizen to FDA: pull diabetes drug Victoza from market immediately. *Public Citizen*. 2012 April 19.

49 Lindeberg M. [Novo Nordisk has sent warnings about the cancer risk with its diabetes drug Victoza to US physicians]. *Berlingske*. 2011 June 14.

50 US Food and Drug Administration. *FDA Approves New Treatment for Type 2 Diabetes*. 2010 Jan 25.

51 Maxmen A. Debate on diabetes drugs gathers pace: petition unveils unnerving reports on potential carcinogenicity of GLP-1 mimics. *Nature*. 2012 April 30.

Psychiatry, the drug industry's paradise

There is probably no other area of medicine in which the academic literature is so at odds with the raw data.

David Healy, psychiatrist[1]

Leaving the determination of whether mental illness exists strictly to the psychiatrists is like leaving the determination of the validity of astrology in the hands of professional astrologers ... people are unlikely to question the underlying premises of their occupations, in which they often have a large financial and emotional stake.

Judi Chamberlin, former mental patient[2]

I have spent most of my professional life evaluating the quality of clinical research, and I believe it is especially poor in psychiatry. The industry-sponsored studies ... are selectively published, tend to be short-term, designed to favor the drug, and show benefits so small that they are unlikely to outweigh the long-term harms.

Marcia Angell, former editor, *New England Journal of Medicine*[3]

ARE WE ALL CRAZY OR WHAT?

Psychiatry is the drug industry's paradise as definitions of psychiatric disorders are vague and easy to manipulate.[2,4] Leading psychiatrists are therefore at high risk of corruption and, indeed, psychiatrists collect more money from drug makers than doctors in any other specialty.[5,6] Those who take most money tend to prescribe antipsychotics to children most often.[5] Psychiatrists are also 'educated' with industry's hospitality more often than any other specialty.[7]

This has dire consequences for the patients. The *Diagnostic and Statistical Manual of Mental Disorders* (DSM) from the American Psychiatric Association (APA) has become infamous. It is now so bad that Allen Frances, who chaired the task force for DSM-IV (which lists 374 different ways to be mentally ill; up from 297 in DSM-III)[2] believes the responsibility for defining psychiatric conditions needs to be taken away from the APA.[4] Frances has warned that DSM-V could unleash multiple new false positive epidemics, not only because of industry money but also because researchers push for greater recognition of their pet conditions. He noted that already the DSM-IV created three false epidemics because the diagnostic criteria were too wide: attention deficit hyperactivity disorder (ADHD), autism and childhood bipolar disorder.

According to Frances, new diagnoses are as dangerous as new drugs: 'We have remarkably casual procedures for defining the nature of conditions, yet they can lead to tens of millions being treated with drugs they may not need, and that may harm them.'[4] Drug regulatory agencies should therefore not only evaluate new drugs but should also oversee how new 'diseases' are being created. The confusion and incompetence is so great that the DSM-IV cannot even define what a mental disorder is.[2] I have highlighted in italics some of the wishy-washy bits of the definition:

> A *clinically significant behavioral or psychological syndrome or pattern* that occurs in an individual and that is associated with present distress (e.g., a painful symptom) or disability (i.e., impairment in one or more important areas of functioning) or with a *significantly increased risk* of suffering death, pain, disability, or an important loss of freedom. In addition, this syndrome or pattern must not be merely an *expectable and culturally sanctioned response* to a particular event, for example, the death of a loved one. Whatever its original cause, *it must currently be considered* a manifestation of a behavioral, psychological, or biological *dysfunction* in the individual. Neither deviant behavior ... nor conflicts that are *primarily* between the individual and society are mental disorders unless the deviance or conflict is a *symptom of a dysfunction* in the individual.

It would be easy to improve on all this ambiguity and subjectivity and arrive at a more meaningful and robust definition. The DSM is a consensus document, which makes it unscientific. The Royal College of Physicians doesn't seek website comments from the public on the diagnosis of breast cancer and 'Real sciences do not decide on the existence and nature of the phenomena they are dealing with via a show of hands with a vested interest and pharmaceutical industry sponsorship.'[8] Homosexuality was listed as a mental disorder till 1974 when 61% of the psychiatrists voted to have it removed, only to retain something called Ego Dystonic Homosexuality for those who felt uncomfortable about others' condemnation of their sexual orientation!

Psychologist Paula Caplan was involved with updating the DSM to its fourth edition and she fought hard to get the silliest ideas out.[2] In 1985, the APA decided to introduce Masochistic Personality Disorder to be used for women who were beaten up by their husbands. Caplan and her colleagues felt the proper response to this should be Macho Personality Disorder for the violent males, but they settled with Delusional Dominating Personality Disorder. They suggested to the APA committee that this would apply if a male fulfilled six of 14 criteria, of which the first was 'Inability to establish and maintain meaningful interpersonal relationships'. The chairman, Allen Frances, asked what the empirical documentation was for this disorder and warned that it would be folly to open the floodgates to new and unsupported diagnoses. An interesting remark considering what was already included in DSM-III.

The people who develop DSM have heavy conflicts of interest and creating many diagnoses means big business in all sorts of ways and fame and power for those at the top.[2] But does it help people to be labelled? Some of us still remember Minimal Brain Damage Dysfunction, which was thrown in the faces of millions of parents, and which could only be harmful, as there was nothing they could do whatever the problem was, if any. Other elastic diagnoses that could be used for most healthy people are Oppositional Defiant Disorder for children and Self-Defeating Personality Disorder for women.

Labelling women with Premenstrual Dysphoric Disorder might prevent them from getting a job or have custody of their children in case of a divorce.[2] When the criteria for this diagnosis were tested, it turned out that they couldn't distinguish between women with severe premenstrual symptoms and other women. Even men gave answers similar to those with severe symptoms. But who cares? The FDA obviously didn't. It approved Eli Lilly's antidepressant Prozac (fluoxetine) for this non-disease, which the US psychiatrists even had the gall to call depression![9] Lilly had the audacity to give the drug another name, Sarafem, which was a repainted Prozac with attractive lavender and pink colours.[10] Pretty ironic to use pink as a symbol for a pill that ruins people's sex lives (see below). Since men have the same symptoms, it would seem okay to treat them, too. In Europe, Lilly was forbidden to promote fluoxetine for something that wasn't considered a disease, and the EMA fiercely criticised the company's trials, which had major deficiencies. The Cochrane review of this non-disease included 40 trials and SSRIs were said to be highly effective.[11] Of course. SSRIs have amphetamine-like effects, and some people feel better when they take speed.

Few psychiatrists are willing to admit that their specialty is out of control and they will continue to tell you that many patients are underdiagnosed. This is their standard defence, but under the glittering surface they know that they and their patients have a big problem. In a 2007 survey, 51% of 108 Danish psychiatrists said that they used too much medicine and only 4% that they used too little.[12] In 2009, sales of drugs for the nervous system in Denmark were so high that one-quarter of the whole population could be in treatment every day,[13] and yet Denmark comes out as the most happy nation on earth in poll after poll despite our terrible weather, which should make people depressed.

In the United States, it's even worse. The most sold drugs in 2009 were antipsychotics, and antidepressants came fourth, after lipid-lowering drugs and proton pump inhibitors (used for stomach problems).[14] It's hard to imagine that so many Americans can be so mentally disturbed that these sales reflect genuine needs, but it gets worse all the time, with an alarming speed. In 1990–92, 12% of the US population aged 18–54 years received treatment for emotional problems, which went up to 20% in 2001–2003.[15] Although there are hundreds of diagnoses in DSM-IV, only half of people who were in treatment met diagnostic criteria for a disorder. In 2012, the US Centers for Disease Control reported that 25% of Americans have a mental illness.[16]

Not even our children have avoided the disease mongering. In New Jersey, one in 30 boys is considered to have autistic spectrum disorder,[16] and about a quarter of the children in American summer camps are medicated for ADHD, mood disorder or other psychiatric problems.[17] *One in four, and we are talking about children!* As early as in the 1990s, a quarter of the children in an elementary school in Iowa were on drugs for ADHD,[18] and in California, the diagnosis rates of ADHD increased sharply as school funding declined. About one-fifth of doctors didn't follow the official protocol when making the diagnosis but rather their personal instinct.[19]

Psychiatry is really elastic and has replaced care with pills. Like SSRIs, drugs for ADHD have amphetamine-like effects.[9] That the children can sit still at school cannot be taken as evidence that the diagnosis was correct; it merely shows that speed has this effect (and many others, including apathy, lack of humour and social isolation).

In 2011, an enterprise – evidently working on behalf of an anonymous drug company – sent a most bizarre invitation to Danish specialists treating children and adolescents for ADHD.[20] The doctors would be divided into two groups for an exercise called Wargames where they should defend their product (two different ADHD medicines) with arguments and a visual presentation. Their efforts would be filmed and the company's anonymous client might be watching from another room what went on. This 'Big brother is watching you' exercise was illegal. Danish doctors are not allowed to help companies market their products.

Drugs for ADHD are dangerous. We don't know much about their long-term harms, but we do know that they can damage the heart in the same way as seen in long-term cocaine addicts and lead to death, even in children.[18] We also know that *the ADHD drugs cause bipolar disorder in about 10% of the children*, which is a serious condition.[21]

In 2010, the US Centers for Disease Control and Prevention published a report stating that 9% of the interviewed adults met the criteria for current depression.[22] The criteria were those listed in DSM-IV and very little was needed. You were depressed if you had had little interest or pleasure in doing things for more than half of the days over the past 2 weeks plus one additional 'symptom', which could be many things; for example:[23]
- trouble falling asleep
- poor appetite or overeating
- being so fidgety or restless that you have been moving around a lot more than usual.

This is insane. How on earth did we get to the point of accepting a system that labels one-tenth of the US adult population as depressed at any one time? Are people who do this to us normal, or should we invent a diagnosis for them, e.g. Compulsive Disease Mongering Disorder? Little pleasure in doing things for eight days out of 14 will happen for most people, no matter how positive, active and outgoing they are. Trouble falling asleep is common; many people overeat (otherwise, we wouldn't have an obesity epidemic); and people might move around more than usual if they succeed with something they badly wanted to achieve.

With such an approach to diagnosis, it's easier to understand why *the rate of depression in the population has increased a thousandfold* since the days when we didn't have antidepressant drugs.[24] According to DSM-IV, I have been depressed many times in my life, but according to myself and those who know me I have never been anywhere near being depressed.

Allen Frances found it alarming that one-tenth of Americans were considered depressed and felt that the prescription of antidepressants is increasingly out of control because it is controlled by drug companies who profit from it being out of control.[25] He also noted that DSM-V will further increase overtreatment with antidepressants, for example by medicalising grief, reducing the threshold for generalised anxiety disorder, and introducing new and highly questionable disorders for mixed anxiety/depression and binge eating. It is really perverse. All of us will experience the death of a close relative, but in DSM-V, bereavement is a depressive disorder if it has lasted more than 2 weeks.[26] In DSM-III, that period of time was set at 1 year, and in DSM-IV it was 2 months. Why not 2 hours in DSM-VI? We should allow people to be unhappy at times – which is completely normal – without giving them a diagnosis of depression.

Over the years, many new disorders have been included and existing disorders exploded, e.g. in DSM-III, anxiety neurosis was split into seven new disorders.[27] Another change was the introduction of a symptom-based approach for diagnosis, which has been criticised for creating diseases, and for classifying normal life distress and sadness as mental disease in need of drugs. The criteria for depression no longer distinguish between a disorder and expected reactions to a situational context, for example the loss of a beloved person or other life crises like divorce, serious disease or loss of job, which are no longer mentioned as exclusion criteria when making the diagnosis. These changes, which are so generous towards the drug industry, could be related to the fact that 100% of the DSM-IV panel members on 'mood disorders' had financial ties to the pharmaceutical industry.[27]

The psychiatrists are running amok. The DSM-V committee have had plans for lowering the diagnostic thresholds for many other conditions, e.g. for ADHD and attenuated psychosis syndrome, which describes experiences common in the general population, but the latter diagnosis was dropped.[28] An international protest has been launched against DSM-V and even the chair of the DSM-III task force, Robert Spitzer, is critical towards the major revisions of personality disorders, which often lack any empirical basis.

After my depressing experience with the DSM-IV criteria for depression, I looked up Psych Central, a large website that has been highly praised by neutral observers and has won awards. It offers many tests, even including one for psychopaths, and its slogan is: 'You're going to be okay, we're here to help.' It's comforting to know that if you break down under the weight of the diagnoses after having tried some of the tests, the website offers immediate access to a psychiatrist. You can read about psychotropic drugs and find out which codes in DSM-IV may be appropriate for you. A little experiment I did suggests that there is a diagnosis for each of us. We were eight perfectly normal and successful people that tried the tests for depression, ADHD and mania, and none of us survived all three tests. Two had depression and four had definite, likely or possibly ADHD. Seven of us suffered from mania; one needed immediate treatment (perhaps because she has written a book critical of the drug industry), three had moderate to severe mania, and three had milder degrees. It's not the least surprising that when therapists have been asked to use DSM criteria, a quarter of healthy people also get a psychiatric diagnosis.[2]

One of the new epidemics is bipolar II.[29] Unlike bipolar I, it has no mania or psychotic features, and the diagnostic criteria are very lenient. There only needs to be one episode of depression, and one episode of hypomania lasting more than 4 days. This opens up the floodgate for treating vast numbers of patients with antipsychotic drugs resulting in tremendous harm at a huge cost; even the very old drug quetiapine cost a staggering £2000 a year in the UK in 2011. The diagnosis of hypomania builds on simplistic questions, one of which is 'I drink more coffee'. In trials, bipolar I and II are mixed together so that one cannot see whether antipsychotics have any effect in bipolar II, which is supposed to be milder. A smart marketing trick.

Bipolar illness in children rose 35-fold in 20 years in the United States.[21] It's not only the loose criteria that cause this disaster; both *SSRIs and ADHD drugs cause bipolar illness*, and both types of drugs may lead to conversion of a depression or ADHD, respectively, into bipolar disorder in one out of 10 young people.[30] However, psychiatrists hail this as 'better' diagnosis, or they add insult to injury by saying that the drug unmasked the diagnosis![21]

Even the characters in *Winnie-the-Pooh* have been found to suffer from psychiatric disorders. For example, little Piglet obviously suffers from generalised anxiety disorder and the donkey Eeyore from a dysthymic disorder.[31]

There is a substantial risk of circular evidence in all of this. If a new class of drugs affect mood, appetite and sleep patterns, depression may be defined by industry-supported psychiatrists as a disease that consists of just that; problems with mood, appetite and sleep patterns.[32]

UK general practitioner Des Spence has described eloquently how psychiatry has become so corrupted:[33]

> *Psychiatry has ... become pharma's goldmine, with a simple business plan. Seek a small group of specialists from a prestigious institution. Pharma becomes the professional kingmaker, funding research for these specialists. Research always reports underdiagnosis and undertreatment, never the opposite. Control all data and make the study duration short. Use the media, plant news stories, and bankroll patient support groups. Pay your specialists large advisory fees. Lobby government. Get your pharma sponsored specialists to advise the government. So now the world view is dominated by a tiny group of specialists with vested interests. Use celebrity endorsements to sprinkle on the marketing magic of emotion. Expand the market by promoting online questionnaires that loosen the diagnostic criteria further. Make the illegitimate legitimate.*

Spence mentions that a small Harvard group of world specialists admitted undisclosed personal payments from drug companies totalling $4.2 million.

A review of 43 studies in ADHD, of which 34 were randomised, supports Spence's kingmaker tale. Very few of the reported adverse drug reactions were called serious, although many children dropped out of the studies because of precisely that: serious adverse drug reactions.[34] A large number of studies were conducted by the same groups of authors and sponsored by the companies manufacturing the drugs. Not a set-up that is likely to tell us the true occurrence of serious harms. Many of the studies are also rigged, either by dropping all children who improve on placebo before the trial starts, or the opposite, studying only children who have tolerated the drug before they are randomised to drug or placebo.[18] Such manipulations are very common in trials of psychotropic drugs, also in trials of SSRIs,[24] and they make people think the drugs are much better than they really are. Some trials even use both types of patient cleansing before they are randomised.[21]

PSYCHIATRISTS AS DRUG PUSHERS

Leading psychiatrists are often highly effective drug pushers. In 1999, Charles Nemeroff and Alan Schatzberg published a psychiatry textbook that was ghost-written by GlaxoSmithKline.[35] In 2006, Nemeroff was first author of a review on the effectiveness of a vagal nerve-stimulating device for treatment of severe depression,[36] a truly weird idea. The paper was ghostwritten and published in the journal, Nemeroff edited,[37] and all authors had financial ties to the device makers but none were revealed.[36] The FDA approved the device based upon a senior manager overruling more than 20 FDA scientists as well as other managers who had reviewed the data and concluded that the device didn't demonstrate a reasonable assurance of safety and effectiveness.

There was also corruption at Emory University where Nemeroff worked and at the closely affiliated hospital, Grady Hospital, but it was kept secret for more than a decade.[38] In 2008, Senator Charles Grassley released a damning report about Nemeroff that showed that one reason why the scam could continue for so long was that the whistle-blowers (at least 15) were ordered psychiatric evaluations at Emory's psychiatric department. Emory's own chosen psychiatrists reportedly wrote up such exams without even examining the targeted doctors or gathering factual evidence, whereafter several of them were fired.[39] (I wonder how these same psychiatrists conduct clinical trials for the drug companies.) At least four of the 'evaluations' were done by Nemeroff himself, which made the processes similar in nature to Stalin's processes in the Soviet Union. The staunchest whistle-blower, who sat at the Conflicts of Interests committee at Emory University, refused to get an 'evaluation' after he had blown the whistle on alleged research-funding fraud and he became the victim of more than 12 years of continuing litigation, which he ultimately won.

In 2000, an antidepressant trial was published in the *New England Journal of Medicine* where the authors had so many conflicts of interest that there wasn't room for them in the journal; instead, they were listed on a website.[40] The conflicts of interest for three psychiatrists I comment on in this book were:

Dr. Nemeroff has been a consultant to or received honoraria from Abbott, AstraZeneca, Bristol-Myers Squibb, Forest Laboratories, Janssen, Eli Lilly, Merck, Mitsubishi, Neurocrine Biosciences, Organon, Otsuka, Pfizer, Pharmacia–Upjohn, Sanofi, SmithKline Beecham, Solvay, and Wyeth–Ayerst. He has received research support from Abbott, AstraZeneca, Bristol-Myers Squibb, Forest Laboratories, Janssen, Eli Lilly, Organon, Pfizer, Pharmacia–Upjohn, SmithKline Beecham, Solvay, and Wyeth–Ayerst.

Dr. Schatzberg has served as a consultant to or received honoraria from Abbott, Bristol-Myers Squibb, Corcept Therapeutics, Forest Laboratories, Janssen, Eli Lilly, Merck, Mitsubishi Pharmaceuticals, Organon, Parke-Davis, Pfizer, Pharmacia–Upjohn, Sanofi, Scirex, SmithKline Beecham, Solvay, and Wyeth–Ayerst. He has received research support from Bristol-Myers Squibb, Pfizer, and SmithKline Beecham. He has equity ownership in Corcept, Merck, Pfizer, and Scirex.

Dr. Keller has served as a consultant to or received honoraria from Pfizer, Bristol-Myers Squibb, Forest Laboratories/Parke-Davis, Wyeth–Ayerst, Merck, Janssen, Eli Lilly, Organon, and Pharmacia–Upjohn. He has received research grants from Wyeth–Ayerst, SmithKline Beecham, Upjohn, Pfizer, Bristol-Myers Squibb, Merck, Forest Laboratories, Zeneca, and Organon. He has served on the advisory board of Wyeth–Ayerst, Pfizer, Bristol-Myers Squibb, Eli Lilly, Forest Laboratories/Parke-Davis, Organon, SmithKline Beecham, Merck, Janssen, Mitsubishi Pharmaceuticals, Zeneca, Scirex, and Otsuka.

This trial gave rise to an editorial with the title: 'Is academic medicine for sale?'[41] One wonders when these people have time for seeing the patients. People who take money from many companies usually argue that they are not in the pocket of industry because they are not dependent on any particular company. Accepting this line of reasoning, it should be quite okay to be a prostitute as long as you make sure you have many customers every day so that you aren't dependent on any particular one.

Psychiatry is in deep crisis. It has not only turned what were previously acute conditions chronic (see below), it has also medicalised normality. Psychotropic drugs are being used for the most bizarre ailments, e.g. a trial showed that escitalopram reduced the daily incidence of hot flushes in menopausal women from 10 to 9.[42] This tiny effect might even be non-existing, as many women may have broken the blind as they can feel the difference between an SSRI and a placebo (*see* Chapter 4).

Considering the many effects psychotropic drugs have,[21,24] their massive use is harmful. For example, a carefully controlled cohort study of depressed people over 65 years of age showed that SSRIs more often lead to falls than older antidepressants or if the depression was left untreated.[43] *For every 28 elderly people treated for 1 year with an SSRI, there was one additional death, compared to no treatment.*

THE CHEMICAL IMBALANCE HOAX

Instead of trying to understand the patients, psychiatry has developed into a checklist exercise,[44] which one could ask a secretary or the patients themselves to do. Diagnoses are often made after brief consultations of 10–15 minutes, after which many patients are told that they need a drug for the rest of their life to fix a 'chemical imbalance' in the brain. Very often, they are also told that this is similar to being a patient with diabetes needing insulin.[21] If this were true, the number of disabled mentally ill would have gone down after we introduced the antipsychotics and antidepressants, but instead, the number of people with psychiatric diagnoses and disability pension has skyrocketed. Worst of all, this has also affected our children. In 1987, just before the SSRIs came on the market, very few children were disabled mentally ill in the United States; 20 years later, it was more than 500 000, which was a 35-fold increase.[21]

WHO studies have shown that the patients fare much better in parts of the world where psychotropic drugs are little used, e.g. in poor countries where only 16% of patients with schizophrenia were regularly maintained on antipsychotics as compared with 61% in rich countries.[21] These positive results have been confirmed in Finland where drug use was restricted so that only 20% of patients with schizophrenia took antipsychotics regularly and two-thirds were never exposed to drugs.[21] In the United States, researchers who arrived at similar results experienced that their funding from the National Institute of Mental Health and elsewhere dried out.[21] The news were not welcomed by the psychiatric leaders.

The chemical imbalance story, which is being told about all psychotropic drugs, even for benzodiazepines ('nerve' or sleeping pills),[21] is a big lie. It has never been documented that any of the large psychiatric diseases is caused by a biochemical defect and there is no biological test that can tell us whether someone has a particular mental disorder.[45] As an example, the idea that depressed patients lack serotonin has been convincingly rejected.[24,46] In fact, some drugs that *decrease* serotonin also work for depression,[24,47] e.g. tianeptine, and the Irish drug regulator banned GlaxoSmithKline from claiming that paroxetine corrects a chemical imbalance. There is a lot else that speaks against the chemical imbalance hoax, e.g. it takes weeks before the drugs work.[48]

> *Psychotropic drugs don't fix a chemical imbalance, they cause it, which is why it is so difficult to come off the drugs again. If taken for more than a few weeks, these drugs create the disease they were intended to cure.*[21,24,49–53]
> *We have turned schizophrenia, ADHD and depression, which were often self-limited diseases in the past, into chronic disorders because of the drugs we use.*[21]

People may get terrible symptoms when they try to stop, both symptoms that resemble the disease and many others they have never experienced before. It is most unfortunate that almost all psychiatrists – and the patients themselves – interpret this as a sign that they still need the drug. They usually don't. They have become dependent, just like a junkie is dependent on heroin or cocaine, and as ADHD drugs and SSRIs have amphetamine effects, *we should view these drugs as narcotics on prescription and use them as little as possible.*

Most psychiatric patients would be better off by not receiving drugs at all,[21] (*see also* Chapter 4 and Chapter 18) and those that need treatment usually only need it for a short time or intermittently. Psychiatrists should consider that other medical specialists, unlike psychiatrists, would be very reluctant to offer long-term symptomatic treatment without knowing what lies behind the symptoms, e.g. if a patient suffers from nausea or headache.[3] However, it requires strong determination, time, patience, and a tapering period to get patients off the drugs and minimise the withdrawal symptoms. If patients have been on drugs for years, the tapering period may go up to a full year. Most psychiatrists choose life-long treatment instead, which is a disaster for many reasons. It keeps the patients locked in the patient role and the drugs change their personality so that they don't learn to cope with life's challenges.[21] It also seems likely that not only antipsychotics but all the drugs can cause permanent brain damage and permanent personality changes, e.g. with tardive dyskinesia, cognitive decline and emotional flatness.[21]

The brain damage has been shown to occur at receptor level and there is nothing strange about this, as this is how the brain works. Hashish, LSD and other brain-active substances may also lead to permanent brain damage and psychosis.

The fact that psychotropic drugs in the long run create the diseases they have a short-term effect on has been brought up again and again over the last 30–40 years, but every time, no matter how strong the new evidence, leading psychiatrists have brushed it under the carpet as quickly as possible.[21] It is too painful and too difficult for them to handle. After they put psychoanalysis behind them – which was terribly unscientific, to the point of Sigmund Freud claiming we're all homosexuals and that those of us who think otherwise are latent homosexuals – they embraced biological psychiatry, which made their specialty look as scientific as internal medicine, which it isn't.

It is unhealthy to perturb normal brain functions with drugs whether they are legal or illegal. Psychotropic drugs can lead to violence, including murder. An analysis of adverse drug events submitted to the FDA between 2004 and 2009 identified 1937 cases of violence, 387 of which were homicide.[54] The violence was particularly often reported for psychotropic drugs (antidepressants, sedatives/hypnotics, ADHD drugs and a smoking cessation drug that also affects brain functions). Antidepressants are being suspected of having a causal role in shootings, but when one of the teenage shooters in the Columbine High School massacre was found to have an antidepressant in his blood, the American Psychiatric Association immediately denounced the notion that there could be a causal relation and added that undiagnosed and untreated mental illness exacts a heavy toll on those who suffer from these disorders as well as those around them.[55] This is sickening. It's marketing speak and standard industry tactic to blame the disease and not the drug, but this is what psychiatrists routinely do, in particular when patients who try to stop experience withdrawal symptoms. Psychotropic drugs, including SSRIs, also increase the risk of traffic crashes.[56]

In the United States, people can be prescribed Nuvigil (armodafinil), which, as the name implies, makes you vigil again. It's approved for shift work disorder. I am not joking, the drug exists. People who get tired at nightshifts now have a disorder. Like so many other psychotropic drugs, Nuvigil has effects like amphetamine and cocaine, so it's yet another narcotic on prescription, and as always, the drug may kill you. It can lead to a life-threatening rash (Stevens-Johnson Syndrome), fatal multi-organ failure, mania, delusions, hallucinations, and suicidal ideation, hospitalisation, and a lot else.[57] I'll stick to my coffee, which won't harm me.

SCREENING FOR PSYCHIATRIC DISORDERS

As indicated above, the sure way of making us all crazy is to screen for mental disorders. A notorious programme in the United States was TeenScreen, which came up with the result that one in five children suffered from a mental disorder, leading to a flurry of discussions about a 'crisis' in children's mental health.[18]

The science related to screening for depression is of appallingly poor quality.[58] For example, only in 5% of studies assessing the false positive and false negative results of screening for depression had the researchers excluded patients who were already diagnosed with depression. This flaw is inexcusable. If you want to know how good ultrasound is to pick up cancers in the stomach in people who look healthy, you don't study people who have already been diagnosed with large cancers with ultrasound, the very technique you want to test.

Despite the fact that the authors of the Cochrane review on screening for depression recommended firmly against screening, after having examined 12 trials with 6000 participants,[59] the Danish authorities – after dutifully quoting the Cochrane review – recommended screening for various poorly defined 'risk' groups. The test to be used has been recommended by the WHO, but it's so poor that for every 100 000 healthy people screened, there will be 36 000 false positive.[60] Many of these 36 000 will get a prescription for an SSRI.

Psychiatrists have already created raging epidemics of psychiatric diagnoses, but when I point out to them how harmful screening is, they won't listen. What's wrong with psychiatrists? Why aren't they evidence-based? If I were to nominate a new psychiatric disorder, it would be ODUFD: *Obsessive Denial of Unwelcome Facts Disorder*. It's very common among doctors, politicians and high-level administrators and there is no cure. University administrators are happy to accept enormous gifts from industry at the same time as they implement stringent conflict of interest policies for their faculty and their relationship with commercial sponsors.[61]

UNHAPPY PILLS

I don't think fraud and lies in research and marketing, corruption of doctors, and the insufficiency of drug regulators have been worse than for the so-called happy pills.[21,24,62] The deceptions start already with the name. The term selective serotonin reuptake inhibitors (SSRIs) was invented by SmithKline Beecham, which in 2000 merged into GlaxoSmithKline. Unfortunately, it's the official scientific name of this class of drugs although there is nothing particularly selective about them. They are not particularly specific either. Most substances that affect the brain, including alcohol, are likely to have an effect on depression similar to that of SSRIs,[24] and alprazolam, for example, an old benzodiazepine, is better than placebo and similarly effective as tricyclic antidepressants, although these drugs are better than SSRIs.[63]

Until 2003, the UK drug regulator propagated the hoax about lack of serotonin as the cause of depression in patient information leaflets.[62] No one knows why SSRIs have the effects they have and there isn't much happiness in the pills. Their most pronounced effect is to cause sexual disturbances. An FDA scientist found out that the companies had hidden sexual problems by blaming the patients rather than the drug, e.g. female anorgasmia was coded as 'Female Genital Disorder'.[62] The companies claimed that only 5% of the patients were sexually disturbed,[24] which is one-tenth of the true occurrence. In a study designed to look at this problem, sexual disturbances developed in 59% of 1022 patients who all had a normal sex life before they started using an antidepressant.[64] The symptoms include decreased libido, delayed orgasm or ejaculation, no orgasm or ejaculation and erectile dysfunction, all at a high rate, and with a low tolerance among 40% of the patients. Some patients yawned during orgasm, which isn't the most fantastic way of building up an intimate relationship. These problems have been overlooked because patients aren't likely to discuss them with their doctor. The drugs should therefore have been marketed as a formidable disrupter of your sex life, but that wouldn't have sold many pills.

In Denmark, sales of SSRIs are now so high that 7% of the entire population can be in treatment with an adult dose every day for their entire life.[27] Or every one of us can be in treatment for 6 years of our lives! It's clear that the drug companies are behind the overtreatment. The sales of SSRIs increased almost linearly by a factor of 18, while the number of products on the market (and therefore the marketing pressure) increased by a factor of 16 (r = 0.97, almost perfect correlation).[27] In 2007, no less than 23 different drug companies marketed 47 different products. This enormous marketing pressure has also been important in the United States. Between 1989 and 2000, the use of SSRIs and similar drugs almost trebled in primary care, with each new agent adding to the aggregate use without a concomitant decrease in previously introduced newer agents.[65]

The patients aren't too happy to take happy pills. In clinical trials, doctors have an incentive to persuade the patients to take the drugs, but in general practice, more than half of the patients stop them again within 2–3 months.[62]

PROZAC, A TERRIBLE ELI LILLY DRUG TURNED INTO A BLOCKBUSTER

The first SSRI was fluoxetine (Prozac), which was marketed in 1988. It's a terrible drug and senior management in Lilly wanted to shelve it.[24] But Lilly had a problem. It was in serious financial trouble, and if Prozac failed, Lilly could 'go down the tubes'.[66–68]

Fluoxetine is such a poor drug that the German drug regulator concluded in its assessment: 'Considering the benefit and the risk, we think this preparation totally unsuitable for the treatment of depression.'[24,69] When Eli Lilly showed some of its data to Swedish psychiatrists, they laughed and didn't think Lilly was serious about seeking approval for the drug,[70] and the FDA noted serious flaws in the trials.[24]

However, to survive as a company, Lilly was determined to make Prozac a success, and it was crucial to get Prozac approved in Sweden, as it would then be easier to get it approved by the FDA. The vice president for Europe left no doubt that the managing director for Sweden, John Virapen, needed to do whatever it took to succeed.

Virapen, who felt his future career at Lilly depended on approval of Prozac, solved his problem with bribery. He launched seeding trials before the drug was approved and invited doctors to the Caribbean for a week, with plenty of relaxation, including 'diving, surfing, sailing, pretty girls and hot nights'.[70] By planting indirect questions to the secretaries of prominent psychiatrists, Virapen found out the identity of the independent expert who was going to examine the clinical documentation for the Swedish drug agency. The expert didn't like fluoxetine at all and just 2 weeks earlier, he had laughed about the idea of ever getting fluoxetine approved. However, already at their second meeting, he suggested $20000 as a reasonable sum for a speedy approval, which, moreover, shouldn't become known to the taxman but was to be handled by Lilly's office in Geneva. He furthermore demanded that Lilly provided a good deal of research money to his department. The money was split so that the second half was to be paid when the drug was approved. This is how the mob operates when it orders a murder.

Next, one of Virapen's associates met with the expert in Göteborg to improve on the registration application. Deaths disappeared in footnotes and it went somewhat like this:

'Five had hallucinations and tried to commit suicide, which four of the test subjects succeeded in doing' was changed into: 'Five of the other test subjects had miscellaneous effects.'

On top of this, the independent expert placed his own personal letter of recommendation. It didn't take long before Virapen received a phone call to start negotiations about what the drug should cost, which meant the drug would be approved. When the price had been settled for a 20 mg dose, a top psychiatrist who had done research with fluoxetine postponed approval as she found that 5 mg was the maximum that should be allowed, and she demanded that the 5 mg dose should be made available. However, Lilly managed to avoid this, which might potentially have reduced its income by 75%.

There weren't that many truly depressed people in the mid-1980s when the criteria for the diagnosis were much more stringent and relevant than today, and fluoxetine was therefore marketed as a *mood lifter*. Isn't that something? A drug with cocaine-like effects is marketed as a mood lifter! What's the difference to street pushers?

The approval in Germany also followed 'unorthodox lobbying methods exercised on independent members of the regulatory authorities'.[70]

After having been so enormously helpful to Lilly, Virapen was fired. This is also like a script from the mob. When the boss has persuaded a lower-ranked person to murder a well-known political figure, it is safest to kill the assassin soon afterwards, as a dead man doesn't talk. The official explanation was that Lilly had certain ethical principles! Two other people who knew about the bribery were also fired without reason. Virapen tried to persecute the corrupt psychiatrist, but that wasn't possible because the psychiatrist wasn't an employee of the health authority. After this affair, the Swedish anticorruption law was amended. The psychiatrist just went on and, ironically, came to work for the court, as a psychiatric assessor for Sweden.

Eli Lilly promoted Prozac illegally for several non-approved ailments, e.g. shyness, eating disorders and low self-esteem, and concealed the increased risk of suicide and violence associated with the drug.[1,24,71] However, in 1990, only 2 years after Prozac came on the market, Martin Teicher et al. described six patients who had become suicidal and reacted in bizarre ways with intense, violent suicidal preoccupation while receiving Prozac, which was something completely new to them.[72] Teicher's observations were ground-breaking and the paper was highly convincing. However, internal Lilly documents revealed later that the FDA worked together with the company on the suicide issue, and Lilly's hired guns among the psychiatrists came in handy while Lilly's own scientist left out information that would have been incriminating for the company at the subsequent 1991 FDA hearings.[1] The chair of the FDA committee, psychiatrist Daniel Casey, brutally interrupted Teicher so that he couldn't present his findings and reasons! He was only allowed to present a few slides while Lilly staff presented many. A few years later, Teicher's wife was offered a job at Lilly as their top scientist in oncology without having applied. This was hardly a coincidence. The standard procedure is to blacklist and haunt critical people and if that doesn't work, to buy them or their close relatives. His wife divorced Teicher and went to work for Lilly.

In 2004, the *BMJ* received a series of internal Lilly documents and studies on Prozac from an anonymous source, which the journal sent to the FDA.[73] These documents were made available in a litigation case in 1994, but were not accessible for the public. They revealed that Lilly officials were aware already in the 1980s that fluoxetine had troubling side effects in terms of suicide attempts and violence and sought to minimise their negative effect on prescribing. Lilly was keen to root out the word 'suicide' altogether from its database record of side effects experienced by patients and its headquarters suggested that, when doctors reported a suicide attempt on Prozac to Lilly, it should be coded as 'overdose' (which is terribly misleading, as it is hardly possible to kill yourself by overdosing Prozac; the suicides occur on *normal* doses), and 'suicidal ideation' should be recorded as 'depression' (blame the disease, not the drug).[68] Two Lilly researchers in Germany were unhappy with these directions: 'I do not think I could explain to the BGA [the German regulator], to a judge, to a reporter or even to my family why we would do this, especially on the sensitive issue of suicide and suicide ideation.'[24,74]

One of the documents the *BMJ* received noted that in clinical trials, 38% of fluoxetine-treated patients reported new activation compared to only 19% of placebo-treated patients. SSRIs often lead to agitation or akathisia, an extreme form of restlessness, which some patients describe as wanting to jump out of their skin, and which increases the risk of suicide.[1,24] Early on, Lilly recommended that in their trials of fluoxetine such patients should also take benzodiazepines,[24] which reduce the symptoms. We therefore don't know what the true side effects are, or even what the true effect on depression is, as benzodiazepines have an effect on depression.

However, when Lilly became interested in showing that its drug, Prozac, led to fewer withdrawal symptoms than its competitors' drugs because of its longer half-life, the result was overwhelming. More than half of the patients on paroxetine and sertraline developed abstinence symptoms within a week when they were switched from active drug to placebo.[62,75] The most frequent symptoms clearly had nothing to do with relapse of the depression but with abstinence: worsened mood, irritability and agitation.

The bias in industry-sponsored trials is really massive. In head-to-head trials where Prozac was the drug of interest, significantly more patients improved on Prozac than in trials where Prozac was the comparator drug.[76]

In 2004, the FDA issued a warning that antidepressants can cause a cluster of activating or stimulating symptoms such as agitation, panic attacks, insomnia and aggressiveness. Such effects were expected, as fluoxetine is similar to cocaine in its effects on serotonin.[73] Interestingly, however, when the EMA in 2000 continued to deny that the use of SSRIs leads to dependence, it nonetheless stated that SSRIs 'have been shown to reduce intake of addictive substances like cocaine and ethanol. The interpretation of this aspect is difficult.'[77] The interpretation is only difficult for those who are so blind that they *will not* see.

In 1989, a man shot eight people dead, wounded another 12 and then killed himself 1 month after he was placed on fluoxetine.[73] Lilly won a nine to three jury verdict and subsequently claimed it was 'proven in a court of law ... that Prozac is safe and effective'. However, the trial judge, who suspected that a secret deal had been struck, pursued Lilly and the plaintiffs, eventually forcing Lilly to admit that it had made a secret settlement with the plaintiffs during the trial. Infuriated by Lilly's actions, the judge ordered the finding changed from a verdict in Lilly's favour to one of 'dismissed as settled with prejudice', saying, 'Lilly sought to buy not just the verdict but the court's judgment as well.'

Lilly also bought FDA panel members. An FDA advisory panel was convened in 1991 to review the fluoxetine data. It concluded that fluoxetine was safe despite the concerns raised by safety officer David Graham and others, which led critics to point out that several of the panellists had financial ties to Lilly.

Throughout the 1990s, while swearing publicly that Prozac didn't increase the risk of suicide or violence, Lilly quietly settled lawsuits out of court and was able to keep the incriminating evidence hidden by obtaining court orders to seal the documents, just as it had done with its best-selling antipsychotic drug, Zyprexa (olanzapine), until a batch of documents was leaked to the press.[71]

Lilly's internal papers disclose a long and successful battle against the idea that Prozac could induce violence or suicide, and they suggest that Lilly had an explicit strategy to blame the disease and not the drug, which some of Lilly's own scientists had reservations about. Some of Lilly's actions appeared fraudulent, e.g. the company excluded 76 of 97 cases of suicidality on Prozac in a post-marketing surveillance study it submitted to the FDA.[78,79]

In 1997, Prozac was the fifth most prescribed drug in the United States.[80] It also became the most complained-about drug, and hundreds of suicides were reported.[21] In relation to lawsuits, David Healy found early drafts of Prozac's package insert that stated that psychosis might be precipitated in susceptible patients by antidepressant therapy.[80] It turned out that Lilly had known since

1978 that Prozac can produce in some people a strange, agitated state of mind that can trigger in them an unstoppable urge to commit suicide or murder.[67] The warning about induction of psychosis wasn't included in the final package insert for the United States, whereas the German drug agency required it. By 1999, the FDA had received reports of over 2000 Prozac-associated suicides and a quarter of the reports specifically referred to agitation and akathisia. As always, the FDA protected the drug and not the patients, as it said that it would not have allowed a company to put a warning about akathisia or suicide on the label; it would have considered it mislabelling![80] The EMA announced in 2006 that parents and doctors should carefully monitor children and youth being treated with fluoxetine and watch out for suicidal tendencies.[70] A fake fix. Children commit suicide whatever the warnings are. Fluoxetine should never have been approved for children, or indeed for any creature, not even dogs (SSRIs are used for 'separation anxiety' in dogs, which is when dogs howl too much when their owner leaves home).

Lilly also kept completed suicides from public view. In 2004, the body of a 19-year-old college student was found hanging by a scarf from a shower rod in an Indianapolis laboratory run by Lilly.[78] She had entered a clinical study as a healthy volunteer in order to help pay her college tuition after having undergone thorough medical testing to screen out depression or suicidal tendencies. She had not taken Prozac but another SSRI, duloxetine (Cymbalta), which Lilly wanted to develop for stress urinary incontinence under the trade name Yentreve. When researchers and the press started asking questions about duloxetine, the FDA didn't scour its database and go public. It kept quiet and gave a legal rationale for its silence:

> Some clinical trial data are considered trade secrets, or commercially protected information.

It is outrageous that a drug regulator puts profits over human lives in this way. Clinical trial data are *not* trade secrets (*see* Chapter 11), and the FDA *must* change its attitudes and bring them on par with those at the EMA. A *BMJ* journalist, Jeanne Lenzer, filed several Freedom of Information Act requests for all safety data related to Cymbalta and Yentreve and received a database that included 41 deaths and 13 suicides among patients taking Cymbalta. Missing from the database was any record of the college student and at least four other volunteers known to have committed suicide while taking Cymbalta for depression.

Lilly admitted that it had never made public at least two of those deaths, and anonymous sources told Lenzer that duloxetine caused suicidal tendencies in patients who took the drug for incontinence and who weren't depressed. Lenzer couldn't get access to these data, as the FDA is prohibited from releasing study data for a drug that fails to win FDA approval, and the FDA didn't approve Yentreve. It cannot be more absurd than this, as the active chemical is the same in Yentreve as in Cymbalta. The United States *must* change their laws so that they serve the public.

The FDA did state later, however, that data from stress urinary incontinence trials had shown that middle-aged women taking duloxetine had a suicide attempt rate of 400 per 100 000 person-years, more than double the rate of about 160 per 100 000 person-years among other women of a similar age. This suggests that SSRIs are not only dangerous in children but also in adults (*see* Chapter 18).

There is one more take-home message from this sad affair. Volunteers, like the dead college student, are told that even if they don't personally benefit from taking a new drug, the scientific knowledge gained from the study will benefit others. The volunteers should be told instead that people will learn about their experience only if it's good news for the company. It's unbelievable and deeply criminal that healthy volunteers can die without anyone knowing about it outside the company.

When Lenzer asked Lilly about Prozac again because the sealed internal Lilly documents had surfaced, Lilly sent her a written statement:[73] 'Prozac has helped to significantly improve millions of lives. It is one of the most studied drugs in the history of medicine, and has been prescribed for more than 50 million people worldwide.'

When drug companies face trouble, they always try to escape by using big numbers. Millions of lives have *not* been improved significantly. In randomised trials, equally many patients stop treatment while on an SSRI as while on placebo, which suggests that, overall, considering benefits and harms together, the drugs are pretty useless.[81] A 2003–2007 study of 7525 patients starting antidepressants, of which two-thirds were SSRIs, showed that already after 2 months, half of the patients had stopped taking the drug.[82] What 50 million people tell us is that millions of people have been harmed, as many of those who continue to take the drug become addicted and cannot stop.

EXERCISE IS A GOOD INTERVENTION

It's not an exaggeration to say that antidepressant research is under total industry control; it supplies randomised pseudo-evidence for multibillion-dollar markets.[83] When we say that 50% improve on placebo and 60% on active drug,[84] it looks better than it really is (*see* Chapter 4). The improvement on the most used scale, Hamilton's depression scale, is so small that the drugs only seem to give a meaningful effect in patients who are rather severely depressed, which is a tiny fraction of all those treated in clinical practice.[85,86] Further, it has never been shown in trials or high-quality observational studies that the use of antidepressant drugs lowers suicide rates. Contrast these facts with a 2013 statement from the president of the American Psychiatric Association, Jeffrey Lieberman:[87]

'As a class, antidepressant medications are highly effective. They alleviate substantial amounts, if not complete symptoms, in 50 to as high as 80% of patients treated who suffer from major depression.'

Any higher bets? With such a monstrous exaggeration, why not go all the way and say the drugs cure 100%?

It would be far better to encourage people to exercise than to take drugs. There are few long-term comparisons between SSRIs and exercise, but those that exist are interesting. In a 4-month trial of 156 patients with major depression, the effect was similar for those randomised to exercise as for those who received sertraline (Zoloft), but 6 months later, only 30% of the patients in the exercise group were depressed, as compared with 52% in the sertraline group and 55% in a group that was randomised to both exercise and sertraline.[88] These differences were seen despite a low treatment contrast: 64% of patients in the exercise group and 66% in the combination group reported that they continued to exercise, but 48% of the sertraline patients also initiated an exercise programme. A Cochrane review of exercise found an effect on depression that was very similar to that reported for SSRIs.[89]

A 24-week randomised trial of 375 patients with social phobia found a similar effect of gradual exposure to the feared symptoms as of sertraline, but during an additional 6-month follow-up, the exposure group continued to improve whereas the patients from the sertraline group did not.[90] Social phobia was a rare disease until the drug companies hijacked it and called it social anxiety disorder. They boosted sales tremendously, aided by PR firms and their whores among psychiatrists and patient organisations.[9] The pool of patients went up from about 2% to 13% – or one in every eight people – handsomely helped by the ludicrous criteria in DSM that broadened over time.

FURTHER LIES ABOUT HAPPY PILLS

SmithKline Beecham, later merged into GlaxoSmithKline, started marketing paroxetine (Paxil or Seroxat) in 1992 and falsely claimed for the next 10 years that it wasn't habit forming.[91] That was pretty misleading considering that, in the original licence application, paroxetine led to withdrawal reactions in 30% of the patients![92] The UK drug regulator also denied there was a problem and failed to warn of the lack of evidence of SSRI effectiveness in mild depression. In 2001, the BBC reported that the World Health Organization had found Paxil to have the hardest withdrawal problems of any antidepressant drug. In 2002, the FDA published a warning, and the International Federation of Pharmaceutical Manufacturers Associations declared the company guilty of misleading the public about paroxetine on US television. In 2003, Glaxo quietly and in small print revised its previous estimate of the risk of withdrawal reactions in the prescribing instructions from 0.2% to 25%,[62] a 100 times increase.

From 2002 onwards, the BBC presented four documentaries about SSRIs in its *Panorama* series, the first one called 'Secrets of Seroxat'. I recommend everyone with an interest in drugs to see them. I started one evening and couldn't stop until I had seen them all. The journalist, Shelley Joffre, cleverly exposed that the Glaxo spokesperson, Alastair Benbow, who is a doctor, lied in front of a running camera. For example, he denied that paroxetine could cause suicidality or self-harm, while he sent data to the drug regulator 1 month later that showed exactly this, and which immediately led to a ban on using the drug in children. The drug regulator also lied when it said that this information was completely new to Glaxo (which had known about it for about 10 years). In addition, the head of the drug agency echoed the drug companies' false assertion that it was the disease, not the drug, that caused the terrible events.

US senator Charles Grassley asked Glaxo for how long the company had known that paroxetine carried a suicide risk.[93] Glaxo wrote back that they 'detected no signal of any possible association between Paxil and suicidality in adult patients until late February 2006'. However, government investigators found that the company had the data back in 1998 and David Healy found evidence in internal company documents that 25% of healthy volunteers experienced agitation and other symptoms of akathisia while taking Paxil.[80] Other studies have found similarly high rates, both in children and adults.[94]

After the first Panorama programme, the public was asked to submit emails to the BBC about their experiences with the drug, and 1374 emails were read by clinical pharmacologist Andrew Herxheimer and researcher Charles Medawar, cofounder of Social Audit. A clear pattern emerged. Though Glaxo had fiercely denied that SSRIs cause dependence and can lead to suicide, it was clear that both claims were wrong. It was also clear that the drugs can lead to hostility and murder, e.g. 'After 3 days on paroxetine, he sat up all night forcing himself to keep still because he wanted to kill everyone in the house.'[62] The richness of the patients' own reports was impressive. For example, many described electric shock sensations in the head and visual problems when they tried to stop; such reactions had been coded by the authorities as dizziness or paraesthesia.

The UK drug regulator's passivity throughout many years made Peter Medawar so frustrated that he suggested that drug agencies be closed down because they were always the last ones to know about the harms of drugs. Because of the revelations from the patients, the UK drug agency now accepts adverse event reports submitted directly by patients to the agency, without having to pass the doctors' obstacles first.

After I started to do research on SSRIs, I have regularly appeared in the media about these drugs and have heard many frightening stories. They are remarkably similar and here is an extract sent to me by a patient who escaped the tyranny of life-long treatment and incompetent psychiatrists:

After a traumatic event (shock, crisis and depression), I was prescribed happy pills without adequate information about possible side effects. A year later, I asked the psychiatrist to help me stopping the drug, as I didn't feel it was helpful ... When I left the psychiatrist, she had convinced me ... that I was undertreated and should have a higher dose ... She warned me against stopping the drug, as it could lead to chronic depression.

During a time when the psychiatrist had long-term sick leave, I had the courage, supported by a psychologist, to taper off the drug. I had been on the drug for 3.5 years and had become more and more lethargic and indifferent to everything. It was like escaping from a cheese-dish cover. Tapering off is not unproblematic, it gives you a lot of abstinence symptoms ...

When the psychiatrist returned after her illness, she was 'insulted' about my decision to stop the drug. However, I was much better, and in reply to my question that I was no longer depressed, she said, 'I don't know.' 'But if I don't want happy pills?' 'Well, then I cannot help you!' was the answer. I have not mentioned the name of the drug, but this psychiatrist had a close relationship to a manufacturer of happy pills.'

People tell me about medical students who are put on happy pills when they have difficulty with their studies, almost always with the fake myth about correcting a chemical imbalance and also comparing this with insulin for diabetes. When the students get abstinence symptoms when they try to stop, they are told that it's not abstinence but the disease that has come back and that they likely need the pills for the rest of their life.

I must admit that this makes me both angry and terribly sad, particularly because we don't seem to learn anything from history. In the 1880s, the UK government didn't think opium use in India resulted in 'any injurious consequences'. In the 1930s, four out of 10 prescriptions contained bromides and the problem of chronic intoxication wasn't recognised, just as – at the same time – addiction to barbiturates wasn't recognised and doctors pointing this out were ignored.[62] It took 40 years – *40 years* – before the addiction problem was finally accepted by the UK Department of Health and it was realised that the reason people continued with barbiturates indefinitely wasn't that they were ill but because they couldn't stop without great suffering.[62] In 1955, the United States produced so many barbiturate pills that 7% of the population could eat a pill every day.[95]

In the 1960s, the doctors believed that benzodiazepines were harmless and prescribed them for almost anything. At the peak of their use, the sales corresponded to a usage in about 10% of the Danish population,[96] which is extraordinary since the effect disappears after a few weeks because of development of tolerance and because the drugs are highly addictive and have many harms. The trials are biased, but when used as sleeping pills – before tolerance sets in and they still work – the increase in sleeping time is 15 minutes in older people with insomnia, whereas adverse cognitive events are five times more common, adverse psychomotor events three times more common and daytime fatigue four times more common.[97] Patients who take such drugs also have a higher risk of falls and motor vehicle crashes, and a study found that the use of benzodiazepines increased the risk of dementia by about 50%.[98] Why would an old person take such a dangerous drug rather than read a book until falling asleep naturally?

The companies denied for decades that benzodiazepines cause dependency and got away with it. Although serious dependency was documented already in 1961, it wasn't generally accepted until more than 20 years later.[27] In 1980, the UK drug regulator concluded, based on submitted reports of adverse events to the agency, that only 28 people became dependent on benzodiazepines from 1960 to 1977.[62] We now know the true number is more likely to have been around 500000, or 20000 times as many!

As doctors and regulators refuse to learn from history, I was happy to fund a PhD student who wanted to carry out the research: *Why is history repeating itself? A study on benzodiazepines and antidepressants (SSRIs).*[99] We found that the definition of substance dependence changed from DSM-III to the DSM-IIIR revision that came out in 1987 where the criteria for dependence were narrowed so that they must include also behavioural, physiological and cognitive manifestations.[51] This substantive change came about after the recognition of benzodiazepine dependence and – very conveniently – just before the SSRIs were marketed in 1988. It was a smokescreen that served to deflect attention from the fact that SSRIs also cause dependence. We found that discontinuation symptoms were described with similar terms for benzodiazepines and SSRIs and were very similar for 37 of 42 identified symptoms described as withdrawal reactions for SSRIs. To call similar problems dependence for benzodiazepines and withdrawal reactions for SSRIs is totally irrational. And for the patients, it's just the same. It's very hard for them to stop either type of drug.

Another similarity to the benzodiazepines is that it took the drug agencies many years after they had the information before they warned about the drugs.[99] The UK regulator misrepresented the data when it described withdrawal reaction after SSRIs as generally rare and mild. An analysis of the reported adverse events by independent researchers showed that the reactions had been classified as moderate in 60% of the cases and as severe in 20% by the same UK regulator that announced to the public that they were mild![52] What they also found was that suicide attempts had often been coded by the companies as non-accidental overdose.

Just like in the 1960s with the benzodiazepines, the companies – assisted by their hired psychiatrist opinion leaders and drug regulators suffering from self-inflicted blindness – have hooked many millions of patients on drugs most of them didn't need. And when people became abstinent, whether on benzodiazepines or on SSRIs, company tactics were just the same: Blame the disease, not the pills.[21,24,62] The companies fiercely denied that their SSRIs could lead to dependency even though they had shown in their own unpublished studies early on that also healthy volunteers become dependent after only a few weeks on the drug.[24]

It's truly amazing that the companies have succeeded to such an extent with their deceptions and shocking that the psychiatrists believe them. SSRIs reduce the number of serotonin receptors in the brain,[21] so when a drug is abruptly removed, the patients will feel badly about it, just like an alcoholic or a smoker will feel terrible if there is no more alcohol or cigarettes around. Therefore, whatever the symptoms are, they *cannot* be interpreted as meaning that the patient is still depressed and in need of the drug. The worst argument I have heard is that the patients are not dependent because they don't crave higher doses. If that were true, smokers are not dependent on nicotine because they don't increase their consumption of cigarettes! It's unbelievable what nonsense professors of psychiatry have told me in order to maintain the level of self-deception in their specialty.

The true risk of relapse of depression for a patient who is no longer depressed is small. We cannot measure how small it is in patients who are in treatment with SSRIs, as they have perturbed the normal equilibrium in the brain. However, it's clear that most of the symptoms that occur after abrupt withdrawal of an SSRI aren't depression symptoms but symptoms of abstinence.[51] Even when slow tapering of SSRIs was attempted after successful behavioural treatment for panic disorder and agoraphobia, which have nothing to do with depression, about half of the patients had withdrawal symptoms.[100] Unfortunately, willing doctors with numerous financial ties to makers of the drugs assist in propagating the delusions in their research, above all Stuart Montgomery from the UK, who seems to interpret all withdrawal symptoms as relapse.[62,101,102] In 2003, a systematic review in the *Lancet* reported that 41% relapsed when they continued with placebo compared to 18% that continued on active drug,[103] but it's plainly wrong to interpret the symptoms that occur after abrupt drug withdrawal as relapse.

Our citizens are drugged to about the same extent today as they were 50 years ago. The decline in the use of benzodiazepines of more than 50% has been compensated by a similar increase in the use of SSRIs (*see* Figure 17.1).[27] SSRIs are used for many of the same conditions as benzodiazepines, and it seems a bit *too* convenient to me that psychiatrists now say that much of what they previously called anxiety – when it was still okay to use benzodiazepines – in reality was depression, so that they can now use SSRIs for the same patients. The change in treatment of anxiety disorders, from benzodiazepines to SSRIs, has happened despite a lack of evidence in support of this change.[27]

We have seen a similar explosion in dubious indications for SSRIs as we previously saw for benzodiazepines, and before that for barbiturates, although all these drugs are addictive.[51,99,104] Until 2003, the UK drug regulator propagated the falsehood that SSRIs are not addictive, but the same year, the World Health Organization published a report that noted that *three SSRIs (fluoxetine, paroxetine and sertraline) were among the top 30 highest-ranking drugs for which drug dependence had ever been reported.*[62]

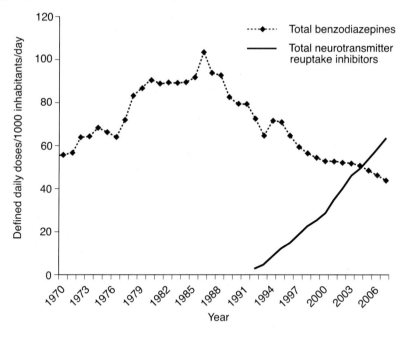

Figure 17.1 Total sales of specific neurotransmitter reuptake inhibitors and of benzodiazepines and benzodiazepine-like drugs 1970–2007, as defined daily doses per 1000 inhabitants per day

REFERENCES

1 Bass A. *Side Effects – a prosecutor, a whistleblower, and a bestselling antidepressant on trial*. Chapel Hill: Algonquin Books; 2008.

2 Caplan PJ. *They Say You're Crazy: how the world's most powerful psychiatrists decide who's normal*. Jackson: Da Capo Press; 1995.

3 Angell M. 'The illusions of psychiatry': an exchange. *New York Rev Books*. 2011 Aug 18.

4 Moynihan R. Medicalization. A new deal on disease definition. *BMJ*. 2011; **342**: d2548.

5 Harris G, Carey B, Roberts J. Psychiatrists, children and drug industry's role. *New York Times*. 2007 May 10.

6 Insel TR. Psychiatrists' relationships with pharmaceutical companies: part of the problem or part of the solution? *JAMA*. 2010; **303**: 1192–3.

7 Moynihan R. Is the relationship between pharma and medical education on the rocks? *BMJ*. 2008; **337**: 484–5.

8 Watts G. More psychiatrists attack plans for DSM-5. *BMJ*. 2012; **344**: e3357.

9 Moynihan R, Cassels A. *Selling Sickness: how the world's biggest pharmaceutical companies are turning us all into patients*. New York: Nation Books; 2005.

10 Boseley S. Prozac, used by 40m people, does not work say scientists. *The Guardian*. 2008 Feb 26.

11 Brown J, O'Brien PMS, Marjoribanks J, *et al*. Selective serotonin reuptake inhibitors for premenstrual syndrome. *Cochrane Database Syst Rev*. 2009; **2**: CD001396.

12 [*Work environment and treatment modalities in Danish psychiatry*]. Nordjyske Medier; 2007.

13 Total sales of medicinal products. Danish Medicines Agency. 2011.

14 IMS Health. *IMS Health Reports U.S. Prescription Sales Grew 5.1 percent in 2009, to $300.3 billion*. Press release. 2010 April 1.

15 Kessler RC, Demler O, Frank RG, *et al*. Prevalence and treatment of mental disorders, 1990 to 2003. *N Engl J Med*. 2005; **352**: 2515–23.

16 Spence D. The psychiatric oligarchs who medicalise normality. *BMJ*. 2012; **344**: e3135.

17 Gross J. Checklist for camp: bug spray, sunscreen, pills. *New York Times*. 2006 July 16.

18 Petersen M. *Our Daily Meds*. New York: Sarah Crichton Books; 2008.

19 Schwarz A. Attention disorder or not, pills to help in school. *New York Times*. 2012 Oct 9.

20 GfK Denmark. [Focus group about treatment of ADHD in children and adolescents]. Letter. 2011 Nov 23.

21 Whitaker R. *Anatomy of an Epidemic*. New York: Broadway Paperbacks; 2010.

22 Morbidity and Mortality Weekly Report. Current depression among adults – United States, 2006 and 2008. *JAMA*. 2010; **304**: 2233–5.

23 The Patient Health Questionnaire (PHQ-9). Available online at: www.agencymeddirectors. wa.gov/Files/depressoverview.pdf (accessed 20 October 2012).

24 Healy D. *Let Them Eat Prozac*. New York: New York University Press; 2004.

25 Frances A. Antidepressant use has gone crazy: bad news from the CDC. *Psychiatric Times*. 2011 Oct 28.

26 Friedman RA. Grief, depression, and the DSM-5. *N Engl J Med*. 2012; **366**: 1855–7.

27 Nielsen M, Gøtzsche P. An analysis of psychotropic drug sales. Increasing sales of selective serotonin reuptake inhibitors are closely related to number of products. *Int J Risk Saf Med*. 2011; **23**: 125–32.

28 Open letter to the DSM-5. Online petition. Available online at: www.ipetitions.com/petition/ dsm5/.

29 Spence D. Bad medicine: bipolar II disorder. *BMJ*. 2011; **342**: d2767.

30 Martin A, Young C, Leckman JF, *et al*. Age effects on antidepressant-induced manic conversion. *Arch Pediatr Adolesc Med*. 2004; **158**: 773–80.

31 Shea SE, Gordon K, Hawkins A, *et al*. Pathology in the Hundred Acre Wood: a neurodevelopmental perspective on A.A. Milne. *CMAJ*. 2000; **163**: 1557–9.

32 The creation of the Prozac myth. *The Guardian*. 2008 Feb 27.

33 Spence D. Bad medicine: adult attention-deficit/hyperactivity disorder. *BMJ*. 2011; **343**: d7244.

34 Aagaard L, Hansen EH. The occurrence of adverse drug reactions reported for attention deficit hyperactivity disorder (ADHD) medications in the pediatric population: a qualitative review of empirical studies. *Neuropsychiatr Dis Treat*. 2011; **7**: 729–44.

35 More fraud from drug giant GlaxoSmithKline companies – court documents show. Blog post. *Child Health Safety*. 2010 Dec 1. Available online at: http://childhealthsafety.wordpress.com/2010/12/01/more-fraud-from-drug-giant-glaxosmithkline-companies/ (accessed 17 July 2013).

36 Rennie D. When evidence isn't: trials, drug companies and the FDA. *J Law Policy*. 2007 July: 991–1012.

37 Nemeroff CB, Mayberg HS, Krahl SE, *et al*. VNS therapy in treatment-resistant depression: clinical evidence and putative neurobiological mechanisms. *Neuropsychopharmacol*. 2006; **31**: 1345–55.

38 Volpe M. Dr Charles Nemeroff and Emory University's culture of corruption. Blog post. *The Provocateur*. 2009 July 10. Available at: http://theeprovocateur.blogspot.co.nz/2009/07/dr-charles-nemeroff-and-emorys-culture.html (accessed 17 July 2013).

39 Nugent T. Profile in courage: A beleaguered whistle-blower physician fights for patients and jobs – and wins. *Opednews*. 2012 Nov 1.

40 Keller MB, McCullough JP, Klein DN, *et al*. A comparison of nefazodone, the cognitive behavioral-analysis system of psychotherapy, and their combination for the treatment of chronic depression. *N Engl J Med*. 2000; **342**: 1462–70.

41 Angell M. Is academic medicine for sale? *N Engl J Med*. 2000; **342**: 1516–8.

42 Larson JC, Ensrud KE, Reed SD, *et al*. Efficacy of escitalopram for hot flashes in healthy menopausal women: a randomized controlled trial. *JAMA*. 2011; **305**: 267–74.

43 Coupland C, Dhiman P, Morriss R, *et al*. Antidepressant use and risk of adverse outcomes in older people: population based cohort study. *BMJ*. 2011; **343**: d4551.

44 McHugh PR, Slavney PR. Mental illness – comprehensive evaluation or checklist? *N Engl J Med*. 2012; **366**: 1853–5.

45 Kleinman A. Rebalancing academic psychiatry: why it needs to happen – and soon. *Br J Psych*. 2012; **201**: 421–2.

46 Lacasse JR, Leo J. Serotonin and depression: a disconnect between the advertisements and the scientific literature. *PLoS Med*. 2005; **2**: e392.

47 Goldacre B. *Bad Pharma*. London: Fourth Estate; 2012.

48 Castrén E. Is mood chemistry? *Nat Rev Neurosci*. 2005; **6**: 241–6.

49 Andrews PW, Kornstein SG, Halberstadt LJ, *et al*. Blue again: perturbational effects of antidepressants suggest monoaminergic homeostasis in major depression. *Front Psychol*. 2011; **2**: 159.

50 Medawar C, Herxheimer A, Bell A, *et al*. Paroxetine, Panorama and user reporting of ADRs: Consumer intelligence matters in clinical practice and post-marketing drug surveillance. *Int J Risk Saf Med*. 2002; **15**: 161–9.

51 Nielsen M, Hansen EH, Gøtzsche PC. What is the difference between dependence and withdrawal reactions? A comparison of benzodiazepines and selective serotonin re-uptake inhibitors. *Addiction*. 2012; **107**: 900–8.

52 Medawar C, Herxheimer A. A comparison of adverse drug reaction reports from professionals and users, relating to risk of dependence and suicidal behaviour with paroxetine. *Int J Risk Saf Med*. 2003/2004; **16**: 5–19.

53 El-Mallakh RS, Gao Y, Jeannie Roberts R. Tardive dysphoria: the role of long term antidepressant use in inducing chronic depression. *Med Hypotheses*. 2011; **76**: 769–73.

54 Moore TJ, Glenmullen J, Furberg CD. Prescription drugs associated with reports of violence towards others. *PLoS One*. 2010; **5**: e15337.

55 Healy D. Reply to D. Wilkinson – Loss of anxiety and increased aggression in a 15-year-old boy taking fluoxetine. *J Psychopharmacol*. 1999; **13**: 421.

56 Orriols L, Delorme B, Gadegbeku B, *et al*. Prescription medicines and the risk of road traffic crashes: a French registry-based study. *PLoS Med*. 2010; **7**: e1000366.

57 *FDA Approved Labeling Text for NDA 21-875/NUVIGIL™ (armodafinil) Tablets*. 2007 June 15. Available online at: www.accessdata.fda.gov/drugsatfda_docs/label/2007/021875lbl.pdf (accessed 17 July 2013).

58 Thombs BD, Arthurs E, El-Baalbaki G, *et al*. Risk of bias from inclusion of patients who already have diagnosis of or are undergoing treatment for depression in diagnostic accuracy studies of screening tools for depression: systematic review. *BMJ*. 2011; **343**: d4825.

59 Gilbody S, House A, Sheldon T. Screening and case finding instruments for depression. *Cochrane Database Syst Rev.* 2005; **4**: CD002792.

60 Lundh A. [Is there evidence for screening for depression]? *Ugeskr Læger.* 2008; **170**: 1479.

61 Brody H. *Hooked: ethics, the medical profession, and the pharmaceutical industry.* Lanham: Rowman & Littlefield; 2008.

62 Medawar C, Hardon A. *Medicines out of Control? Antidepressants and the conspiracy of goodwill.* Netherlands: Aksant Academic Publishers; 2004.

63 van Marwijk H, Allick G, Wegman F, *et al.* Alprazolam for depression. *Cochrane Database Syst Rev.* 2012; **7**: CD007139.

64 Montejo A, Llorca G, Izquierdo J, *et al.* Incidence of sexual dysfunction associated with antidepressant agents: a prospective multicenter study of 1022 outpatients. Spanish Working Group for the study of psychotropic-related sexual dysfunction. *J Clin Psychiatry.* 2001; **62**(Suppl. 3): 10–21.

65 Pirraglia PA, Stafford RS, Singer DE. Trends in prescribing of selective serotonin reuptake inhibitors and other newer antidepressant agents in adult primary care. *Prim Care Companion J Clin Psychiatry.* 2003; **5**: 153–7.

66 Brownlee S. *Overtreated: why too much medicine is making us sicker and poorer.* New York: Bloomsbury; 2007.

67 Boseley S. They said it was safe. *The Guardian.* 1999 Oct 30.

68 Healy D. *Pharmageddon.* Berkeley: University of California Press; 2012.

69 Internal Eli Lilly memo. Bad Homburg. 1984 May 25.

70 Virapen J. *Side Effects: death.* College Station: Virtualbookworm.com Publishing; 2010.

71 Pringle E. Eli Lilly hides data: Zyprexa, Evista, Prozac risk. *Conspiracy Planet.* Available online at: www.conspiracyplanet.com/channel.cfm?channelid=55&contentid=4181&page=2 (accessed 28 June 2012).

72 Teicher MH, Glod C, Cole JO. Emergence of intense suicidal preoccupation during fluoxetine treatment. *Am J Psychiatry.* 1990; **147**: 207–10.

73 Lenzer J. FDA to review 'missing' drug company documents. *BMJ.* 2005; **330**: 7.

74 Bouchy C. Internal Eli Lilly memo. 1990 Nov 13.

75 Rosenbaum JF, Fava M, Hoog SL, *et al.* Selective serotonin reuptake inhibitor discontinuation syndrome: a randomized clinical trial. *Biol Psychiatry.* 1998; **44**: 77–87.

76 Barbui C, Cipriani A, Brambilla P, *et al.* 'Wish bias' in antidepressant drug trials? *J Clin Psychopharmacol.* 2004; **24**: 126–30.

77 European Medicines Agency (1999/2000). EMEA/CPMP/2775/99.

78 Lenzer J. Drug secrets: what the FDA isn't telling. *Slate.* 2005 Sept 27.

79 Lenzer J. Secret US report surfaces on antidepressants in children. *BMJ.* 2004; **329**: 307.

80 Jurand SH. Lawsuits over antidepressants claim the drug is worse than the disease. American Association for Justice. 2003 Mar 1. Available online at: www.thefreelibrary.com/_/print/PrintArticle.aspx?id=99601757 (accessed 23 December 2012).

81 Barbui C, Furukawa TA, Cipriani A. Effectiveness of paroxetine in the treatment of acute major depression in adults: a systematic re-examination of published and unpublished data from randomized trials. *CMAJ.* 2008; **178**: 296–305.

82 Serna MC, Cruz I, Real J, *et al.* Duration and adherence of antidepressant treatment (2003 to 2007) based on prescription database. *Eur Psychiatry.* 2010; **25**: 206–13.

83 Ioannidis JPA. Ranking antidepressants. *Lancet.* 2009; **373**: 1759–60.

84 Laughren TP. Overview for December 13 Meeting of Psychopharmacologic Drugs Advisory Committee (PDAC). 2006 Nov 16. Available online at: www.fda.gov/ohrms/dockets/ac/06/briefing/2006-4272b1-01-FDA.pdf (accessed 22 October 2012).

85 Fournier JC, DeRubeis RJ, Hollon SD, *et al.* Antidepressant drug effects and depression severity. A patient-level meta-analysis, *JAMA.* 2010; **303**: 47–53.

86 DeRubeis, Fournier JC. Depression severity and effect of antidepressant medications. *JAMA.* 2010; **303**: 1599.

87 Johnson LA. Pfizer disputes claim against antidepressant. *USA Today.* 2013 Jan 31.

88 Babyak M, Blumenthal JA, Herman S, *et al.* Exercise treatment for major depression: maintenance of therapeutic benefit at 10 months. *Psychosom Med.* 2000 Sep–Oct; **62**: 633–8.

89 Rimer J, Dwan K, Lawlor DA, *et al*. Exercise for depression. *Cochrane Database Syst Rev.* 2012; 7: CD004366.

90 Haug TT, Blomhoff S, Hellstrøm K, *et al*. Exposure therapy and sertraline in social phobia: 1-year follow-up of a randomised controlled trial. *Br J Psychiatry.* 2003; **182**: 312–18.

91 Wikipedia. GlaxoSmithKline. Available online at: http://en.wikipedia.org/wiki/GlaxoSmithKline (accessed 20 June 2012).

92 Herxheimer A. Turbulence in UK medicines regulation: A stink about SSRI antidepressants that isn't going away. In: Glavanis K, O'Donovan O, editors. *Power, Politics and Pharmaceuticals: drug regulation in Ireland in the global context.* Cork: Cork University Press; 2008.

93 Grassley CE. Paxil. Speech at the US Senate. 2008 June 11.

94 Riddle MA, King RA, Hardin MT, *et al*. Behavioral side effects of fluoxetine in children and adolescents. *J Child Adolesc Psychopharmacol.* 1990/1991; **1**: 193–8.

95 Brynner R, Stephens T. *Dark Remedy: the impact of thalidomide and its revival as a vital medicine.* New York: Perseus Publishing; 2001.

96 Hansen EH, Gyldmark M. [Psychotropic drug use. Distribution and development]. Copenhagen: Sundhedsstyrelsen; 1990.

97 Glass J, Lanctôt KL, Herrmann N, *et al*. Sedative hypnotics in older people with insomnia: meta-analysis of risks and benefits. *BMJ.* 2005; **331**: 1169–73.

98 de Gage SB, Bégaud B, Bazin F, *et al*. Benzodiazepine use and risk of dementia: prospective population based study. *BMJ.* 2012; **345**: e6231.

99 Nielsen M. Selective Serotonin Reuptake Inhibitors (SSRI) – sales, withdrawal reactions and how drug regulators reacted to this with benzodiazepines as comparator [PhD thesis]. Copenhagen: University of Copenhagen; 2013.

100 Fava GA, Bernardi M, Tomba E, *et al*. Effects of gradual discontinuation of selective serotonin reuptake inhibitors in panic disorder with agoraphobia. *Int J Neuropsychopharmacol.* 2007; **10**: 835–8.

101 Medawar C. The antidepressant web – marketing depression and making medicines work. *Int J Risk Saf Med.* 1997; **10**: 75–126.

102 Montgomery SA, Dunbar G. Paroxetine is better than placebo in relapse prevention and the prophylaxis of recurrent depression. *Int Clin Psychopharmacol.* 1993 Fall; 8(3): 189–95.

103 Geddes JR, Carney SM, Davies C, *et al*. Relapse prevention with antidepressant drug treatment in depressive disorders: a systematic review. *Lancet.* 2003; **361**: 653–61.

104 House of Commons Health Committee. *The Influence of the Pharmaceutical Industry. Fourth Report of Session 2004–05.* Available online at: www.publications.parliament.uk/pa/cm200405/cmselect/cmhealth/42/42.pdf (accessed 26 April 2005).

Pushing children into
suicide with happy pills

GLAXO STUDY 329

In 2001, GlaxoSmithKline published a trial in children and adolescents, study 329.[1] This study reported that Paxil (Seroxat) was effective with minimal side effects, and it was widely believed and cited, no less than 184 times by 2010, which is remarkable. However, the trial was fraudulent. We know this because the Attorney General of New York State sued the company in 2004 for repeated and persistent consumer fraud in relation to concealing harms of Paxil,[2] which opened the company's archives as part of a settlement.

Glaxo lied to its sales force, telling them that trial 329 showed 'REMARKABLE Efficacy and Safety',[3] while the company admitted in internal documents that the study didn't show Paxil was effective. The study was negative for efficacy on all eight protocol-specified outcomes and positive for harm. These indisputable facts were washed away with extensive data manipulations, so that the published paper, which – although it was ghostwritten – had 22 'authors', ended up reporting positive effects.[3,4] The data massage produced four statistically significant effects after splitting the data in various ways, and it was clear that many variations were tried before the data confessed. The paper didn't leave any trace of the torture; in fact, it falsely stated that the new outcomes were declared a priori.

For harms, the manipulations were even worse. The internal unpublished study report that became available through litigation showed that at least eight children became suicidal on Paxil versus one on placebo. This was a serious and statistically significant harm of Paxil (P = 0.035). There were 11 serious adverse effects in total among 93 children treated with Paxil and two among 87 children treated with placebo, which was also significant (P = 0.01, my calculation; the paper didn't say that this difference was statistically significant). This means that for every 10 children treated with Paxil instead of placebo, there was one more serious adverse event (the inverse of the risk difference, 11/93 – 2/87, is 10). However, the abstract of the paper ended thus:

'**Conclusions:** Paroxetine is generally well tolerated and effective for major depression in adolescents.'

An early draft of the paper prepared for *JAMA* didn't discuss serious adverse effects at all! *JAMA* rejected the paper, and later drafts mentioned that worsening depression, emotional lability, headache and hostility were considered related or possibly related to treatment. The published paper did mention the serious adverse effects, but only headache in one patient was considered by the treating investigator to be related to paroxetine treatment. I have my doubts about whether the treating investigators really made these decisions. As the adverse events were reported to the company and appeared in earlier drafts, it's more likely that it was people employed by Glaxo that interpreted the drug's harms so generously. In the published paper, five cases of suicidal thoughts and behaviour were listed as 'emotional lability' and three additional cases of suicidal ideation or self-harm were called 'hospitalisation'.

At least three adolescents threatened or attempted suicide, but this wasn't described in the paper. Its first author, Martin Keller, wrote that they were terminated from the study because of non-compliance.[2] There were other issues the published paper said nothing about. For one of the suicidal teenagers, the treating psychiatrist asked a researcher involved with the study to break the blind, which he refused although the protocol provided for this. Another 'non-compliant' teenager ingested 82 tablets of paracetamol, which is a deadly dose. Most curiously, another teenager was enrolled with the same trial number as the suicidal one, although this should be impossible, but perhaps the new patient took what remained of the study drug? This raises the uncomfortable question whether some patients who had fared badly were excluded from the trial. When the FDA demanded the company to review the data again, there were four additional cases of intentional self-injury, suicidal ideation or suicide attempt, all on paroxetine.

Keller is some character. He double-billed his travel expenses, which were reimbursed both by his university and the drug sponsor. Further, the Massachusetts Department of Mental Health had paid Brown's psychiatry department, which Keller chaired, hundreds of thousands of dollars to fund research that wasn't being conducted. Keller himself received hundreds of thousands of dollars from drug companies every year that he didn't disclose. A social worker found a computer disc in the hallway and opened it to see to whom she should return it. She realised that adolescents were listed as if they had been enrolled in a study, which wasn't true. It seemed they were made up, which would have been tempting given that $25000 was offered by the drug company for each vulnerable teenager. The president of a chapter of the National Alliance for the Mentally Ill, supposed to be a patient advocacy group but heavily supported by big pharma, lectured for patients and their relatives on drug company money, which he didn't reveal, and the honoraria were whitewashed.[2]

Keller never admitted there was anything wrong with the way he reported study 329. And his misdeeds didn't harm his career. His department has received $50 million in research funding and a spokesperson from Brown said that 'Brown takes seriously the integrity of its scientific research. Dr Keller's research regarding Paxil complied with Brown's research standards.' Well, thanks for letting us know that, with such ethical standards, we should never apply for a job at Brown's.

The role of the journal, *Journal of the American Academy of Child and Adolescent Psychiatry*, was similarly depressing. Although the journal's editors were shown evidence that the article misrepresented the science, they refused to convey this information to the medical community and to retract the article, thereby jeopardising their scientific standing and moral responsibility to prescribers and patients.[4] An explanation for this passivity can likely be found by following the money that goes to the journal's owner.

What caused the greatest public uproar was that Glaxo pushed its drug for use in children, although it not only didn't work in children, it was also very harmful, and it wasn't even approved for use in children. The illegal marketing involved withholding trials showing Paxil was ineffective.[5] An internal company document showed that the company knew what it was doing: 'It would be commercially unacceptable to include a statement that efficacy had not been demonstrated, as this would undermine the profile of paroxetine.'[4]

The ruthless marketing worked. From 1998 to 2001, five million prescriptions a year were being written for Paxil and Zoloft for children and adolescents.[6] We should remember that there are real tragedies behind the numbers and real people who have paid with their lives for the companies' unscrupulous lies, frauds and crimes:[7]

> Matt Miller was unhappy. Having moved to a new neighborhood and a new school, Matt was thrust into unknown territory without his support system of old friends with whom he had grown up. That summer, Matt was prescribed Zoloft … and was told to call his doctor in a week. On a Sunday night, after taking his seventh pill, Matt went to his bedroom closet, where there was a hook just a little higher than he was tall. Matt hung himself, having to lift his legs off the floor and hold himself there until he passed out. He was only thirteen years old.

Jeremy Lown, a teenager, suffered from Tourette's syndrome. To treat his uncontrollable tics and verbal outbursts, his neurologist prescribed Prozac. Three weeks after starting the medication, Jeremy hanged himself in the woods behind his house.[8]

Candace, a 12-year-old girl, was prescribed Zoloft because she suffered from anxiety. She was a happy child that had never been depressed or had suicidal ideation. She hanged herself after 4 days.[9]

Vicky Hartman was given a sample pack of Zoloft by her child's doctor. She didn't suffer from any mental disorder but mentioned she needed a 'pick-me-up' to help with stress. Soon after starting the medication, she shot her husband and herself.[8]

A man hanged himself after taking Prozac, which his cardiologist had prescribed for chest pain, and a woman shot herself after taking the Prozac her family doctor had prescribed for migraine.

Twenty-year-old student Justin Cheslek had trouble sleeping and was prescribed sleeping pills by his doctor.[10] A few days later, he complained to the doctor that the pills made him feel groggy and 'depressed'. The doctor gave him Paxil, and Justin told his mother that Paxil made him feel awful, wound up, jumpy and unable to sit still or concentrate. Two weeks later, the doctor gave him another SSRI, Effexor (venlafaxine), which caused a seizure after the first tablet. Justin still felt 'really, really bad' and 3 weeks after he took his first Paxil tablet, he hanged himself. Justin had no history of depression and if he hadn't used the term 'depressed', he might not have been prescribed SSRIs. He just had trouble sleeping. In the days before his death, Justin described a feeling of wanting to jump out of his skin, a symptom typical of akathisia, which may lead to suicide.

In November 2010, Nancy and Shaun McCartney's 18-year-old son, Brennan, went to their family doctor with a chest cold.[11] The extroverted high school student mentioned feeling sad over breaking up with a girl he'd been seeing for 3 months. He left with a script for an antibiotic and a sample pack of Cipralex. Nancy expressed concern, as Brennan had no history of depression, but he assured her the doctor had said it would help. On the fourth day, Brennan seemed agitated when he left the house and he failed to come home. The next day his body was found. He had hung himself in a local park. Nancy wanted to warn other Canadians about Cipralex and submitted an adverse reaction report, and when she noticed a typo on her entry, she called the Vigilance Branch requesting a correction. She also asked for an updated copy but was told she'd have to file an access to information request. Seven months later, anyone searching Cipralex on MedEffect would find 317 reports, including five suicides, 12 suicide attempts and many references to suicidal ideation, but not Nancy's submission. When the journalist writing about the tragedy asked Health Canada why, its spokesperson responded weeks later saying the entry was in the database and provided a screen grab. However, subsequent searches using the same terms failed to find it. It's unbelievable. Not even suicides reported to the authorities may be traceable in their records.

Here is an example that the advertising of prescription drugs to the public, which is legal in the United States, can kill healthy people who don't need them:[12]

> Ten years ago my irrepressible teenage daughter Caitlin returned from holiday with relatives in the US, where prescription drugs are widely advertised; she saw an ad for an antidepressant drug called Prozac and wanted to try it. She went to our local GP and it took her 8 minutes to get the prescription. Sixty-three days later, during which time she descended into unprecedented chaos, including neural twitches, violent nightmares and self-harm, she hanged herself.

CONCEALING SUICIDES AND SUICIDE ATTEMPTS IN CLINICAL TRIALS

I shall explore here what the true risks of suicide and suicidality with SSRIs are. They are certainly much larger than what the drug companies have told us. David Healy performed a study in 20 healthy volunteers – all with no history of depression or other mental illness – and to his big surprise two of them became suicidal when they received sertraline.[13] One of them was on her way out the door to kill herself in front of a train or a car when a phone call saved her. Both volunteers remained disturbed several months later and seriously questioned the stability of their personalities. Pfizer's own studies in healthy volunteers had shown similar deleterious effects, but most of these data are hidden in company files.[13]

FDA reviewers and independent researchers found that the big companies had concealed cases of suicidal thoughts and acts by labelling them 'emotional lability'.[13-15] However, the FDA bosses suppressed this information. When safety officer Andrew Mosholder concluded that SSRIs cause increased suicidality among teenagers, the FDA prevented him from presenting his findings at an advisory meeting and suppressed his report. When the report was leaked, the FDA's reaction was to do a criminal investigation into the leak.[16,17]

There were other problems. In data submitted by GlaxoSmithKline to the FDA in the late 1980s and early 1990s, the company had included suicide attempts from the washout period before the patients were randomised in the results for the placebo arms of trials, but not from the paroxetine arms. A Harvard psychiatrist, Joseph Glenmullen, who studied the released papers for the lawyers, said that it's virtually impossible that Glaxo simply misunderstood the data. Martin Brecher, the FDA scientist who reviewed paroxetine's safety, said that this use of the washout data was scientifically illegitimate.[18] Indeed. I believe it's fraud.

David Healy wrote in 2002[19] that, based on data he had obtained from the FDA, three of five suicide attempts on placebo in a sertraline trial[20] had occurred during washout rather than while on placebo and that two suicides and three of six attempts on placebo in a paroxetine trial[20] had also occurred in the washout period. Healy's observations weren't denied by Pfizer and Glaxo,[21,22] but Glaxo again provided a glaring example that their lies are not of this world:[22]

> *The 'drug' v. 'true placebo' analysis Dr Healy describes is not only scientifically invalid, but also misleading. Major depressive disorder is a potentially very serious illness associated with substantial morbidity, mortality, suicidal ideation, suicide attempts and completed suicide. Unwarranted conclusions about the use and risk of antidepressants, including paroxetine, do a disservice to patients and physicians.*

So, should we trust people who deliberately hide suicidal harms of their drug and hide trials that showed no effect and make billions out of their frauds, who are only responsible to their shareholders, and who nonetheless wants us to believe that patient welfare is their primary concern? Or should we trust an academic like Healy whose job it is to take care of the patients?

At least three companies, Glaxo, Lilly and Pfizer, added cases of suicide and suicide attempts in patients to the placebo arm of their trials, although they didn't occur while the patients were randomised to placebo.[13,19,23-25] These omissions can be important for the companies in court cases. For example, a man on paroxetine had murdered his wife, daughter and granddaughter and committed suicide, but in its defence, Glaxo said that its trials didn't show an increased risk of suicide on paroxetine.[26]

The pervasive scientific misconduct has distorted seriously our perception of the benefits and harms of SSRIs. As an example, a 2004 systematic review showed that, when unpublished trials were included, a favourable risk–benefit profile changed to an unfavourable one for several of the SSRIs.[27] Also in 2004, a researcher used the full reports of Glaxo's trials that were made available on the internet as a result of litigation, and he found in his meta-analysis that paroxetine increased significantly suicidal tendencies, odds ratio 2.77 (95% confidence interval 1.03 to 7.41).[14] He included three trials, among them the unpublished study 377, which didn't show that paroxetine was better than placebo (Glaxo had stated in an internal document that 'There are no plans to publish data from Study 377.')[28] He also included the infamous study 329. He described that an 11-year-old boy who threatened to harm himself and was hospitalised was coded as a case of exacerbated depression, and that a 14-year-old boy who had harmed himself and expressed hopelessness and possible suicide thoughts and was hospitalised was coded as a case of aggression.

It is widely believed that SSRIs only increase suicidal behaviour in people below 25 years of age, but this is not correct. A 2006 FDA analysis of 372 placebo-controlled trials of SSRIs and similar drugs involving 100 000 patients found that up to about 40 years of age, the drugs increased suicidal behaviour, and in older patients, they decreased it (see Figure 18.1).[29] However, as explained below, it is much worse than this. A major weakness of the FDA study is that the agency asked the companies to adjudicate possibly suicide-related adverse events and send them to the FDA, which didn't verify whether they were correct or whether some had been left out. We already know that the companies have cheated shamelessly when publishing suicidal events. Why should they not continue cheating when they know that the FDA doesn't check what they are doing? Furthermore, collection of adverse events was limited to within one day of stopping randomised treatment, although stopping an SSRI increases the risk of suicidality for several days or weeks. This rule therefore also seriously underestimated the harms of SSRIs.

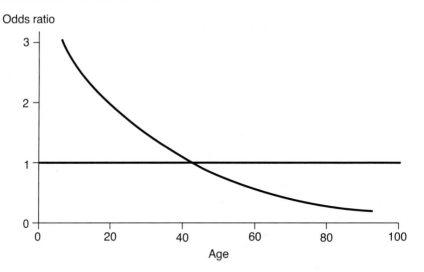

Figure 18.1 FDA meta-analysis of 372 placebo-controlled trials of SSRIs and similar drugs involving nearly 100 000 patients. Odds ratios for suicidal behaviour for active drug relative to placebo by age

Other data show that the huge FDA analysis *cannot* be reliable. An internal Lilly memo from 1984 reported that the German drug agency described two suicides and 16 suicide attempts among only 1427 patients on fluoxetine in clinical trials even though patients at risk of suicide were excluded from the trials.[30] A memo from Lilly Germany listed nine suicides in 6993 patients on fluoxetine in the trials.[31] In contrast, there were only five suicides in total in FDA's analysis of 52 960 patients on SSRI drugs, or one per 10 000 patients, although one would have expected 74 and 68, respectively, based on the two Lilly reports, or 13 per 10 000 patients.

Many suicides are missing in the FDA analysis. In a 1995 meta-analysis, there were five suicides on paroxetine in 2963 patients,[32] which is 17 per 10 000 patients. This meta-analysis wrongly reported two suicides on placebo, which had occurred in the washout period. The UK drug regulator was much more careful than the FDA and did not only search for suicide terms in the documents but also read text in case report forms and narratives.[33] *They showed that paroxetine was harmful in adults with major depressive disorder.* There were 11 suicide attempts on paroxetine (3455 patients) and only one on placebo (1978 patients), P = 0.058 for the difference. I wonder why no suicides were reported, as we would have expected six on paroxetine.

A 2005 meta-analysis that built on data in a report the UK drug regulator had made found nine suicides in 23 804 patients,[34] or four per 10 000. This was an unusually low rate, and it has been shown that the companies underreported the suicide risk.[35] There were other oddities; the researchers found that non-fatal self-harm and suicidality were seriously underreported compared to the reported suicides.

A 2005 meta-analysis of published trials including 87 650 patients conducted by independent researchers included all ages and found double as many suicide attempts on drug than on placebo.[36] Even so, they found that many suicide attempts must have been missing, e.g. by asking the investigators, some of whom responded that there were suicide attempts they had not reported, while others replied that they didn't even look for them in their trials. There were other issues related to trial design that likely led to underestimation of suicide attempts, e.g. events occurring shortly after active treatment is stopped might very well be caused by the drug but were not counted.

It is abundantly clear that suicides, suicidality and violence caused by SSRIs are grossly underestimated,[37] and we also know the reasons. First, there is outright fraud. Second, many suicidal events have been coded as something else. Third, the drug industry has taken great care to bias its trials by only recruiting people at very low risk of committing suicide. Fourth, the companies have urged the investigators to use benzodiazepines in addition to the trial drugs, which blunt some of the violent reactions that would otherwise have occurred. Fifth, some trials have run-in periods on active drug, and patients who don't tolerate it aren't randomised, which comes close to scientific misconduct, as it artificially minimises the occurrence of suicidality. Sixth, and perhaps the worst of all the biases, events occurring shortly after active treatment is stopped, e.g. because the patients feel very badly, might very well be suicidal events caused by the drug but are often not registered. Seventh, many trials are buried in company archives and these are not the most positive ones.

Given what I have just described above, and earlier, e.g. that middle-aged women who use duloxetine for urinary incontinence have a suicide attempt rate that is more than double the rate among other women of a similar age, my take on all this is:

SSRIs likely increase the risk of suicide at all ages. These drugs are immensely harmful.

LUNDBECK'S EVERGREENING OF CITALOPRAM

Lundbeck launched citalopram (Cipramil or Celexa) in 1989. It became one of the most widely used SSRIs and provided the company with most of its income. That was a risky situation to be in but Lundbeck was lucky. Citalopram is a stereoisomer and consists of two halves, which are mirror images of each other, but only one of them is active.

Lundbeck patented the active half before the old patent ran out and called the rejuvenated me-again drug escitalopram (Cipralex or Lexapro), which it launched in 2002. When the patent for citalopram expired, generics of Cipramil entered the market at much lower prices, but the price of Cipralex continued to be very high. When I checked the Danish prices in 2009, Cipralex cost 19 times as much for a daily dose as Cipramil. This enormous price difference should have deterred the doctors from using Cipralex, but it didn't. The sales of Cipralex were six times higher in monetary terms than the sales of citalopram both at hospitals and in primary care. I calculated that if all patients had received the cheapest citalopram instead of Cipralex or other SSRIs, Danish taxpayers could have saved around €30 million a year, or 87% of the total amount spent on SSRIs.

How is it possible for doctors to have such a blatant disregard for the public purse to which we all contribute and why can it continue year after year? The old recipe with a blend of money and hyped research seems infallible. A psychiatrist described vividly that when Lundbeck launched Cipralex in 2002, most of the Danish psychiatrists (she did say most, although there are more than a thousand psychiatrists in Denmark) were invited to a meeting in Paris. That meeting seems to have been enjoyable, 'with expensive lecturers – of course from Lundbeck's own "stable" – luxurious hotel and gourmet food. A so-called whore trip. Under influence? No, of course not, a doctor doesn't get influenced, right?'[38]

When the patent of Cipramil was expiring, Jack M Gorman published an article in a special supplement of *CNS Spectrums*, a neuropsychiatric journal he edits.[39] The article concluded that escitalopram may have a faster onset of action and greater overall effect than citalopram'[40] Gorman was a paid consultant to Forest that marketed both drugs in North America, and Forest paid Medworks Media, the publisher of *CNS Spectrums*, to print the article. At the same time, *Medical Letter*, an independent drug bulletin with no advertising, also reviewed the two drugs and found no difference between them.[41]

On one of the occasions where I was invited to give a lecture for Danish psychiatrists, I expressed my doubts that a drug could be better than itself to a person sitting close to me at the lunch table. She was a chemist working at Lundbeck and didn't agree. She sent me a copy of Gorman's paper, which on page 2 says: 'Brought to you by an unrestricted educational grant from Forest Pharmaceuticals, Inc.' Oh no, I thought I would never accept 'an unrestricted educational grant' from a drug company, not even in the form of a reprint, but here it was. All three authors worked for Forest, Gorman as a consultant and the others in the company. The paper was a meta-analysis of three trials that compared the two drugs with placebo.

What am I supposed to make out of a paper published in a bought supplement to a journal edited by a person who is also bought by the company? Nothing, I would say. We cannot trust the drug industry, and a paper published this way is nothing but an advertisement. There are so many ways a trial can be manipulated, and in SSRI trials it's particularly crucial how the statistician deals with dropped out patients and other missing values.[42] On top of this, Lundbeck was in a pretty desperate situation. I therefore wouldn't believe anything unless I got access to the raw data and analysed them myself.

But it isn't necessary to go to such lengths. What Forest published was small differences between the two drugs and between active drugs and placebo (*see* Figure 18.2). After 8 weeks, the difference between the two drugs was 1, on a scale that goes from 0 to 60, and the difference between active drugs and placebo was 3. Obviously, a difference of 1 on a 60-point scale has no importance for the patients. Furthermore, as explained in Chapter 4, it doesn't take much unblinding before we find a difference of 3 between active drugs and placebo, even if the drugs have no effect on depression. There is therefore no good reason to use a drug that is 19 times more expensive than itself.

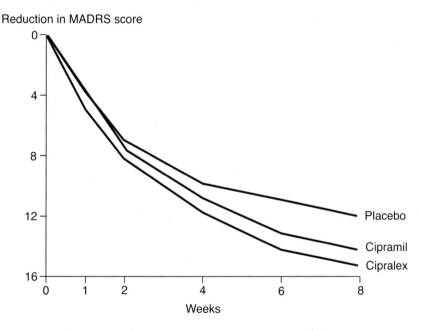

Figure 18.2 Change from baseline in MADRS score throughout 8 weeks; the scale goes from 0 to 60. Redrawn

The official task of the government-funded Danish Institute for Rational Drug Therapy is to inform Danish doctors about drugs in an evidence-based fashion. In 2002, the institute reviewed the clinical documentation for Lundbeck's me-again drug, escitalopram, and informed Danish doctors that it didn't have clear advantages over the old drug, which contained the same active substance.[43] Lundbeck complained loudly about this in the press and said it was beyond the institute's competence to give statements that could affect the international competition and damage Danish drug exports.[44]

Although it *wasn't* beyond the institute's competence to give recommendations about new drugs, whatever the consequences for drug exports, the institute was reprimanded by the minister of health and it declined to comment when asked by a journalist, for pretty obvious reasons. The Danish drug industry has tried for years to get political backing for closing down the institute, which is a thorn in its flesh, as it reduces sales of expensive drugs, but it hasn't succeeded.

It seems that our highly praised governmental institute is only allowed to tell the truth about imported drugs, not about drugs we export. An untenable position that shows that *principles are only valid as long as they don't cost too much.*

Two years after these events, the institute announced that escitalopram was better than citalopram and might be tried if the effect of citalopram hadn't been satisfactory.[45] The institute must have stepped on its toes to find a politically correct way to express themselves.[46] Its information to doctors now stated that they should usually choose the cheapest SSRI, as there are no major differences between the drugs. About escitalopram it said that 'Two studies have shown that the effect of escitalopram comes somewhat faster than that of venlafaxine and citalopram, but with about the same maximum effect', and 'In a single study it was made likely in a subgroup analysis that escitalopram is a little better in severe depression than venlafaxine and citalopram.'

I had a big laugh when I saw the four references in support of these statements. Paper is grateful, as we say; it doesn't protest, no matter what you write on it. One of the academic authors was Stuart Montgomery, who concealed that he worked for Pfizer helping the company to get sertraline approved at the same time as he worked for the UK drug regulator that approved the drug (*see* Chapter 10). I laughed again when an employee from the institute was interviewed in the TV news. She was pressured by the journalist who asked her if she couldn't imagine any situation where it *might* be an advantage that the drug worked faster. Yes, she said, if a patient was about to throw herself out the window! She learned the hard way how to deal with journalists. Jokes won't do on the news, particularly not if they are about patients. It was doubly ironic, as it has never been demonstrated that SSRIs decrease the risk of suicide; they seem to increase the risk (see above).

Four independent reviews of the evidence – by the FDA, the American advisory group Micromedex, the Stockholm Medical Council and the Danish institute – concluded that escitalopram offers no significant benefit over its predecessor.[47] The Cochrane review on escitalopram says that it's better than citalopram but warns against this finding because of potential sponsorship bias.[48] The trials were performed by Lundbeck and many negative antidepressant trials never get published. Furthermore, the reporting of the outcomes in the included studies was often unclear or incomplete. Analyses made by disinterested parties who have access to the data, such as scientists working at drug agencies, have repeatedly found that there are no important differences in benefits and harms of the various

SSRIs, whereas what gets published is seriously misleading.[29,42,49] Comprehensive reviews by other researchers have also failed to find important differences.[50]

In 2003, Lundbeck breached the UK industry code of practice in its advertising.[51] The company breached the code on five counts, notably by claiming that 'Cipralex is significantly more effective than Cipramil in treating depression'. The company also attributed adverse effects to citalopram in its literature on escitalopram that weren't mentioned in promotional material for citalopram. This confirms the adage that it's surprising how quickly a good drug becomes a bad drug when a more expensive drug comes around. The UK advertising campaign was intensive and highly successful, as escitalopram rapidly gained market share.

Lundbeck's CEO, Erik Sprunk-Jansen, retired in 2003 and started a company selling herbal medicine. One of the products is Masculine, which 'Spices up your love life', and is said to give extra energy that strengthens the lust and blood circulation,[52] typical mumbo-jumbo pep talk for alternative medicine. It doesn't seem to matter much what drug pushers sell, as long as they sell *something*.

In 2011, we asked Lundbeck for unpublished trials of its antidepressant drugs, which we needed for our research on suicidality, but we were told that the company, as a matter of principle, doesn't hand out the clinical documentation that forms the basis for marketing authorisation. The same year, Lundbeck's new CEO, Ulf Wiinberg, denied in an interview that the increase in suicidal events with happy pills in children and adolescents means that the drugs increase the risk of suicide.[53] He even stated that treatment of depression in children and adolescents *decreases* the suicide risk, in violation of the labelling that warns that the drugs may increase the risk of suicide. Why does any doctor trust what the companies tell them?

Events in America were also interesting. In 2001, Lundbeck's American partner Forest had performed a trial of citalopram (Celexa) for compulsive shopping disorder (I'm not joking), and Good Morning America told the viewers that this new disorder could affect as many as 20 million Americans of which 90% were women.[54] Gorman appeared as an expert in the programme and said that 80% of the compulsive shoppers had slowed their purchases on Celexa. The ensuing flurry of publicity forced the APA to say it had no intention of adding such a disorder to the DSM.

In 2010, the US Justice Department announced that Forest had pleaded guilty to charges relating to obstruction of justice and the illegal promotion of citalopram (Celexa) and escitalopram (Lexapro) for use in treating children and adolescents with depression.[55] Forest agreed to pay more than $313 million to resolve criminal and civil liability arising from these matters and also faced numerous court cases from parents to children who had either committed suicide or had tried.[56] There were also charges that the company launched seeding studies, which were marketing efforts to promote the drugs' use. Two whistle-blowers would receive approximately $14 million, and Forest signed a Corporate Integrity Agreement.[55,57] Six years earlier, a Forest executive had testified before Congress that Forest followed the law and had not promoted Celexa and Lexapro to children, although Forest had illegally done exactly that.[58]

The government mentioned that Forest publicised and circulated the positive results of a double-blind, placebo-controlled Forest study in 2004 on the use of Celexa in adolescents while, at the same time, failed to discuss the negative results of a contemporaneous double-blind, placebo-controlled Lundbeck study on the use of Celexa in adolescents, finished in 2002 in Europe but only mentioned in a textbook in Danish in 2003 in a single line of a chart.[59] For 3 years, Forest executives didn't disclose those results within the company or to outside researchers who published results on Celexa, and the existence of the Lundbeck study first came to public light when the *New York Times* published an article about it. Only then did Forest acknowledge the study as well as another, earlier trial that also failed to show any benefits of Lexapro as a depression treatment for children.[55,57]

Forest's official excuse for not mentioning the negative trials was that 'there was no citable public reference for the authors to examine'.[59] But drug makers often announce trials with positive results without waiting for the results to be published, e.g. Forest issued a news release that highlighted the outcome of the positive Celexa trial already in 2001, shortly after the trial's completion.

Forest had 19 000 advisory board members[58] and used illegal kickbacks to induce physicians and others to prescribe Celexa and Lexapro, which allegedly included cash payments disguised as grants or consulting fees, expensive meals and lavish entertainment. On one occasion, Forest paid physicians five hundred dollars to dine at one of the most expensive restaurants in Manhattan and called them consultants – for the evening it seemed, and they didn't do any consulting.[54] Vermont officials found that Forest's payments to doctors in 2008 were surpassed only by those of Eli Lilly, Pfizer, Novartis and Merck – companies with annual sales that were five to 10 times larger than Forest's.[60]

What was Lundbeck's reaction to the crimes? 'We know Forest is a decent and ethically responsible firm and we are therefore certain that this is an isolated error.'[56] Perhaps this confidence in Forest's business ethics was related to the fact that Lexapro sold for $2.3 billion in 2008.[57] At any rate, we do know something about what it means to be 'a decent and ethically responsible firm'. In 2009, the US Senate released documents it had requested from Forest.[61] They start out by saying that Forest will communicate that Lexapro offers superior efficacy and tolerability over all SSRIs, which is pure fantasy.

We are also told that the antidepressant market is the most heavily detailed category in the drug industry and that the sales mirror the promotional effort. Forest will develop ghostwritten articles for 'thought leaders', which will 'allow us to fold Lexapro messages', and will also use thought leaders at sponsored symposia, which will be published in supplements to medical journals to 'help disseminate relevant Lexapro data and messages to key target audiences'.

The thought leaders, advisors and Lexapro investigators will be kept informed by monthly mailings, and Forest will use the consultant services of thought leaders and advisors to obtain critical feedback and recommendations on 'educational and promotional strategies and tactics'. Forest recruited about 2000 psychiatrists and primary care physicians whom the company trained to 'serve as faculty for the Lexapro Speakers' Bureau Program'. It was obligatory that speakers used the slide kit prepared by Forest.

The documents include details of a huge programme of phase IV studies (seeding trials it seems) and describe that investigator grants would cover the costs of 'Thought Leader Initiated Phase IV studies with Lexapro'. The outcome of all these studies seemed to have been determined beforehand, even before the studies started, as key messages were listed for each study:

- Escitalopram has the lowest potential for drug interactions
- Escitalopram has an excellent dosing profile
- Escitalopram represents a new more selective and/or potent generation of SSRIs
- Escitalopram is an effective first-line treatment for depression
- Escitalopram has a favourable side-effect profile
- Escitalopram has improved side-effect, drug interaction and safety profiles resulting from the removal of the inactive moiety, the R-enantiomer
- Escitalopram is a refinement of citalopram in terms of antidepressant effect and tolerability.

Forest provided 'unrestricted grants' to professional societies, e.g. the American Psychiatric Association, so that they could develop 'reasonable practice' guidelines. What was meant by this was 'to improve the percent of patients who adhere to the full duration of therapy'. Forest became a corporate sponsor of the American College of Physicians 'which provides additional marketing opportunities', and this organisation was also involved with developing the 'reasonable practice' guidelines.

I could throw up. Total corruption of academic medicine resulting in immense harms to patients who cannot get off the drug once they have adhered to 'the full duration of therapy'. So this is a 'decent and ethically responsible firm',[56] right?

ANTIPSYCHOTIC DRUGS

Antipsychotics are dangerous drugs that should only be used if there is a compelling reason, and preferably as short-term therapy at a low dose because the drugs produce severe and permanent brain damage. As explained above, even most patients with schizophrenia can avoid the drugs and it results in much better long-term outcomes than if they are treated and substantial financial savings as well.[21]

Antipsychotics increase the risk of dying substantially through a variety of mechanisms, which include suicide, cardiac arrhythmias, diabetes and major weight gains.[9]

The drug companies have caused tremendous harm by their widespread illegal and aggressive promotion of the drugs for off-label use (*see* Chapter 3). The legal use is also increasing, e.g. in children, the use of antipsychotics went up eight-fold between 1993–1998 and 2005–2009, and it doubled in adults.[62]

The story of antipsychotics has many similarities to that of the SSRIs. The clinical research wasn't aimed at clarifying the role of the new drugs for clinicians and patients but was driven by marketing strategy, and new drugs were much hyped although large, independent government-funded trials found they weren't better than old drugs[63–65] (*see also* Chapter 9). A trial of 498 patients with a first-episode schizophrenia found no difference in discontinuation rates between four newer drugs and haloperidol.[65] Discontinuation rate is a sound outcome, as it combines perceptions of benefits and harms of the drugs. The study was funded by three drug companies but they were kept at arm's length.

Antipsychotics are standard treatment for bipolar disorder, which is mainly iatrogenic, caused by SSRIs and ADHD drugs, and they are also used for depression when treatment with an antidepressant is not enough. We now see advertisements, e.g. for AstraZeneca, about combination therapy for depression, and there are even preparations that combine the drugs in the same pill, e.g. Symbyax from Lilly, which contains Prozac (fluoxetine) and Zyprexa (olanzapine),[48] two of the worst psychotropic drugs ever invented.

Like for the SSRIs, there are many perverse trials supporting antipsychotics for virtually everything. In 2011, an AstraZeneca trial studying whether quetiapine could prevent the development of psychosis in people as young as 15 years 'at risk' of psychosis was stopped after protests that it was unethical.[66] There is no good reason to believe that these drugs can prevent psychosis, in fact, they *cause* psychosis in the long run (see above);[21] and most people 'at risk' would never have developed psychosis.

A 2009 meta-analysis of 150 trials with 21 533 patients showed that psychiatrists had been duped for 20 years.[63,67] The drug industry invented catchy but entirely misleading terms such as 'second generation antipsychotics' and 'atypical antipsychotics', but there is nothing special about the new drugs, and as they are widely heterogeneous, it's wrong to divide them into two classes.

It's remarkable that it was possible to show in a meta-analysis of published trials that new drugs aren't better than old ones, as the research literature is so flawed. Haloperidol is the comparator in most of the trials, and their design is often flawed, using too high doses or too quick dose increases for haloperidol and other old drugs, resulting in a false claim that a new drug is similarly effective but better tolerated.[68] An analysis of 2000 trials in schizophrenia revealed a disaster area of poor-quality research that didn't even improve over time, and with 640 different instruments to measure the outcome; 369 of these mostly homemade scales were only used once![69]

Unsurprisingly, an internal Pfizer memorandum shows that the flaws are introduced deliberately:[70]

> If we were going to have to increase dothiepin dosage from 75 mg to 100 mg, we should do so at 1 week rather than at 2 weeks, which would result in a high drop-out rate on dothiepin due to side effects. By 2 weeks, patients have learnt to live with side effects.

ZYPREXA, ANOTHER TERRIBLE ELI LILLY DRUG TURNED INTO A BLOCKBUSTER

The deceptions worked, as always. Everybody wants a 'modern' drug, whatever that means, and this bad habit is extremely costly, even when the 'modern' drug is only an old drug in disguise. Olanzapine was an old substance and the patent was running out, but Lilly got a new patent by showing that it produced less elevation of cholesterol in dogs than a never-marketed drug![9] This was totally ludicrous, and in fact, olanzapine raises cholesterol more than most other drugs. It could therefore have been marketed as a cholesterol-raising drug, but that wouldn't have made Zyprexa a blockbuster with sales of around $5 billion per year for more than a decade.[9]

A Cochrane review from 2005 reported that the largest trial with olanzapine had been published 142 times in papers and conference abstracts.[71] I am not kidding, it was the same trial in 142 publications. The carpet bombing also included criminal activities (*see* Chapter 3), and the aggressive marketing made Zyprexa the most widely used antipsychotic drug in the world, although it isn't any better than far cheaper alternatives. In 2005, Zyprexa was Lilly's top-selling drug at $4.2 billion.[72]

Money, marketing and lies ensured that doctors didn't use the old cheap drugs. In 2002, the sales of Zyprexa were 54 times larger than the sales for haloperidol in Denmark, amounting to a staggering €30 million a year, although our country is very small. There was no excuse for this. Two years earlier, a meta-analysis was published in the *BMJ* that concluded that 'the new drugs have no unequivocal advantages for first line use'.[73]

The last time I checked the price for Zyprexa, it cost seven times as much as haloperidol. It's irresponsible to waste so much money, and patient organisations contribute to this. They only know what the drug firms have told them, or what the psychiatrists have told them, which is about the same, as the psychiatrists also generally only know what the drug firms have told them. It was therefore not surprising when the chairman of an organisation for psychiatric patients in 2001 called it unethical that Danish psychiatrists in her view were too slow to use the newer antipsychotics such as Zyprexa and Risperdal (risperidone).[74] A researcher explained that many patients on Zyprexa increased their body weight by 15–25 kg during a few months, that there was a risk of diabetes, and that increased cholesterol was commonly seen. He also commented on the adverse effects of Risperdal and said that the likely reason that the chairman wanted these drugs to be used much more was that the adverse effects were little known. Wise words indeed.

In Chapter 3, I described that Lilly agreed to pay more than $1.4 billion for illegal marketing for numerous off-label uses including Alzheimer's, depression and dementia, and Zyprexa was pushed particularly hard in children and the elderly, although the harms of the drug are substantial, inducing heart failure, pneumonia, considerable weight gain and diabetes.[75] In 2006, internal Lilly documents were leaked to the *New York Times*, which demonstrate the extent to which the company downplayed the risks of its drug.[72,76] Lilly's chief scientist, Alan Breier, told employees in 1999 that 'weight gain and possible hyperglycemia is a major threat to the long-term success of this critically important molecule', but the company didn't discuss with outsiders that a 1999 study, disclosed in the documents, found that blood sugar levels in the patients increased steadily for 3 years.[76] Lilly instigated legal action against a number of doctors, lawyers, journalists and activists to stop them from publishing the incriminating leaked documents on the internet, and after the injunction, they disappeared.

In 2007, Lilly still maintained that 'numerous studies ... have not found that

Zyprexa causes diabetes', even though Zyprexa and similar drugs since 2003 on their label had carried an FDA warning that hyperglycaemia had been reported. Lilly's own studies showed that 30% of the patients gained at least 10 kg in weight after a year on the drug, and both psychiatrists and endocrinologists said that Zyprexa caused many more patients to become diabetic than other drugs.[76]

Zyprexa is likely more harmful than many other antipsychotics.[77] In 2001, Lilly's best-selling antidepressant Prozac was running out of patent and the company was desperate to somehow fool people into using Zyprexa also for mood disorders and called it a mood-stabiliser rather than an antipsychotic. It doesn't stabilise the mood, and it was also a challenge that general practitioners were worried about the harms of antipsychotics, but Lilly was determined to 'change their paradigm'. The internal documents say it all. In psychiatry, it doesn't really matter which drugs you have, as most drugs can be used more or less for everything, and psychiatrists are easily amenable for manipulation, even in the way they define and name their diseases.

Let's estimate how many people Lilly has killed with Zyprexa. In 2007, it was reported that more than 20 million people had taken Zyprexa.[78] A meta-analysis of the randomised trials of olanzapine and similar drugs given to patients with Alzheimer's disease or dementia showed that 3.5% died on drug and 2.3% on placebo (P = 0.02).[79] Thus, for every 100 patients treated, there was one additional death on the drug. Elderly patients are often treated with several drugs and are more vulnerable to their harms, which means that the death rate is likely higher than in younger patients. However, the reviewed trials generally ran for only 10–12 weeks, and most patients in real life are treated for years. Further, drugs like Zyprexa are most used in the elderly, and as deaths are often underreported in trials, the true death rate is likely higher than shown in the meta-analysis. One death in a hundred therefore seems a reasonable estimate to use. I therefore estimate that 200 000 of the 20 million patients treated with Zyprexa have been killed because of the drug's harms. What is particularly saddening is that many of these patients shouldn't have been treated with Zyprexa.

As Zyprexa is not the only drug, the death toll must be much higher than this. AstraZeneca silenced a trial that showed that quetiapine (Seroquel) led to high rates of treatment discontinuations and significant weight increases while the company at the same time presented data at European and US meetings that indicated that the drug *helped* psychotic patients *lose* weight.[80] Speakers Slide Kit and at least one journal article stated that quetiapine didn't increase body weight while internal data showed that 18% of the patients had a weight gain of at least 7%.[77] AstraZeneca propagated other lies.[77] It presented a meta-analysis of four trials showing that quetiapine had better effect than haloperidol, but internal documents released through litigation showed it was exactly the opposite: quetiapine was *less* effective than haloperidol.

THE BOTTOM LINE OF PSYCHOTROPIC DRUGS

How come we have allowed drug companies to lie so much, commit habitual crime and kill hundreds of thousands of patients, and yet we do nothing? Why don't we put those responsible in jail? Why are many people still against allowing citizens to get access to all the raw data from all clinical trials and why are they against scrapping the whole system and only allow publicly employed academics to test drugs in patients, independently of the drug industry?

I know some excellent psychiatrists who help their patients a lot, e.g. David Healy uses watchful waiting before giving drugs to first-episode patients.[21] I also know that some drugs can be helpful sometimes for some patients. And I am not 'antipsychiatry' in any way. But my studies in this area lead me to a very uncomfortable conclusion:

Our citizens would be far better off if we removed all the psychotropic drugs from the market, as doctors are unable to handle them. It is inescapable that their availability creates more harm than good.

REFERENCES

1 Keller MB, Ryan ND, Strober M, *et al.* Efficacy of paroxetine in the treatment of adolescent major depression: a randomized, controlled trial. *J Am Acad Child Adolesc Psychiatry.* 2001; **40**: 762–72.

2 Bass A. *Side Effects – a prosecutor, a whistleblower, and a bestselling antidepressant on trial.* Chapel Hill: Algonquin Books; 2008.

3 Jureidini JN, McHenry LB, Mansfield PR. Clinical trials and drug promotion: selective reporting of study 329. *Int J Risk Safety Med.* 2008; **20**: 73–81.

4 Jureidini JN, McHenry LB. Conflicted medical journals and the failure of trust. *Accountability in Research.* 2001; **18**: 45–54.

5 More fraud from drug giant GlaxoSmithKline companies – court documents show. *Child Health Safety.* 2010 Dec 1.

6 Moynihan R, Cassels A. *Selling Sickness: how the world's biggest pharmaceutical companies are turning us all into patients.* New York: Nation Books; 2005.

7 Boyce J. Disclosure of clinical trial data: why exemption 4 of the freedom of information act should be restored. *Duke Law & Technology Review.* 2005; **3**.

8 Jurand SH. *Lawsuits over Antidepressants Claim the Drug is worse than the Disease.* American Association for Justice. 2003 Mar 1. Available online at: www.thefreelibrary.com/_/print/PrintArticle.aspx?id=99601757 (accessed 23 Dec 2012).

9 Healy D. *Pharmageddon.* Berkeley: University of California Press; 2012.

10 Brownlee S. *Overtreated: why too much medicine is making us sicker and poorer.* New York: Bloomsbury; 2007.

11 Kingston A. A national embarrassment. *Maclean's Magazine.* 2012 Oct 17.

12 The creation of the Prozac myth. *The Guardian.* 2008 Feb 27.

13 Healy D. *Let Them Eat Prozac.* New York: New York University Press; 2004.

14 Furukawa TA. All clinical trials must be reported in detail and made publicly available. *Lancet.* 2004; **329**: 626.

15 Harris G. Merck says it will post the results of all drug trials. *New York Times.* 2004 Sept 6.

16 Lenzer J. Secret US report surfaces on antidepressants in children. *BMJ.* 2004; **329**: 307.

17 Lenzer J. Crisis deepens at the US Food and Drug Administration. *BMJ.* 2004; **329**: 1308.

18 Giles J. Did GSK trial data mask Paxil suicide risk? *New Scientist.* 2008 Feb 8.

19 Healy D. SSRIs and deliberate self-harm. *Br J Psychiatry.* 2002; **180**: 547.

20 Khan A, Warner HA, Brown WA. Symptom reduction and suicide risk in patients treated with placebo in antidepressant clinical trials: an analysis of the Food and Drug Administration database. *Arch Gen Psychiatry.* 2000; **57**: 311–17.

21 Power N, Lloyd K. Response from Pfizer. *Br J Psychiatry.* 2002; **180**: 547–8.

22 Rockhold F, Metz A, Traber P. Response from GlaxoSmithKline. *Br J Psychiatry.* 2002; **180**: 548.

23 Healy D. Did regulators fail over selective serotonin reuptake inhibitors? *BMJ.* 2006; **333**: 92–5.

24 Healy D, Cattell D. Interface between authorship, industry and science in the domain of thera-peutics. *Br J Psychiatry.* 2003; **183**: 22–7.

25 Lenzer J. FDA to review 'missing' drug company documents. *BMJ.* 2005; **330**: 7.

26 Boseley S. Scandal of scientists who take money for papers ghostwritten by drug companies. *The Guardian.* 2002 Feb 7.

27 Whittington CJ, Kendall T, Fonagy P, *et al.* Selective serotonin reuptake inhibitors in childhood depression: systematic review of published versus unpublished data. *Lancet.* 2004; **363**: 1341–5.

28 *Seroxat/Paxil Adolescent Depression. Position piece on the phase III clinical studies.* GlaxoSmithKline document. 1998 Oct.

29 Laughren TP. *Overview for December 13 Meeting of Psychopharmacologic Drugs Advisory Committee (PDAC).* 2006 Nov 16. Available online at: www.fda.gov/ohrms/dockets/ac/06/briefing/2006-4272b1-01-FDA.pdf (accessed 22 October 2012).

30 Internal Eli Lilly memo. Bad Homburg. 1984 May 25.

31 Eli Lilly memo. *Suicide Report for BGA.* Bad Homburg. 1990 Aug 3.

32 Montgomery SA, Dunner DL, Dunbar GC. Reduction of suicidal thoughts with paroxetine in comparison with reference antidepressants and placebo. *Eur Neuropsychopharmacol.* 1995; **5**: 5–13.

33 GlaxoSmithKline. *Briefing Document. Paroxetine adult suicidality analysis: major depressive disorder and non-major depressive disorder.* 2006 April 5.

34 Gunnell D, Saperia J, Ashby D. Selective serotonin reuptake inhibitors (SSRIs) and suicide in adults: meta-analysis of drug company data from placebo controlled, randomised controlled trials submitted to the MHRA's safety review. *BMJ.* 2005; **330**: 385.

35 Healy DT. Risk of suicide. *BMJ.* 2005 Feb 18. Available online at: www.bmj.com/content/330/7488/385?tab=responses (accessed 18 December 2012).

36 Fergusson D, Doucette S, Glass KC, *et al.* Association between suicide attempts and selective serotonin reuptake inhibitors: systematic review of randomised controlled trials. *BMJ.* 2005; **330**: 396.

37 Menzies KB. *2006 PDAC Regarding the Results of FDA's Ongoing Meta-Analysis of Suicidality Data from Adult Antidepressant Trials.* FDA. 2006 Dec 1.

38 Schelin EM. [Healthy skepticism is the best medicine]. *Ugeskr Læger.* 2010; **172**: 3361.

39 Lexchin J, Light DW. Commercial influence and the content of medical journals. *BMJ.* 2006; **332**: 1444–7.

40 Gorman JM, Korotzer A, Su G. Efficacy comparison of escitalopram and citalopram in the treatment of major depressive disorder: pooled analysis of placebo-controlled trials. *CNS Spectr.* 2002; 7(4 Suppl. 1): 40–4.

41 Escitalopram (Lexapro) for depression. *Medical Letter.* 2002; **44**: 83–4.

42 Melander H, Ahlqvist-Rastad J, Meijer G, *et al.* Evidence b(i)ased medicine – selective reporting from studies sponsored by pharmaceutical industry: review of studies in new drug applications. *BMJ.* 2003; **326**: 1171–3.

43 Carlsen LT. [A difficult balance]. *Tænk + Test.* 2003; **32**: 30–3.

44 Lindberg M. [Interesting regard for exports]. *Dagens Medicin.* 2002 Nov 29.

45 [The Danish Drug Agency gives Lundbeck hindwind]. *Politiken.* 2004 Sept 13.

46 [Treatment with antidepressants]. Danish Institute for Rational Drug Therapy. 2004 Sept 10.

47 Dyer O. Lundbeck broke advertising rules. *BMJ.* 2003; **326**: 1004.

48 Cipriani A, Santilli C, Furukawa TA, *et al.* Escitalopram versus other antidepressive agents for depression. *Cochrane Database Syst Rev.* 2009; **2**: CD006532.

49 Turner EH, Matthews AM, Linardatos E, *et al.* Selective publication of antidepressant trials and its influence on apparent efficacy. *N Engl J Med.* 2008; **358**: 252–60.

50 Gartlehner G, Hansen RA, Morgan LC, *et al.* Comparative benefits and harms of second-generation antidepressants for treating major depressive disorder: an updated meta-analysis. *Ann Intern Med.* 2011; **155**: 772–85.

51 Dyer O. Lundbeck broke advertising rules. *BMJ.* 2003; **326**: 1004.

52 Masculine. Available online at: www.sprunk-jansen.com/da (accessed 2012 October 28).

53 Svansø VL. [Lundbeck needs to fight for the company's image]. *Berlingske.* 2011 May 14.

54 Petersen M. *Our Daily Meds.* New York: Sarah Crichton Books; 2008.

55 US Department of Justice. *Drug Maker Forest Pleads Guilty; to pay more than $313 million to resolve criminal charges and False Claims Act allegations.* 2010 Sept 15.

56 Hyltoft V. [Lundbeck partner in settlement about suicides]. *Berlingske.* 2011 Feb 8.

57 Meier B, Carey B. Drug maker is accused of fraud. *New York Times.* 2009 Feb 25.

58 Edwards J. Suit vs. Forest Labs names execs linked to alleged lies about Lexapro, Celexa. *CBS News, Moneywatch.* 2009 Feb 26.

59 Meier B. A medical journal quandary: how to report on drug trials. *New York Times.* 2004 June 21.

60 Harris G. Document details plan to promote costly drug. *New York Times.* 2009 Sept 1.

61 US Senate, Committee on Finance. Letter about Lexapro documents. 2009 Aug 12. Available online at: www.nytimes.com/packages/pdf/politics/20090831MEDICARE/20090831_MEDICARE.pdf (accessed 2011).

62 Olfson M, Blanco C, Liu SM, *et al.* National trends in the office-based treatment of children, adolescents, and adults with antipsychotics. *Arch Gen Psychiatry.* 2012; Aug 6: 1–10.

63 Tyrer P, Kendall T. The spurious advance of antipsychotic drug therapy. *Lancet.* 2009; **373**: 4–5.

64 Rosenheck RA. Pharmacotherapy of first-episode schizophrenia. *Lancet.* 2008; **371**: 1048–9.

65 Kahn RS, Fleischhacker WW, Boter H, *et al.* Effectiveness of antipsychotic drugs in first-episode schizophrenia and schizophreniform disorder: an open randomised clinical trial. *Lancet.* 2008; **371**: 1085–97.

66 Stark J. McGorry aborts teen drug trial. *Sydney Morning Herald.* 2011 Aug 21.

67 Leucht S, Corves C, Arbter D, *et al.* Second-generation versus first-generation antipsychotic drugs for schizophrenia: a meta-analysis. *Lancet.* 2009; **373**: 31–41.

68 Safer DJ. Design and reporting modifications in industry-sponsored comparative psychopharmacology trials. *J Nerv Ment Dis.* 2002; **190**: 583–92.

69 Thornley B, Adams C. Content and quality of 2000 controlled trials in schizophrenia over 50 years. *BMJ.* 1998; **317**: 1181–4.

70 Pfizer memorandum. 1989 April 26.

71 Duggan L, Fenton M, Rathbone J, *et al.* Olanzapine for schizophrenia. *Cochrane Database Syst Rev.* 2005; **2**: CD001359.

72 Lenzer J. Drug company tries to suppress internal memos. *BMJ.* 2007; **334**: 59.

73 Geddes J, Freemantle N, Harrison P, *et al.* Atypical antipsychotics in the treatment of schizophrenia: systematic overview and meta-regression analysis. *BMJ.* 2000; **321**: 1371–6.

74 Larsen N-E. [New medicine has considerable adverse effects]. *Dagens Medicin.* 2001 Sept 27.

75 Sheller SA. The Largest Pharma Fraud Whistleblower Case in US history totaling $1.4 billion. Press release. 2009 Jan 15. Available online at: www.reuters.com/article/2009/01/15/idUS182128+15-Jan-2009+PRN20090115 (accessed 17 July 2013).

76 Berenson A. Eli Lilly said to play down risk of top pill. *New York Times.* 2006 Dec 17.

77 Spielmans GI, Parry PI. From evidence-based medicine to marketing-based medicine: evidence from internal industry documents. *Bioethical Inquiry.* 2010. DOI 10.1007/s11673-010-9208-8.

78 Dyer O. Lilly investigated in US over the marketing of olanzapine. *BMJ.* 2007; **334**: 171.

79 Schneider LS, Dagerman KS, Insel P. Risk of death with atypical antipsychotic drug treatment for dementia: meta-analysis of randomized placebo-controlled trials. *JAMA.* 2005; **294**: 1934–43.

80 McGauran N, Wieseler B, Kreis J, *et al.* Reporting bias in medical research – a narrative review. *Trials.* 2010; **11**: 37.

Intimidation, threats and violence to protect sales

I came to realize that, by comparison with the reality, my story was as tame as a holiday postcard.

John le Carré, *The Constant Gardener*

It takes great courage to become a whistle-blower. Healthcare is so corrupt that those who expose drug companies' criminal acts become pariahs. They disturb the lucrative status quo where people around them benefit handsomely from industry money: colleagues and bosses, the hospital, the university, the specialist society, the medical association and some politicians.

A whistle-blower may even have the whole state against him, as happened for Stanley Adams when he reported Roche's vitamin cartel to the European Commission in 1973.[1] Willi Schlieder, Director-General for Competition at the Commission, leaked Adams' name to Roche and he ended up in a Swiss prison, charged – and later convicted – with crimes against the state by giving economic information to a foreign power. Roche seems to have orchestrated the police interrogations and when Adams' wife was told he could face 20 years in prison, she committed suicide. Adams was treated as a spy, court proceedings were held in secret, and he wasn't even allowed to attend his wife's funeral. The Swiss courts were completely resistant to the argument that Adams had done nothing wrong because Switzerland had broken its free trade agreement with the EU, which specified that violations of free competition should be reported.

It is only in the United States that whistle-blowers may get rewarded to a substantial degree that allows them not to worry – at least not financially – that they might never get a job again. However, whistle-blowers are not motivated by possible financial bounty, but by their conscience, e.g. 'I didn't want to be responsible for somebody dying.'[2] Some companies have ethical guidelines urging people to report irregularities internally and sometimes the leadership is happy to get such information, as they might want to take action. But that's the exception. All the companies I have studied engage deliberately in criminal activities, and in the United States, there is a log of nearly a thousand healthcare *qui tam* cases (in which whistle-blowers with direct knowledge of the alleged fraud initiate the litigation on behalf of the government), and the Justice Department has suggested that the problem may get worse.[2]

It's a pretty bad idea to tell a company about its crimes, just like it's a bad idea to tell a gangster that you have observed his unlawful activities. Peter Rost, a global vice president of marketing for Pfizer turned whistle-blower, has explained that 'Pharmacia's lawyer clearly thought that anyone who tried to resolve potential criminal acts within the company and keep his job was a mental case.'[3] Most whistle-blowers who have contacted the company have been subjected to various pressures and sometimes seriously threatened, e.g. 'Even if they find something the company will throw you under the bus and prove that you were a loose cannon and the only person doing it.'[2] The company violence also extends to other companies: 'I was fired ... Then I took a job. Then somehow [company name not revealed] called the job. Then I was fired.'

There are many similarities to mob crimes. Those who threaten the income from the crimes are exposed to violence, the difference being that in the drug industry, the violence is not of a physical but psychological nature, which can be equally devastating. This violence includes intimidation, instigation of fear, threats of firing or legal proceedings, actual firing and litigation, unfounded accusations of scientific misconduct, and other attempts at defamation and destruction of research careers. The manoeuvres are often carried out by the industry's lawyers,[4-16] and private detectives may be involved.[16,17]

It is highly stressful to become a whistle-blower and cases take 5 years, on average.[2] Peter Rost has described how things went for 233 people who blew the whistle on fraud:[3] 90% were fired or demoted, 27% faced lawsuits, 26% had to seek psychiatric or physical care, 25% suffered alcohol abuse, 17% lost their homes, 15% got divorced, 10% attempted suicide and 8% went bankrupt. But in spite of all this, only 16% said that they wouldn't blow the whistle again.

Thalidomide

Private detectives kept an eye on physicians who criticised thalidomide,[17] and when a physician had found 14 cases of extremely rare birth defects related to the drug, Grünenthal threatened him with legal action and sent letters to about 70 000 German doctors declaring that thalidomide was a safe drug, although the company – in addition to the birth defects – had reports of about 2000 cases of serious and irreversible nerve damage they kept quiet about. Grünenthal harassed the alert doctor for the next 10 years. An FDA scientist that refused to approve thalidomide for the US market was also harassed and intimidated, not only by the company but also by her bosses at the FDA.

The immense power of big pharma is illustrated by the thalidomide court cases. They started in 1965 in Södertälje, the home town of Scandinavia's biggest drug company, Astra. Astra had manufactured thalidomide, but the lawyer had enormous difficulty finding experts who were willing to testify against Astra.[17] In the United States, the company that had distributed thalidomide even though it wasn't approved by the FDA had hired every expert there was on birth defects to prevent them from testifying for the victims.

In Germany, the court cases were a complete farce. The company's lawyers argued that it wasn't against the law to damage a fetus, as it had no legal rights. Maybe they should have thought about the malformed children, or about the millions of people the Nazis had murdered shortly before this that were also considered to be subhuman and of no value. Three years into the trial, Grünenthal threatened journalists for what they had written and the trial ended with a ridiculously small settlement, about $11 000 for each deformed baby. No guilty verdict was ever rendered, no personal responsibility was assigned, and no one went to prison.

The United Kingdom behaved like a dictatorship state. The journalists weren't allowed to write about the court cases and people at the highest positions in the country, including the prime minister, were more interested in defending the company and its shareholders than in helping the victims. After a stalemate that lasted for 10 years, the national scandal couldn't be held back any longer and the company, Distillers, which also sold liquor, faced a public boycott. A chain of 260 stores actually did boycott Distillers, and Ralph Nader announced that if the victims didn't get a similar compensation as in the United States, a US boycott would be launched. It took 16 years before the incriminating evidence that had been described in an article the *Sunday Times* was forbidden to print finally came to public knowledge. This was only because the affair ended in the European Court where Prime Minister Margaret Thatcher was asked to explain the mysteries of English law, the rationale of which no one on the continent could understand. The European Commission issued a report that contained the *Sunday Times'* unpublished article in an appendix. It is difficult to understand that the UK censorship happened in a European country. As in Germany, no one was found guilty and no one was even charged with a crime.

Other cases

It is not only the politicians that rather consistently fail to act on industry's crimes, apart from a few outspoken ones in the United States. The chiefs at the whistle-blower's home institution also prefer to look the other way, as they have their own interests to protect.[18] Merck selectively targeted doctors who raised questions about Vioxx and pressured some of them through deans and department chairs, often with the hint of loss of funding.[19] A few days after Eric Topol had testified for a federal jury that Merck's former chair, Raymond Gilmartin, had called the chair of the clinic's board of trustees to complain about Topol's views on Vioxx, his titles as provost and chief academic officer at the medical school in Cleveland were removed.[20]

Lawsuits against Merck have uncovered details about how the company systematically persecuted critical doctors and tried to win opinion leaders over on their side.[5] A spreadsheet contained information about named doctors and the Merck people who were responsible for haunting them, and an email said: 'We may need to seek them out and destroy them where they live',[21] as if Merck had started a rat extermination campaign. There was detailed information about each doctor's influence and of Merck's plans and outcomes of the harassments, e.g. 'NEUTRALIZED' and 'DISCREDIT'. Some examples are shown in Table 19.1. An invitation to a 'thought-leader event' is like George Orwell's thought police, which was the secret police of Oceania in his novel *1984*. It seems that Merck had problems both when doctors were honest, like a doctor who would 'only present data for approved products or information from peer-reviewed literature', and when they were *too* dishonest, e.g. 'frankly would not want this type of person speaking for my product'.

Table 19.1 Quotes from internal Merck spreadsheet concerning doctors who were critical towards Vioxx

'Strong recommendation to discredit him'

'Visit from a high-level senior team not necessary'

'Needs to be on a larger clinical trial with VIOXX'

'invitation to Merck thought-leader event'

'He will be a good advocate once we have some published data for him to review'

'He is being developed by G. Foster/T. Williams'

'Invite to consultant meetings'

'He is in the Searle camp and speaks for them'

'Most influential rheumatologist in the state of South Carolina'

'somewhat argumentative at the Board Meeting but has been treated well by Merck'

'held off acceptance of Celebrex on formulary at Oschner pending approval of VIOXX'

'National impact; speaking extensively for Searle/Pfizer (200 days this year)'

'numerous reports of biased and inaccurate presentations' (when speaking for other firms)

'loose cannon, written transcript of a talk was like an advertisement for Arthrotec'

'will only present data for approved products or information from peer-reviewed literature'

'would be offended if offered a seed study'

'is very influential and will have a strong effect on PCP prescribing habits'

I have given many examples that show senior staff in drug agencies can behave just as badly as bought deans and department chairs (*see* Chapter 10). When associate director in the FDA's Office of Drug Safety, David Graham, had shown that Vioxx increases serious coronary heart disease, his study was pulled at the last minute from the *Lancet* after Steven Galson, director of the FDA's Center for Drug Evaluation and Research, had raised allegations of scientific misconduct with the editor, which Graham's supervisors knew were untrue when they raised them.[22,23] The study was later published,[24] but just a week before Merck withdrew Vioxx from the market, senior people at the FDA questioned why Graham studied the harms of Vioxx, as FDA had no regulatory problems with it, and they also wanted him to stop, saying he had done 'junk science'.[22]

There were hearings at Congress after Merck pulled the drug, but Graham's superiors tried to prevent his testimony by telling Senator Grassley that Graham was a liar, a cheat, and a bully not worth listening to.[22] Graham needed congressional protection to keep his job after threats, abuse, intimidation and lies that culminated in his sacking from the agency.[6,22] Fearing for his job, Graham had contacted a public interest group, the Government Accountability Project, which uncovered what had happened.[25] People who had claimed to be anonymous whistle-blowers and had accused Graham of bullying them turned out to be higher-ups at the FDA management! The FDA flunked every test of credibility while Graham passed all of them. An email showed that an FDA director promised to notify Merck before Graham's findings became public so that Merck could prepare for the media attention.[26] That left no doubt about whose side the FDA was on. Hearings were also held at the FDA, but the agency barred the participation of one of its own experts, Curt Furberg, after he had criticised Pfizer for having withheld data that showed that valdecoxib, which was later taken off the market, increased cardiovascular events, which Pfizer had denied.[27,28]

Considering these events, it's not surprising that the *Lancet* concluded: 'with Vioxx, Merck and the FDA acted out of ruthless, short-sighted, and irresponsible self-interest.'[29] The COX-2 inhibitors have taught us a lesson, not only about fraud but also about threats. When the *Lancet* raised questions with the authors over a paper on COX-2 inhibitors, the drug company (not named) sponsoring the research telephoned *Lancet*'s editor, Richard Horton, asking him to 'stop being so critical', adding 'If you carry on like this we are going to pull the paper, and that means no income for the journal.'[30]

Pfizer threatened a Danish physician, Preben Holme Jørgensen, with litigation after he had stated in an interview in a newspaper – in accordance with the facts – that it was dishonest and unethical that the company had published only some of the data from its CLASS trial of celecoxib (*see* Chapter 14).[31,32] Outraged by Pfizer's conduct, many of Jørgensen's colleagues declared publicly that they would boycott Pfizer. Pfizer dropped the charge against Jørgensen but wrote to doctors and in a press release that Jørgensen was misquoted in the newspaper. This was a lie; Jørgensen was not misquoted. Pfizer also complained to the press council alleging that the newspaper's criticism of Pfizer was 'undocumented', which was also a lie. The press council ruled that the newspaper had done nothing wrong. All the wrongdoing was Pfizer's.

The threats can be particularly malignant when scientists have found lethal harms with marketed drugs that the companies have successfully concealed. Such threats have included frightening telephone calls from the company warning that 'very bad things could happen', cars waiting near the researcher's home through the night, a ghoulish funeral gift, or an anonymous letter containing a picture of the researcher's young daughter leaving home to go to school.[4] Not much difference to organised gang crime there.

Journalists have often been threatened with reprisals.[16] A lawyer phoned a journalist who had written critically about the drug industry based on my research and said he called on behalf of a friend. He was interested in knowing how she had gotten access to documents that the company considered strictly confidential. He wouldn't reveal who his client was. He called again and threatened her by saying that journalists who are critical towards the drug industry may lose everything, their family, friends and job. The journalist got very scared and didn't sleep much that night.

Even researchers who have contracts giving them permission to publish, or who do not collaborate with the industry at all, may face legal threats if they wish to publish papers that don't fit with the industry's propaganda machine.[33] Immune Response filed a $7 million legal action against the University of

California after researchers published negative findings from a clinical trial of an AIDS vaccine, having refused to let the company insert its own misleading analysis in the report. This occurred despite the fact that the contract gave the researchers permission to publish. The company also tried to prevent publication by withholding some of the data.[34]

Two British dermatologists had a similar experience. They wrote a detailed review on evening primrose oil for atopic dermatitis. Out of courtesy, they showed a copy of the peer-reviewed article to the manufacturers, who threatened legal action. The article was never published, despite getting to proof stage, and it took another 12 years before the drug agency withdrew the marketing authorisation for evening primrose oil.[35]

A Canadian researcher wrote that all proton pump inhibitors are essentially equivalent in her draft guidelines, which she sent to the companies as a courtesy. AstraZeneca, which sold Losec, called for retraction of the guidelines claiming they were unlawful and threatened legal proceedings. How can guidelines be unlawful? The Ministry of Health didn't promise to pay for her legal fees.[7]

In Germany, the president for the Society of General Practice wrote a paper with a colleague from the Drug Commission at the German Medical Association where they also concluded that the proton pump inhibitors were the same.[33] Their paper was accepted for publication in *Zeitschrift für Allgemeinmedizin* (*Journal of General Practice*), but is was pulled in the last minute and caused a delay for that particular issue. The editors forgot to change the list of contents where the paper they censored still appears, but inside they published an advertisement. The journal gave in to the pressure from big pharma, which the authors considered intellectual bankruptcy.

No doubt about that. We must resist pressures and threats. And we should never show anything to drug companies as a courtesy before it is out in the public domain. The threats are bluff most of the time anyway.

But not always. When a Canadian health technology assessment concluded that the various statins had largely the same effect, Bristol-Myers Squibb sued the agency claiming 'negligent misstatements'.[36] Although the agency won the case, the legal costs amounted to 13% of its annual budget whereas this sum amounted to one day of sales revenues for Bristol-Myers Squibb's statin. Their lawsuit was a type of abuse of power called SLAPP (strategic lawsuits against public participation).

A Danish researcher who was critical towards giving women hormones around menopause received letters with threats of legal action from drug companies,[8] even though it was well documented at the time that the drugs are harmful. When another Danish researcher published convincing data on two occasions showing that the newer contraception pills, Yaz or Yasmin, result in more blood clots than older pills, he was fiercely attacked by colleagues on Bayer payroll, and studies that didn't show the newer pills were dangerous were also financed by Bayer.[9]

In 2008, one of my colleagues, Jens Lundgren, received a death threat at the international AIDS congress in Mexico City in an SMS sent a few hours before he presented data showing that GlaxoSmithKline's £600 million drug, abacavir, almost doubles the risk of heart attacks.[10,11] The pressures had already been immense after he published his results in the *Lancet* 4 months earlier, and Lundgren described how 'We were completely crushed in the GSK media machine when our study came out'. The organisers had also received threats, and as soon as Lundgren had finished his talk, he was escorted to the airport with eight bodyguards. Three years earlier, the international drug-monitoring centre operated by the WHO in Uppsala had warned Glaxo about the heart problems, but the company downplayed the warning and sent a reply that was in effect a no-reply. To coincide with the *Lancet* publication, Glaxo issued a statement to its investors that downplayed the association between abacavir and heart attacks, saying that the findings were unexpected and that no possible biological mechanism to explain it had been found. Glaxo didn't mention in its statement that the company had been warned 3 years earlier, or that the company's own research on animals had found that abacavir is associated with myocardial degeneration in the heart tissue of rats and mice.

In 2012, other Danish researchers came in trouble. They had shown in a publicly funded trial that hydroxyethyl starch, a plasma expander used in patients with severe sepsis, kills the patients, compared to giving them a much cheaper balanced salt solution.[12] When the study was published in the *New England Journal of Medicine*, a letter was promptly sent by the lawyers for Fresenius Kabi AG.[13] The lawyers wrote that 'Fresenius Kabi AG is prepared to take all appropriate legal action to recover the economic losses it has suffered (and will continue to suffer) as a result of the false information you and your colleagues have reported' and called for immediate withdrawal of the paper and correction to be made within 2 days. This was ludicrous. The researchers had written 'HES 130/0.4' in their paper but should have written 'HES 130/0.42' Did you notice the difference? If we round 0.42 to one less decimal, we'll get 0.4, won't we? The issue is that these two designations refer to two slightly different versions of hydroxyethyl starch, sold by two different companies, and the researchers had not studied Fresenius' product but the other one.

The 0.4 refers to the degree of molar substitution,[13] which can vary in the same bottle from 0.38 to 0.45 for Fresenius' product and from 0.40 to 0.44 for the product they had studied.[15] This means that the two products must be considered equivalent, but Fresenius was determined to defend its product even though hydroxyethyl starch kills the patients.

The lawyers' letter noted that 'This error is misleading readers of the article and causing them to mistakenly attribute to the Voluven product the negative effects reported to have been found with Tetraspan, resulting in significant harm to Fresenius Kabi's reputation and economic damage through lost sales.' Pretty ludicrous again, as both the abstract and the methods section mentioned the product that had been tested, Tetraspan, and not Voluven.

There was an outrage in the press and the hospital declared that it would support the researchers in case of legal proceedings. The researchers didn't retract their paper but published an erratum,[14] which resolved the case.

The whole affair was hair-splitting *ad absurdum*. If I call a person John, although his name is Mike, I make an error, but if I say that Mike's height is 1.8 m rather than 1.82 m, I don't make an error. I merely use a lesser degree of precision, which is not lawyers' business. In the media, Fresenius Kabi's reputation, which the company seemed so anxious to protect, was completely lost. Its methods were described as sending a gang of thugs.

In 2000, psychiatrist David Healy from Wales was urged to apply for a post at the Centre for Addiction and Mental Health (CAMH) at the University of Toronto by chief physician David Goldbloom.[37] Two months after Healy had accepted the post, he gave at lecture at a conference arranged by his new centre where he mentioned that Eli Lilly's antidepressant, Prozac (fluoxetine) – the best-selling drug of all time[37] – may cause suicide. A week later, Healy received an email from Goldbloom, saying:

> Essentially, we believe that it is not a good fit between you and the role as leader of an academic program in mood and anxiety disorders at the centre and in relation to the university ... This view was solidified by your recent appearance at the centre in the context of an academic lecture. While you are held in high regard as a scholar of the history of modern psychiatry, we do not feel your approach is compatible with the goals for development of the academic and clinical resource that we have.

The decision to rescind Healy's job offer caused uproar in Canadian academic circles because Lilly had donated $1.5 million to the centre. James Turk, executive director of the Canadian Association of University Teachers, explained that 'Development is a euphemism here for fundraising. I read that as meaning your appointment will make it more difficult to raise the money that we need to pursue our programmes.'[37] An international group of physicians that included two Nobel Prize winners published an open letter to the president of the university where they wrote that 'To have sullied Dr Healy's reputation by withdrawing the job offer is an affront to the standards of free speech and academic freedom.'[38]

The stakes were huge. Lilly made $2.6 billion from Prozac in 2000 alone and had just succeeded in getting the drug renamed and repackaged as Sarafem, for severe premenstrual tension, which would keep the profits rolling in until 2007, although the patent for Prozac was just about to expire.[37] Healy's findings weren't new. Six months earlier, Healy had published his concerns in the *Hastings Center Report*, which caused Eli Lilly to withdraw its support to the Hastings Center.[38] Industry money is everywhere, like a metastatic cancer that threatens to kill our societies as we know them and our free speech.

Healy suspects that Charles Nemeroff (*see* Chapter 17) was behind his rescindment.[37] Nemeroff had strong links, including shareholdings, to manufacturers of SSRIs that had been involved in court cases where Healy was an expert witness. Nemeroff was present at the Toronto meeting and announced at another psychiatric gathering the next day that Healy had lost his job, before Healy knew it himself. Nemeroff was hostile to Healy's work and had berated him a year earlier over Healy's study that showed that two out of 20 healthy volunteers became suicidal on sertraline.[39] According to Healy, Nemeroff had stated that Healy had no right publishing material like that, and that it was immaterial what psychiatrists did, as the companies were answerable to their shareholders and profit was the bottom line.

David Healy has written more than anybody else about the outrageous frauds big pharma has committed in their research and marketing of SSRIs. He describes how he has run into a legal wall with publishers with about 10 of his papers, even with the journal *Index on Censorship*, which self-censored.[40] Another author who wrote a book about the risks of suicide and homicide made Lilly threaten to sue him in 50 different countries.

Planting industry friends in the auditorium works like spies under dictatorship rule who report their observations about enemies of the state. Under a freedom of information request, Healy saw a document from Lilly about informants 'to monitor what he says and see whether he can be sued'. Lilly seems also to have threatened to pull out of its business in the United Kingdom if Zyprexa wasn't featured prominently in NICE guidelines!

Nancy Olivieri from the Hospital for Sick Children, the University of Toronto, was fired after having communicated her concerns about the harms of a drug she was investigating. The university was negotiating a donation of $20 million from Apotex, the company involved, and Apotex sued her for breaching a confidentiality clause she had signed when she started her research.[38,41]

What both cases at the University of Toronto illustrate is the danger that can arise from university reliance upon industry 'philantropy'.[38] When career success for deans and other higher-ups is measured in significant part by their ability of raise vast sums of money from corporate donors, whistle-blowers and other critics of drugs cannot expect much support.

Another university affair took place in the United Kingdom in 2005 at the University of Sheffield. Aubrey Blumsohn, the lead author of two papers on Actonel (risedronate), an osteoporosis drug marketed by Procter & Gamble, was prevented from seeing the full data that were to be published in his name,[42] although he had concerns about the interpretation of the data.[43] The research dean at the university, Richard Eastell, who was on the company's advisory board and had attracted grants from the company to the university of £1.6 million in recent years, advised caution.[44]

But only towards the company it seemed. He didn't proceed cautiously towards Blumsohn, who was suspended from his university post 2 years later after he had threatened to speak to medical journalists about the issue.[43,44] Blumsohn taped secretly a conversation with Eastell where Eastell said, 'The only thing that we have to watch all the time is our relationship with P & G.' Procter & Gamble had told Blumsohn that a ghostwriter was familiar with the 'key messages' they wanted to convey about the drug.

Procter & Gamble's defence for not sharing the data was pathetic and even ironic. They said that by doing so, they would lose the opportunity to demonstrate their ability to be 'a true partner in scientific endeavours'. In contrast, Blumsohn had stated in a letter to Eastell that 'no self-respecting scientist could ever be expected to publish findings based on data to which they do not have free and full access'. Eastell had some sympathy with this view, as questions had been raised about how much of the data on the drug's performance he himself had seen in the past in relation to papers he had his name on. Eastell later had to admit that the statement – that he and the other authors had seen all the data – was wrong, and he was subjected to a General Medical Council hearing about this falsehood.[45]

When, after numerous approaches, Blumsohn was finally allowed to see limited data, including the key graphs, 40% of the data had been left out and 'everything we'd been told was just nonsense'.

Blumsohn was suspended on the grounds that 'his conduct over these past months amounts to and constitutes conduct that is quite incompatible with the duties of office'. The university could equally well have copied the text David Healy received when he was kicked out of Toronto. In plain language, both pompous messages mean: 'If you are not willing to prostitute yourself to the interests of big pharma, just as we do, you are not welcome here.'

UK cardiologist Peter Wilmshurst was instrumental in setting up a trial studying whether closure of the foramen ovale in the heart with a medical device would help patients with migraine.[46] The results were disappointing even though they were positively biased, as the implanting cardiologists were also the ones to determine whether the hole in the heart had been successfully closed. The steering committee for the trial was unhappy that there wasn't an independent assessment of the outcome, but it was overruled by NMT, the trial sponsor.

Independently of each other, Wilmshurst and another cardiologist assessed the outcome and both came to much more negative results than what was published in *Circulation* in March 2008 with Andrew Dowson as first author. Dowson owned shares in NMT but had assured the ethics committee in writing that he didn't own shares, and he also gave his affiliation as a well-known hospital although he had treated his patients in private practice. Dowson also published a paper with Wilmshurst as co-author that Wilmshurst had never seen.[47]

In the *Circulation* paper, there were only four residual shunts whereas the two assessors had identified 27 and 33 residual shunts, respectively. When the paper was accepted for publication, Wilmshurst and another colleague, who together had contributed more than 30% of the patients and had written a substantial part of the paper, refused to sign the journal's copyright agreement because it said that they had seen the data and took responsibility for their integrity. They had only seen the data analysis, not the data.

Wilmshurst's name didn't appear anywhere in the published paper, not even in the acknowledgements, although his work had inspired the study, he had been joint principal investigator, had taken a major role in designing the trial, had written much of the paper, and had been a member of the steering committee. In contrast, a prominent cardiologist, who died before the trial began, appeared as author, a rare but genuine type of ghost author so to speak. He also co-authored a letter in *Circulation* 5 years after his death in reply to criticism of the trial, even though Wilmshurst had told the editors that he was dead.

After Wilmshurst had mentioned the problems with the trial at a congress and had given an interview, he was sued by NMT for slander and libel in the High Court in London, although the company was American. England has the worst libel laws in the world, which don't protect the whistle-blower but the perpetrator. Simon Singh wrote in *The Guardian* in 2008 that the British Chiropractic Association happily promotes bogus treatments, as the association claims that their members can help treat children with colic, sleeping and feeding problems, frequent ear infections, asthma and prolonged crying.[48] He had to spend 44 solid weeks on a libel action and wrote afterwards that 'in terms of free speech and access to information, our nation would become the European equivalent of China'.[49] He also wrote that Wilmshurst was put under immense stress when he received legal papers on Friday, 21 December 2007 at 5.09 p.m., 9 minutes after most solicitors closed for their Christmas holiday. It was not until the New Year that Wilmshurst was able to get any legal advice. Already 9 months after the *Circulation* paper, Wilmshurst had run up legal bills of nearly £60 000;[50] the lawsuit only ended because NMT went bankrupt.

When the incoming president of the American Diabetes Association, John Buse, had spoken out with his concerns about rosiglitazone's cardiovascular safety in 1999, employees of SmithKline Beecham had told him that 'there were some in the company who felt that my actions were scurrilous enough to attempt to hold me liable for a loss in market capitalisation [share value]'.[51] A US Senate report showed that after Buse had raised questions at a symposium, GlaxoSmithKline's chairman for research and development, Tadataka Yamada, had suggested either 'to sue him for knowingly defaming our product even after we have set him straight on the facts' or to 'launch a well planned offensive on behalf of Avandia'.[52] Yamada telephoned the chairman of Buse's department.

Glaxo prepared and required Buse to sign a letter claiming that he was no longer worried about cardiovascular risks associated with Avandia.[53] It would be interesting to know what made Buse sign the letter contrasting his own conviction, but after he had signed it, Glaxo officials unscrupulously began referring to it as Buse's 'retraction letter' to curry favour with a financial consulting company that was evaluating Glaxo's products for investors.

The company intimidated other physicians raising uncomfortable questions.[54] A doctor in Maryland became alarmed in 1999 after several of her patients on Avandia developed symptoms of congestive heart failure, and a review of the records for all the patients showed an unexpectedly high percentage with this problem.[55] She alerted the manufacturer to the problem, but the company sent a letter to the chief of staff at the hospital telling him that she should not be permitted to talk about the problem since congestive heart failure was not proved to be an effect of the drug. The doctor felt 'highly intimidated' by the letter and what she perceived as an implicit threat of a lawsuit. She had planned to publish her findings, but after the hospital received the letter, one of her intended co-authors, an epidemiologist, stopped responding to her emails, effectively killing publication.

In 2006, as previously noted, we published a rather uncontroversial study in *JAMA* that compared industry trial protocols with published reports and found that the academics generally had their hands tied in their collaborations with the drug industry, which wasn't revealed in any of the publications.[56] When I translated our paper into Danish and published it in the *Ugeskrift for Læger (Journal of the Danish Medical Association)*,[57] The Danish Association of the Pharmaceutical Industry said in a newspaper that it was 'shaken and enraged about the criticism' that it could not recognise. Although the Association knows very well what its member companies write in their protocols and therefore that our findings were correct, in contrast to its public statement, the Association nevertheless harassed us by filing a groundless case alleging we had committed scientific misconduct by deliberately distorting the data. The Association copied some of its letters to the management at the Rigshospitalet, where four of us worked, and to the Copenhagen Hospital Corporation, the Central Scientific-Ethics Committee, the Danish Medical Association, the Danish Drug Agency, the Ministry of Health, the Ministry of Science, and the Journal of the Danish Medical Association. They spared our Queen and Prime Minister, but even after we had been acquitted, the Association continued to insist we were guilty of misconduct. The lies never stop. We described the affair in a paper, but *BMJ*'s lawyer was worried about possible litigation, and our paper was therefore transformed into an article written by a journalist.[58]

REFERENCES

1 Adams S. *Roche versus Adams*. London: J. Cape; 1984.
2 Kesselheim AS, Studdert DM, Mello MM. Whistle-blowers' experiences in fraud litigation against pharmaceutical companies. *N Engl J Med*. 2010; **362**: 1832–9.
3 Rost P. *The Whistleblower: confessions of a healthcare hitman*. New York: Soft Skull Press; 2006.
4 Mundy A. *Dispensing with the Truth*. New York: St. Martin's Press; 2001.
5 Drug Industry Document Archive. University of California, San Francisco. Available online at: http://dida.library.ucsf.edu/search?query=argumentative (accessed 21 September 2012).
6 Day M. Don't blame it all on the bogey. *BMJ*. 2007; **334**: 1250–1.
7 Shuchman M. Drug company threatens legal action over Canadian guidelines. *BMJ*. 1999; **319**: 1388.
8 Tougaard H, Hundevadt K. [The golden promises of the gynaecologists]. *Jyllandsposten*. 2004 Jan 18.
9 Villesen K. [The drug companies earn fortunes while raising doubt]. *Information*. 2011 Dec 9.
10 Glaxo 'downplayed' warning on heart-attack risk from AIDS drug. *The Independent*. 2008 May 12.
11 Brix SM. [Researcher receives death threats]. *Universitetsavisen*. 2008; **14**: 5.
12 Perner A, Haase N, Guttormsen AB, *et al*. Hydroxyethyl Starch 130/0.42 versus Ringer's acetate in severe sepsis. *N Engl J Med*. 2012; **367**: 124–34.
13 Klawitter U, Stief M. Demand for correction of article entitled 'Hydroxyethyl Starch 130/0.4 versus Ringer's Acetate in Severe Sepsis' (published online on June 27, 2012). Letter. 2012 July 9.
14 Corrections. *N Engl J Med*. 2012; **367**: 481.
15 Kupferschmidt K. Squabble Over NEJM paper puts spotlight on antishock drug. *ScienceInsider*. 2012 Aug 2.
16 Braithwaite J. *Corporate Crime in the Pharmaceutical Industry*. London: Routledge & Kegan Paul; 1984.
17 Brynner R, Stephens T. *Dark Remedy: the impact of thalidomide and its revival as a vital medicine*. New York: Perseus Publishing; 2001.
18 Kassirer JP. *On the Take: how medicine's complicity with big business can endanger your health*. Oxford: Oxford University Press; 2005.
19 Fries JF. Letter to Raymond Gilmartin re: physician intimidation. 9 Jan, 2001. Merck. Bates No MRK-ABH0002204 to MRK-ABH0002207. Available online at: www.vioxxdocuments.com/Documents/Krumholz_Vioxx/Fries2001.pdf (accessed 10 October 2007).
20 Wood S. Eric Topol loses provost/chief academic officer titles at Cleveland Clinic and Lerner College. *Heartwire*. 2005 Dec 12.
21 Rout M. Vioxx maker Merck and Co drew up doctor hit list. *The Australian*. 2009 April 1.

22 Blowing the whistle on the FDA: an interview with David Graham. *Multinational Monitor*. 2004; **25**(12).

23 Lenzer J. Crisis deepens at the US Food and Drug Administration. *BMJ*. 2004; **329**: 1308.

24 Graham DJ, Campen D, Hui R, *et al.* Risk of acute myocardial infarction and sudden cardiac death in patients treated with cyclo-oxygenase 2 selective and non-selective non-steroidal anti-inflammatory drugs: nested case-control study. *Lancet*. 2005; **365**: 475–81.

25 Lenzer J. Public interest group accuses FDA of trying to discredit whistleblower. *BMJ*. 2004; **329**: 1255.

26 Lenzer J. US government agency to investigate FDA over rofecoxib. *BMJ*. 2004; **329**: 935.

27 Lenzer J. FDA bars own expert from evaluating risks of painkillers. *BMJ*. 2004; **329**: 1203.

28 Lenzer J. Pfizer criticised over delay in admitting drug's problems. *BMJ*. 2004; **329**: 935.

29 Horton R. Vioxx, the implosion of Merck, and aftershocks at the FDA. *Lancet* 2004; **364**: 1995–6.

30 Eaton L. Editor claims drug companies have a 'parasitic' relationship with journals. *BMJ*. 2005; **330**; 9.

31 Andersen NV, Drachmann H. [Pharmaceutical giant blacklisted]. *Politiken*. 2004 Mar 25.

32 [Verdict in the Press Council in case 2004-6-45]. *Pressenævnet*. 2004 Aug 18.

33 Grill M. *Kranke Geschäfte: wie die Pharmaindustrie uns manipuliert.* Hamburg: Rowohlt Verlag; 2007.

34 Mello MM, Clarridge BR, Studdert DM. Academic medical centers' standards for clinical-trial agreements with industry. *N Engl J Med.* 2005; **352**: 2202–10.

35 Williams HC. Evening primrose oil for atopic dermatitis. *BMJ*. 2003; **327**: 1358–9.

36 Brody H. *Hooked: ethics, the medical profession, and the pharmaceutical industry.* Lanham: Rowman & Littlefield; 2008.

37 Boseley S. Bitter pill. *The Guardian.* 2001 May 7.

38 Schafer A. Biomedical conflicts of interest: a defence of the sequestration thesis – learning from the cases of Nancy Olivieri and David Healy. *J Med Ethics.* 2004; **30**: 8–24.

39 Healy D. *Let Them Eat Prozac.* New York: New York University Press; 2004.

40 Healy D. Medical partisans? Why doctors need conflicting interests. *Aust N Z J Psychiatry.* 2012; **46**: 704–7.

41 Baylis F. The Olivieri debacle: where were the heroes of bioethics? *J Med Ethics.* 2004; **30**: 44–9.

42 Dyer C. Aubrey Blumsohn, academic who took on industry. *BMJ*. 2010; **340**: 22–3.

43 Revill J. Doctor accuses drug giant of 'unethical' secrecy. *Observer.* 2005 Dec 4.

44 Revill J. How the drugs giant and a lone academic went to war. *Observer.* 2005 Dec 4.

45 Dyer C. Professor to face GMC over his claim to have seen full trial data. *BMJ*. 2009; **339**: 774–5.

46 Gornall J. A very public break-up. *BMJ*. 2010; **340**: 180–3.

47 Wilmshurst P. The effects of the libel laws on science – a personal experience. *Radical Statistics.* 2011: **104**: 13–23.

48 Wikipedia. Simon Singh. Available online at: http://en.wikipedia.org/wiki/Simon_Singh (accessed 17 June 2010).

49 Singh S. This is goodbye. *The Guardian.* 2010 March 12.

50 Dyer C. Charity sets up fund to defend researcher being sued for libel. *BMJ*. 2008; **337**: 1313.

51 Tanne JH. FDA places 'black box' warning on antidiabetes drugs. *BMJ*. 2007; **334**: 1237.

52 Burton B. Diabetes expert accuses drug company of 'intimidation'. *BMJ*. 2007; **335**: 1113.

53 Cohen D. Drug study secrecy puts lives at risk. *Index on Censorship.* 2011 Nov 29.

54 DeAngelis CD, Fontanarosa PB. Ensuring integrity in industry-sponsored research. *JAMA*. 2010; **303**: 1196–8.

55 Lenzer J, Brownlee S. Reckless medicine. *Discover.* 2010; **11**: 64–76.

56 Gøtzsche PC, Hróbjartsson A, Johansen HK, *et al.* Constraints on publication rights in industry-initiated clinical trials. *JAMA*. 2006; **295**: 1645–6.

57 Gøtzsche PC, Hróbjartsson A, Johansen HK, *et al.* [Constraints on publication rights in industry-initiated clinical trials: secondary publication]. *Ugeskr Læger.* 2006; **168**: 2467–9.

58 Gornall J. Research transparency: industry attack on academics. *BMJ*. 2009; **338**: 626–8.

Busting the industry myths

The drug industry's myths about their activities and motives have been repeated so often that they are widely believed by doctors, politicians and the general public. As they are an impediment for creating a rational healthcare system, devoid of corruption, I shall debunk the worst of them before suggesting reforms in the next chapter.

Myth 1: Drugs are expensive because of the high discovery and development costs

The former CEO of Merck, Raymond Gilmartin, has admitted that this is a myth: 'The price of medicines isn't determined by their research costs. Instead, it is determined by their value in preventing and treating disease.'[1] Gilmartin forgot to mention that prices of drugs not only reflect what society is willing to pay but also how good the companies are at keeping competition at bay. Anti-competitive activities are widespread,[2,3] and price fixing is common.[4-6]

We often hear that is costs $800 million (in 2000 dollars) to bring a new drug to the market, but this is false. It is based on flawed methods, debatable accounting theory and premised on blind faith in confidential information supplied by the drug industry to its economic consultants at two universities who were paid by the same industry.[1,3,7] The true cost is likely to be below $100 million.[3]

Zidovudine, the first AIDS drug, was synthesised at the Michigan Cancer Foundation in 1964.[3] It cost Burroughs Wellcome very little to develop it, but the company nevertheless charged $10000 per year for one patient in 1987.[1] It was a clear abuse of a monopoly situation, with desperately ill patients demanding the drug, whatever its cost. When Abbott in 2003 suddenly increased the price of its AIDS drug, ritonavir, by 400%, the invention of which had been supported by millions of dollars of taxpayers' money, it caused an outrage and hundreds of doctors decided to boycott all Abbott's products whenever possible.[8]

A similar example is imatinib (Glivec or Gleevec), which is very effective against chronic myeloid leukaemia. Novartis had synthesised it but wasn't interested in it until a haematologist researched it and found out it was highly effective. Again, development costs were minimal, but that didn't prevent Novartis from charging $25000 for a year's treatment in 2002.[3]

Taxol is one of our most useful cancer drugs. It was derived from the bark of the Pacific yew tree and later synthesised by NIH-funded scientists.[1] The drug was handed over to Bristol-Myers Squibb who, despite minimal development costs, took $10000 to $20000 for a year's treatment in 1993. When the patent ran out, the company sued everyone that planned to market a cheaper generic.[9]

Twenty-nine US states sued Bristol-Myers Squibb for violating antitrust laws, but while all this went along before the case was settled at a cost of only $135 million for the company, it gained revenues of more than $5 billion.

After several companies marketing generic versions of citalopram for some reason had withdrawn their products from the Danish market in 2010, the price for the drug suddenly increased by a factor of 12. The companies that increased the price declined to comment.[10]

Another curious example was when all companies marketing generic simvastatin, used by about 6% of all Danes, suddenly multiplied the price of the 40 mg dose by eight.[11] The 40 mg dose was the most commonly used one. The drug was also available at a 20 mg dose at only a fifth of the price, but according to the law, the pharmacies are not allowed to hand out the cheap dose and tell the patient to take two tablets instead of one. Although the five companies raised the price to exactly the same level, to the second decimal, they denied price fixing, and the authorities launched a trenching (investigation).[12] This dirty trick would cost Danish taxpayers an additional €63 million annually for an off-patent drug.

Schering bought a hormone from another company for use in women with menopausal symptoms and sold the drug with a mark-up of 7000%,[4] and when Librium and Valium were patented, Roche sold them in Colombia for 65 times the price on the European market.[6] In 2006, the US Federal Trade Commission opened a court case against Lundbeck, alleging that the company had taken advantage of a monopoly situation to milk seriously ill infants.[13] Lundbeck had bought a US company, which had increased the price of an old, life-saving drug, indomethacin, by 1300% after having bought it from Merck. There weren't any development costs behind these price explosions.

For many years, the obstetricians had used a natural hormone for preventing premature birth, progesterone, which came on the market more than 50 years ago.[14] The pharmacies prepared it for the doctors and it cost about $10–$20 per injection. When KV Pharmaceutical won US government approval to exclusively sell the drug, known as Makena, the price went up to $1500 a dose, an increase of 75 to 150 times. The company bullshittingly declared that 'These moms deserve the opportunity to have the benefits of an FDA-approved Makena', while doctors said that the deal was likely to lead to more premature births (and therefore also to more permanently brain-damaged children), as many women would be unable to afford the drug. Some doctors said they were happy getting the cheaper version from compounding pharmacies, but the company responded by sending cease-and-desist letters to compounding pharmacies, telling them they could face FDA enforcement actions if they kept making the drug.

We are jointly responsible for the complicated society we have created, where we depend on each other and benefit from specialisation. But when drug companies charge copious amounts for their drugs, they make a mockery of their obligations towards the patients, the taxpayers, our societies and our joint assets to such an extent that they out themselves outside society, just like street criminals do. It is theft.

Researchers have shown that the yearly cost per patient is inversely related to the prevalence of the disease. Italian researchers went a step further and developed a simple formula that fitted surprisingly well with the data they had for 17 cancer drugs:[15]

$$\text{yearly cost per patient} = \text{€2 million} \cdot e^{-0.004 \cdot \text{number of patients}} + \text{€10 000}$$

Thus, the annual cost per patient for a drug where there are 900 patients in Italy will be about €60 000.

Accordingly, drugs for patients with rare enzyme deficiencies are monstrously expensive, e.g. $600 000 a year for treating Gaucher's disease,[16] although all research and early development was done entirely by NIH-funded scientists.[1]

A final blow to the myth that drug prices reflect the high research and development costs is: What can then be said about the much higher costs for sales promotion?[3] Those who pay for the drugs also pay for this extravagant marketing. If new drugs were as good as the industry wants us to believe they are, there wouldn't be much need for pushing them and for bribing doctors into using them.

Myth 2: If we don't use expensive drugs, innovation will dry out

This myth is widely believed by politicians and doctors, although it is totally ludicrous. Would these believers be ready to pay 20 times more for their new car just because the car dealer tells them that by so doing, we'll get better cars in future?

According to Marcia Angell, former editor of the *New England Journal of Medicine*, the drug industry insists that they should be essentially left alone without societal control and they also threaten our societies: 'Don't mess with us. Do nothing about our obscene profits. Do nothing about these unsustainable increases in prices, or else we will not give you your miracle cures.'[17] Usually, companies say: 'If we don't spend our money on research, we'll die.' Drug companies say: 'If we don't get *your* money to spend on research, *you'll* die.'[7]

Only religious leaders are smarter. They promise we'll be rewarded *after* we've died, which makes complaints impossible. The industry's promises are also false, indeed so false, that the cause–effect relationship is the reverse. Since the 1980s, profits in the drug industry have skyrocketed (*see* Chapter 5), but in the same period, fewer and fewer innovative drugs have come onto the market.[3] La Revue Prescrire gives an award every year to the most important breakthrough, la Pilule d'Or (the Golden Pill), but couldn't find a worthy candidate for 2012. Or 2011. Or 2010.

In 2011, the Danish regions suggested to create an institute like the National Institute for Health and Care Excellence (NICE) in the United Kingdom, as we cannot afford everything on offer. However, a conservative speaker on health in Parliament didn't want to prioritise drugs and argued it would slow down the development of new drugs if we introduced a maximum we would pay for the drugs.[18] The regions furthermore suggested that new drugs should be tested against existing and often cheaper drugs before they could be approved. This enraged the director of The Danish Association of the Pharmaceutical Industry, Ida Sofie Jensen, who said it was 'pathetic if not shameless that Danish regions again showed their industry-hostile attitudes. The regions blame the drug industry for their poor economy.'[19] The chairman for the regions responded calmly that the drug industry is one of the most profitable of all industries, and that he hoped the industry's ritual tribal dance would soon be over. The fact is that the cost of drugs at Danish hospitals trebled in just 8 years. The year before, the Danish government removed the reimbursement for some drugs that were far too expensive and not any better than cheap drugs of the same type. In response to this, Ida Sofie Jensen displayed another tribal dance: 'The authorities refuse to pay for progress in medicines. We fear this will stop the development of new drugs.'[20] In contrast, a health economist remarked that the move might give the industry an incentive to search for real breakthroughs instead of me-too drugs. That's exactly the point. Innovation has dried out because it's more lucrative for industry to develop me-too products than to do innovative research. Patients will benefit if we remove this incentive.

All over the world, apart from the United States under Republican rule, governments try to contain drug costs. An article from 2011 reported that the Czech Republic would introduce maximum prices for drugs that were reimbursed and limit the use of very expensive drugs at the university hospitals; in Germany, a price ceiling was introduced with the aim of saving €2 billion annually; in the United Kingdom, the government required that the industry reduce its prices, aiming at saving €6 billion annually; and in Australia, the government removed reimbursement for 162 drugs and planned to cut the prices for 1600 drugs by 27%.[21] China, Hungary, Bulgaria and Slovakia also had cost-saving plans.

The way New Zealand has contained its spending on drugs is impressive and simple.[22] In 1993, it was decided to subsidise drugs in the same class (e.g. NSAIDs or SSRIs) that had similar effect with the same amount, whatever the price of the drug was (reference pricing). In addition, drug companies negotiate with the drug agency over price and other conditions for access. The policy had dramatic effects. Statins were provided at half the cost compared to Australia, and the price of generic drugs was less than a quarter of the price in Canada. The community drug budget increased at an annual rate of only 2%, compared with 15% before the new policy, and at the same time, public coverage was improved. Although there are only 4.4 million inhabitants in the country, the annual savings amounted to about €1 billion.

Myth 3: Savings are greater than costs for expensive drugs

At a meeting with the drug industry where this argument was put forward, the director of the Danish National Board of Health said that it was curious that no matter how expensive a new drug was, the company was always able to provide a pharmacoeconomic analysis that showed that the savings in terms of less sick-leave, premature retirement, and whatever else, were greater than the costs for the drug. Economy is a very soft discipline, and you can get almost any result you want depending on the assumptions you put into the model. It is hard to imagine a greater conflict of interest than when a drug company concocts a pharmacoeconomic analysis of its own drug, or asks an economist to do it for hire. The outcome is never negative for the company.

Myth 4: Breakthroughs come from industry-funded research

An often-heard argument is that none of our drugs were invented by the former socialist countries east of the Iron Curtain. That proves nothing. There was so much else that didn't work out in these countries under dictatorship rule. The misconception is huge. Virtually all the basic science that enables modern medicine to move forward takes place in the non-profit sector, at universities, research institutes and government laboratories.[23] A US Congress report from 2000 noted that 'Of the 21 most important drugs introduced between 1965 and 1992, 15 were developed using knowledge and techniques from federally funded research.' Other studies have found the same, e.g. at least 80% of 35 major drugs were based on scientific discoveries made by public-sector research institutions.[24] The National Cancer Institute played the lead role in the development of 50 of 58 new cancer drugs approved by the FDA between 1955 and 2001.[7]

Three of the most important discoveries in the 20th century – penicillin, insulin and the polio vaccine – all came from publicly funded laboratories. The NIH conducted an investigation on the five top-selling drugs in 1995, Zantac (ranitidine, for ulcers), Zovirax (acyclovir, for herpes), Capoten (captopril, for high blood pressure), Vasotec (enalapril, for high blood pressure) and Prozac (fluoxetine, for depression), and found that 16 of the key 17 scientific papers leading to the discovery and development of these drugs came from outside the industry.[3]

The picture is very consistent. The first breakthrough in AIDS also came from public research and the US government spent double as much on research as all the drug companies taken together.[7] The typical story is that drug companies invest relatively little in the real breakthroughs, but when they take over from publicly funded research, they sell the drug at an exorbitant price, as they have a monopoly. In addition, they routinely lie about the research and often steal the credit for the drug and claim they found it themselves.[7] The much-touted public–private partnerships fall totally apart when the private part constantly runs away with all the money and all the credit, making the rest of society look like a fool or a victim of robbery.

Drug companies spend only 1% of revenues on basic research to discover new molecules, net of taxpayer subsidies, and more than four-fifths of all funds for basic research to discover new drugs and vaccines come from public sources.[25]

An important reason why most breakthroughs come from publicly funded research is that capitalism and curiousness go very badly together. It takes time to be curious, and senior people in drug companies don't have the patience. They want a quick return on their investments, which will help them advance to even more lucrative positions in other companies. Managers are therefore likely to shut down a particular line of research if there hasn't been progress after a couple of years.

Psychologists have shown that money is a poor motivator, in contrast to giving people something meaningful to do, and scientists are radically different from managers. The salary isn't important. What matters is solving the puzzles and contributing something of importance to the world. As an example, it took more than 20 years for an indefatigable scientist, Eugene Goldwasser, to find and purify the first small vial of human erythropoietin.[7]

Myth 5: Drug companies compete in a free market

This myth is used successfully to decrease regulation in the mistaken belief that market forces will solve all problems. There can be no free market for products that are heavily subsidised by taxpayers' money and when fraud and crimes are widespread.

When I worked in the industry, I was surprised to find out how the price of drugs is determined. Sales managers produced what they called a sales budget for the coming years, but I wondered how they could make a budget for money they didn't have but only hoped to get. However, once it had been made, it was important to live up to it; otherwise, uncomfortable questions would be asked, and people would be unhappy. There is a simple solution when sales aren't going well: to increase the price for the drug and agree with your main competitors to increase their prices by the same amount, which will make everybody happy. It's illegal but very difficult to prove and therefore common. Even I have seen it happen, although I have never been responsible for a sales budget.

Myth 6: Public–industry partnerships are beneficial for patients

This myth never dies and we saw one of the most shameless examples in 2012. The Association of the British Pharmaceutical Industry (ABPI) issued a new guideline to promote collaboration with doctors.[26,27] It talked about shared aims and objectives and urged healthcare professionals not to be 'tempted to accept the negative myths about cooperating with industry'. Endorsed by many, including the British Medical Association, the Royal College of General Practitioners, the Academy of Medical Royal Colleges and the Department of Health, the *Lancet*'s logo was used to support outrageous claims such as 'Industry plays a valid and important role in the provision of medical education' and 'Medical representatives can be a useful resource for healthcare professionals'.

Under a heading called 'The facts', the guideline starts with two untrue statements: 'Opportunities may be missed or even rejected because of misconceptions stemming from historical practices that are no longer acceptable, or the actions of a few individuals that are not typical of the working relationship between healthcare professionals and the industry.'

These practices are *not* historical and they are *not* atypical. Further, the guideline is said to 'Reflect the industry's determination to ensure that relationships with healthcare professionals are based on integrity, honesty, knowledge, appropriate behaviours, transparency and trust.' We are also told that 'All trials are subject to rigorous scrutiny ... the results of controlled clinical trials are made available in the public domain ... ABPI Code of Practice requires disclosure of details of clinical trials.' The reality is that we never see details of clinical trials, loads of results are buried and effectively sealed in company archives as effectively as if it were nuclear waste, and the trials are never subjected to rigorous scrutiny, as the ethics committees don't do it and don't have the expertise to do it.

The guidance's claims that 'Undertaken appropriately, working with industry will not harm objectivity of clinical decision-making' and that regulations ensure that professional and ethical standards are upheld – are at odds with everything we know about the subject. We are also told that 'Pharmaceutical industry investment is the source of most of the scientific breakthroughs and innovations in medicines … typically costs £550 million to do all the work necessary before a medicine can be licensed for use.'

I have never seen so much bullshit and lies crammed in one place before. Partnerships *can* occasionally be beneficial for both sides, but, overall, it's immensely harmful for patients that the establishment embraces the industry's ways with its drugs. The idea that public health and the drug industry have a common agenda is PR fiction, and the UK healthcare system is already at an ethical bottom level. In 2012, the UK government announced that general practitioners will be expected to work with drug companies to work out how to treat their patients.[28] The ABPI's guide, supported by the Department of Health, says that 'Popular areas for joint working you may wish to consider include identification of undiagnosed patients, reviewing uncontrolled patients, improving patient adherence to medicines and treatment pathway redesign.' This includes inviting salespersons to go through the GPs' patient lists and pick out those they think should receive the company's drugs.

The British must live on another planet than I do. They should read Chapter 12 about Neurotin for everything where salespeople also sat with doctors and their patients and suggested what they should do. What we should do is the exact opposite. Identify overdiagnosed and overtreated patients, take patients off most or all of their drugs, and teach them that a life without drugs is possible for most of us.

In his book *Bad Pharma*, Ben Goldacre writes that the silverbacks – the great and good of British medicine – know full well what the problems with all this are but have decided to be unconcerned, thereby, like the regulators, they actively conspire in the secrecy about what drug companies are really doing to public health.[28] It is hard to imagine a worse betrayal than this. If I were a GP in the UK, I would get another job or leave the country.

Also in 2012, The International Diabetes Federation, an umbrella organisation of more than 200 diabetes associations in over 160 countries, started a partnership with Nestlé, which intensely markets energy-dense confectionery and sugar-sweetened beverages.[29] Nestlé has caused many deaths in the developing world because of its unethical promotion of infant formula, which needs addition of clean water that is often not available. Perhaps our lung associations should follow the fashion and partner with the tobacco industry? Why not? Politicians might acclaim it.

Myth 7: Drug trials are done to improve the treatment of patients

PR material and collaborative agreements between doctors' associations and industry associations propagate this myth.[30] However, no matter what the drug industry says about working for patients, they have no more responsibility to oversee the public's health than the fast-food industry has to oversee the public's diet.[31] And they are not genuinely interested in it. Either a study is designed to maximise sales or it is designed to determine the best way to prevent or treat a particular health problem.

When patients are recruited for trials, a benefit of participation that is almost always described in the consent document is that the research participant will contribute to scientific knowledge, which will in turn contribute positively to the care of other patients. However, as I explained in Chapter 5, this social contract with patients is broken. Trials are done for marketing purposes, and unwelcome results are kept secret or are distorted before they get published, although their availability would have improved the treatment of patients.

Another myth is that the industry would have no point in cheating, as it would always be detected and influence sales negatively. One of the persons who told me this conducted clinical trials for a Danish drug company. He was convinced he was right and was proud of his job. Good for him, but he wasn't the one who analysed the data and made decisions about how they should be interpreted and whether they were so harmful for profits that they would never see the light of day outside the company. As I have documented in this book, the truth is that companies cheat a lot because it can rarely be detected without having access to the raw data and because it pays off.

Myth 8: We need many drugs of the same type because patients vary in their response

I have heard this argument countless times from doctors who have listened to the pep talks of drug salespeople without reflecting much on whether it was true or not. In rare cases, it could be true, but I have not seen convincing data that confirm it. One of the trials that purported to show that patients reacted differently was a crossover trial where patients with rheumatoid arthritis tried four different drugs and told the investigators which period they preferred.[32] This doesn't prove anything, as the severity of the pain fluctuates. To be sure that the preferences aren't just random noise, we would need to expose the same patients to the same drugs more than once.

Myth 9: Don't use generic drugs, as their potency varies

Pfizer once claimed that its own tests of generic products that contained the same active substance as Pfizer's drug against dizziness had shown that 10 of 17 generic products failed to meet potency standards.[6] Contrast this with the fact that drug agencies ensure that generic products are bioequivalent with the original drug by requiring comparative studies in human volunteers that measure the concentrations of the active substance in the blood.

Many doctors believe in this nonsense, which has been consistently rejected whenever researchers without conflicts of interest did the bioavailability studies.

Myth 10: The industry pays for continuing medical education because the public purse won't

If true, this would be an act of immense generosity, as it is expensive and affects most doctors. As I have explained in Chapter 8, it is so clear what this is all about that not even the drug industry's representative bodies deny it but admit that this is how they do business. Three of the largest US advertising agencies handling pharmaceutical accounts invest in contract research organisations and prepare 'educational' packages for the drug industry.[3]

As Marcia Angell said in an interview, the companies perpetrate a gigantic fiction that they somehow are not only in the business of selling drugs, but are also in the medical education business.[17] Their investors expect them to make as high profits as they possibly can by selling drugs. But they have managed to make a lot of people believe that they are also somehow educating them. That can't be. It's as though you look to beer companies to educate you about alcoholism. There is also the conflict of interest. Drug companies might 'educate' doctors about drugs as long as they're talking about the benefits, but are they going to say, 'Our drug isn't really very good; the other company makes a better drug?' No. It doesn't happen.

REFERENCES

1 Angell M. *The Truth about the Drug Companies: how they deceive us and what to do about it.* New York: Random House; 2004.
2 Federal Trade Commission. *Generic Drug Entry Prior to Patent Expiration: an FTC study.* 2002, July. Available online at: www.ftc.gov/os/2002/07/genericdrugstudy.pdf (accessed 1 November 2007).
3 Relman AS, Angell M. America's other drug problem: how the drug industry distorts medicine and politics. *The New Republic.* 2002 Dec 16: 27–41.
4 Braithwaite J. *Corporate Crime in the Pharmaceutical Industry.* London: Routledge & Kegan Paul; 1984.
5 Adams S. *Roche versus Adams.* London: J. Cape; 1984.
6 Clinard MB, Yeager PC. *Corporate Crime.* New Brunswick: Transaction Publishers; 2006.
7 Goozner M. *The $800 Million Pill: the truth behind the cost of new drugs.* Berkeley: University of California Press; 2005.
8 Nelson R. Debate over ritonavir price increase gains momentum. *Lancet.* 2004; **363**: 1369.
9 Brody H. *Hooked: ethics, the medical profession, and the pharmaceutical industry.* Lanham: Rowman & Littlefield; 2008.
10 Hemmingsen MA. [Antidepressant medicine increases by 1200 percent in three months]. *Dagens Medicin.* 2010 Sept 17.
11 Andersen L. [Drug prices will be trenched]. *Jyllandsposten.* 2007 March 30.
12 Dilling S. [Price for cholesterol lowering drug explodes]. *Politiken.* 2007 March 28.
13 Svansø VL. [Lundbeck purchase costs a court case]. *Berlingske.* 2009 Feb 21.
14 Drug company granted monopoly – price of drug increases 15000%. *Pioneer Press.* 2011 March 14.
15 Messori A, Cicchetti A, Patregani L. Relating price determination to disease prevalence. *BMJ.* 2010; **341**: 417–18.
16 Cuatrecasas P. Drug discovery in jeopardy. *J Clin Invest.* 2006; **116**: 2837–42.
17 PBS. The Other Drug War. Interview with Marcia Angell. 2002 Nov 26. Available online at: www.pbs.org/wgbh/pages/frontline/shows/other/interviews/angell.html (accessed 4 April 2005).
18 Steenberger A, Larsen K, Bundgaard B. [The minister of health wishes to discuss prioritisation with the regions]. *Ugeskr Læger.* 2011; **173**: 472.
19 Svansø VL, Hyltoft V. [The regions at war with the drug industry]. *Berlingske.* 2011 Feb 3.
20 Quotations. *Ugeskr Læger.* 2010; **172**: 1568.
21 Svansø VL, Hyltoft V. [Drug industry under pressure]. *Berlingske.* 2011 Feb 3.
22 Cumming J, Mays N, Daubé J. How New Zealand has contained expenditure on drugs. *BMJ.* 2010; **340**: 1224–7.
23 Mintzberg H. Patent nonsense: evidence tells of an industry out of social control. *CMAJ.* 2006; **175**: 374.

24 Stevens AJ, Jensen JJ, Wyller K, *et al*. The role of public-sector research in the discovery of drugs and vaccines. *N Engl J Med*. 2011; **364**: 535–41.

25 Light DW, Lexchin JR. Pharmaceutical research and development: what do we get for all that money? *BMJ*. 2012; **344**: e4348.

26 The Association of the British Pharmaceutical Industry. *Guidance on Collaboration between Healthcare Professionals and the Pharmaceutical Industry*. 2012 March 29. Available online at: www.abpi.org.uk/our-work/library/guidelines/Pages/collaboration-guidance.aspx (accessed 27 December 2012).

27 Braillon A, Bewley S, Herxheimer A, *et al*. Marketing versus evidence-based medicine. *Lancet*. 2012; **380**: 340.

28 Goldacre B. *Bad Pharma*. London: Fourth Estate; 2012.

29 Beran D, Capewell S, de Courten M, *et al*. The International Diabetes Federation: losing its credibility by partnering with Nestlé? *Lancet*. 2012; **380**: 805.

30 Danish Association of the Pharmaceutical Industry. [Revised collaborative agreement between the Medical Association and the Danish Association of the Pharmaceutical Industry about clinical trials and non-intervention studies]. 2010 June 1.

31 Abramson J. *Overdo$ed America: the broken promise of American medicine*. New York: HarperCollins; 2004.

32 Huskisson EC, Woolf DL, Balme HW, *et al*. Four new anti-inflammatory drugs: responses and variations. *Br Med J*. 1976; **1**: 1048–9.

General system failure calls for a revolution

I find it hard to imagine that a system this corrupt can be a good thing, or that it is worth the vast amounts of money spent on it.

Marcia Angell, former editor, *New England Journal of Medicine*[1]

If an improvement in human health was our primary aim, some of the billions currently invested in expensive drugs to lower cholesterol of the worried well might be far more efficiently spent on enhanced campaigns to reduce smoking, increase physical activity, and improve diet.

Moynihan and Cassels, in *Selling Sickness*[2]

OUR DRUGS KILL US

Our drugs kill us on a horrific scale. This is unequivocal proof that we have created a system that is out of control. Good data are available,[3-5] and what I have made out of the various studies is that around 100 000 people die each year in the United States because of the drugs they take even though they take them correctly. Another 100 000 die because of errors, such as too high dose or use of a drug despite contraindications. A carefully done Norwegian study found that 9% of those who died in hospital died directly because of the drugs they were given, and another 9% indirectly.[6] Since about one-third of deaths occur in hospitals, these percentages also correspond to about 200 000 Americans dying every year. The European Commission has estimated that adverse reactions kill about 200 000 EU citizens annually (at a cost of €79 billion),[7] which is somewhat less than the two other estimates, as there are about 60% more people in the EU than in the United States. In 2010, heart disease killed 600 000 Americans, cancer 575 000, and chronic lower respiratory disease came third with 140 000 deaths.[8] This means that in the United States and Europe:

drugs are the third leading cause of death after heart disease and cancer.

The true number of drug deaths is likely higher. In hospital records and coroners' reports, deaths linked to prescription drugs are often considered to be from natural or unknown causes, as they may be impossible to trace. For example, many drugs cause cardiac arrhythmia, which is a major cause of death in people treated with antipsychotic drugs. In previous chapters, I have estimated drug deaths in relation to some particular drugs, not in any way systematically selected, but the data support the finding that drugs are a major killer:

- The use of inferior drugs for hypertension is estimated to have caused heart failure in 40 000 patients in the United States (p. 100)
- At the peak of their use, anti-arrhythmic drugs were likely causing about 50 000 deaths every year in the United States (p. 126)
- By 2004, rofecoxib had likely caused about 120 000 deaths worldwide because of thrombosis (p. 161)
- By 2004, celecoxib had likely caused about 75 000 deaths worldwide because of thrombosis (p. 167)
- NSAIDs likely causes about 20 000 deaths every year in the United States because of ulcer complications (p. 169)
- By 2007, olanzapine had likely killed about 200 000 people worldwide (p. 232).

In addition to all the deaths, millions of people experience serious, disabling drug injuries every year.[9] It is always difficult to separate causes of death, as several causes may contribute. Tobacco results in many deaths from heart disease and cancer, and if we look at tobacco as a separate cause, it comes up to about 440 000 deaths each year in the United States.[10] Thus, the number of drug deaths is roughly half of the number of tobacco deaths.

The main reasons for the deaths are far too permissive drug regulation, over-medicalisation, polypharmacy, too little knowledge about the harms of drugs, and thousands of warnings that no doctor can possibly master. Human errors abound in a system that is far too complicated for the human brain to handle. Imagine if airline pilots had thousands of little buttons in the cockpit at their disposal and that, furthermore, these buttons interacted in unpredictable ways if several were switched on simultaneously, analogous to a patient who is on several drugs.

What we need are radical changes. Most importantly, we need to demedicalise our societies with the same reasoning that no one would dare to fly if the pilots' actions had unpredictable effects. Every one of us can contribute to demedicalisation by being conservative about drugs. If you don't absolutely need a drug, then don't take it. We rarely need drugs. We are rarely in situations where a drug may save our life, or where a drug could make a major difference to our lives. Most of the time, the drugs don't have any positive effect on us (*see* Chapter 4). A systematic review showed that stopping antihypertensive and psychotropic drugs in the elderly generally went very well, and for the latter group of drugs it resulted in fewer falls and improved cognition.[11]

Selling drugs to healthy people who don't need them is how the industry has boosted its profits. It's like a cancer that has grown uncontrollably in society for many years now, which is nourished to a large extent by organised crime, scientific dishonesty, outrageous lies and bribery. We need to stop this.[12]

Journal editors know where the evil comes from. According to Drummond Rennie, deputy editor of *JAMA*, 'The pharmaceutical companies, by their arrogant behaviour and their naked disregard for the well-being of the public, have lost our trust. The FDA, by spinelessly knuckling under to every whim of the drug companies, has thrown away its high reputation, and in so doing, forfeited our trust.'[13] Rennie has also noted that, as soon as they left their posts as editor-in-chief of the *New England Journal of Medicine* and *BMJ*, Jerome Kassirer, Marcia Angell and Richard Smith each bemoaned the appalling influence of drug company money on the morals and practices of their profession in a book.[1,14,15]

In contrast, our politicians understand so little that they usually only make the situation worse when they act. Keeping people healthy is not a priority in America's profit-driven system, which thrives when people are ill.[12] The propaganda has made nearly half of all Americans believe that the United States has the best healthcare in the world, albeit with a clear political divide (68% of the Republicans and 32% of Democrats).[16] The beliefs that what is good for big pharma is also good for the people and that market forces will solve all problems are contradicted by the facts. The Unites States has the most ineffective healthcare system in the developed world.[17,18] The three countries with the lowest healthy life expectancies, Hungary, Poland and Slovakia, are former communist countries (see Figure 21.1). The Unites States has a relatively low healthy life

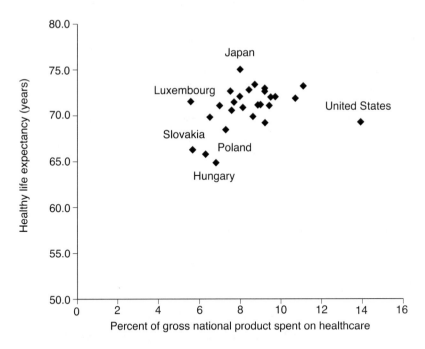

Figure 21.1 Healthy life expectancy in relation to the amount spent on healthcare in developed countries (in percent of the gross national product)

Data were available for Australia, Austria, Belgium, Canada, Czech Republic, Denmark, Finland, France, Germany, Greece, Hungary, Iceland, Ireland, Italy, Japan, Luxembourg, Netherlands, New Zealand, Norway, Poland, Portugal, Slovakia, Spain, Sweden, Switzerland, United Kingdom and the United States.

expectancy despite the fact that this country uses far more resources than any other country. A 2008 report from the Commonwealth Fund found that the Unites States ranked last among 19 industrialised countries across a range of measures of healthcare.[19] The report estimated that if the United States attained the same performance indicators achieved in other industrialised countries, at least 100 000 lives and at least $100 billion could be saved every year, and it tied much of the problem to a weak base of primary care doctors. A study that compared 3075 US counties found that every 20% increase in primary care physicians was associated with a 6% reduction in total mortality.[20] The relative position of the United States on health indicators among OECD countries also worsened in the period where the proportion of specialists increased.

The waste in the United States is gigantic. In relation to the size of the population, the Unites States spent 2.7 times more on drugs than European countries in 2000, and yet – or perhaps because of this – the outcome is much worse.[21]

The data in Figure 21.1 are about 10 years old; currently, the Unites States is even worse off than in the figure, as it spends about 18% of its GDP on healthcare,[22] about double as much as in other industrialised countries. The health disadvantage of Americans is not only because of extreme income inequalities and widespread poverty. It is also seen among those with a health insurance, a college education, higher incomes and healthy behaviours. Even for deaths considered amenable to health care, Americans fare poorly. The decline in amenable mortality in 19 industrialised countries averaged 16% over a 5-year period, whereas it was only 4% for the United States.[23] What is also striking in Figure 21.1 is that there isn't any relation between the amount of money spent on healthcare and life expectancy.

The United Kingdom has come to resemble the United States more and more, as it has moved towards greater privatisation of healthcare. Its healthy life expectancy is lower than in most other European countries, and its prevalence of chronic disease and disability lies between that in the Unites States and the rest of Europe.[24]

Such sobering facts tell us so clearly that capitalism and privatisation impact negatively on public health and they explain why the vast majority of European doctors are left wing when it comes to healthcare. We feel nervous about profit taking any role in the caring professions, even those of us who might be right wing for other political issues. We love our public health service, which US politicians scornfully call socialised medicine.

HOW MUCH MEDICINE DO WE REALLY NEED AND AT WHAT COST?

We waste huge amounts of money on drugs where the patients would have been better off without them. Hypertension is a good example that one cannot just look at the benefits of prevention. When investigators asked how it went for 75 patients with controlled hypertension, their doctors said they had all improved, whereas only 36 of the patients felt they had improved and only one of the relatives said so. The questionnaire completed by the relatives rated 22 of the patients to have suffered severe adverse changes: undue preoccupation with sickness; decline in energy, general activity and sexual activity; and irritability. The reason why all the doctors were satisfied was that none of their patients had made complaints![25]

Screening for hypertension doesn't seem to have any beneficial effects,[26] whereas it may have untoward consequences. A 1984 study of Canadian steel workers showed that those labelled as patients with hypertension through screening had increased absenteeism from work and suffered a decline in marital adjustment, and in the fifth year after screening they earned $1093 less than colleagues who 5 years earlier had comparable wages.[27] This effect on income was seen even in those who didn't take their antihypertensive drug.

We should also consider that the arteries become more rigid with advancing age and that lowering blood pressure in the elderly may lead to vertigo and falls. In a study where the elderly were their own control, start of antihypertensive medication increased the risk of hip fracture by 43%.[28] A quarter of those who suffer a hip fracture die within 1 year,[29] e.g. from pneumonia or thrombosis caused by immobilisation. A professor emeritus of cardiology said: Let's not turn elderly people into patients but let's allow them to enjoy being healthy (i.e. free from drugs).[30]

It can be life-saving to treat seriously elevated blood pressure and the adverse effects of the drugs we use are therefore a minor issue. However, harms of drugs are usually the same for patients who are seriously ill as for those who are not. The benefit–harm balance may therefore change from beneficial to harmful, as we move towards treating people who are healthy but happen to have an elevated risk factor. It's very costly to treat all these healthy people and give them an insurance that their risk of some unhappy event will be a little less if they take the drug for the rest of their lives. As no one subsidises the insurance on our house or car, we could discuss whether it's reasonable to use taxpayer money on drug insurance. Economists use a concept called willingness to pay. If it costs €3000 to treat one person in 5 years prophylactically and this prevents one untoward event for every 30 people treated, what would a person then decide if he was to pay himself for the drug insurance? Would all 30 happily pay the €3000 for a chance of one in 30 to win in the lottery while enduring the side effects of the drug for 5 years? I am pretty sure some would prefer to use the money for a vacation or something else, at least I would.

If we used medicines rationally, we would have much healthier populations, at a fraction of the expenditure we currently have on drugs. In 2012, the top 50 companies sold $610 billion in human prescription pharmaceuticals.[31] I have little doubt that we could easily save 95% of this, which are annual savings of $580 billion, as many of our highly used drugs are 20 times more expensive than equally good alternatives, and as we are so much overtreated. Imagine what we could do for $580 billion. Only 17 countries in the world have a GDP greater than this.

I don't think I exaggerate. Others have estimated that more than $200 billion may be wasted on unnecessary treatment every year in the United States,[32] and although this waste includes treatments other than drugs and poor administration, it's of the same order of magnitude as my estimate, and yet it refers to only one country.

FOR-PROFIT IS THE WRONG MODEL

Although the drug industry already suffers from corporate obesity, it pushes its drugs to medicate us even more. In 2002, a report from the European Federation of Pharmaceutical Companies identified 20 diseases and conditions for which they thought potentially achievable benefits were not achieved.[33] The report warned against undertreatment over 98 pages, but none of its 184 citations were to systematic reviews, although there were many for each of the conditions discussed that could have dampened the hype. For each disease, positive studies were quoted and negative studies were ignored. Not a single study of overtreatment was quoted.

Providers of goods and systems also get their share of the cake. Healthcare and pharmaceutical executives were four of the top 10 best-paid executives in the United States in 2010. The top earner, John Hammergren, was chief executive of the drug distributor McKesson Corp., with total remuneration of $145 million.[34] If the poor guy were to be fired, he would receive $469 million in severance pay, or 10 000 times as much as the median US household income. What can one say about such obscenity? Well, at least we can see what's wrong with the United States' culture of unlimited greed and cheating.[35] The average ratio between CEO compensation and employee is about 13:1 in Germany and 11:1 in Japan. It was also 11:1 in the United States in 1970 but is now a staggering 531:1. The US bonus system creates a minimal incentive for innovation and a huge incentive for fraud. In large drug firms, the value of unexercised stock options held by the top executives is often larger than $50 million, which creates an incentive to increase the stock prices and then 'take the money and run'.[35]

Unfortunately, the Americans seem unwilling to solve their most fundamental problems. This hit the rest of the world with the global financial crisis in 2008 after all brakes on high-risk investments had been removed by foolish politicians guided by equally foolish economists who believe the market will solve all problems and regulate itself. I'm sure we'll soon run into a worse global recession than in 2008, again caused by the United States. This is a bit odd, since so many Americans are devout Christians. The Bible warns against unlimited greed in so many places that it cannot be overlooked.

Here is an example of the consequences of the perverse incentives we have.[36] Aventis developed a drug against cancer, eflornithine, but it didn't work for cancer, whereas it was highly effective for sleeping sickness. Since patients with sleeping sickness are generally poor, Aventis discontinued making the drug. Later, it turned out that eflornithine was an effective depilatory. The drug went back into production and was now made available to Africans with sleeping sickness at little or no cost, the only reason being that many women in the Western world want to remove facial hair.

The control of medical practice by market economics does not serve the needs of the patients very well and is not compatible with an ethically based profession.[37] Business imperatives to make profits do not produce the social benefits claimed by market advocates. Research in the United States has consistently found higher costs, lower quality of care, and higher rates of medical complications and death in for-profit facilities than in public facilities; even billing fraud is far more common in for-profit hospitals than in not-for-profit hospitals.[37] Our universities have also jumped on the bandwagon with their university–industry partnerships and obsession with patents. This is detrimental for public-interest science, e.g. studies of occupational hazards and many other types of non-drug prevention of disease have no commercial interest.[38]

It is inherently immoral that drugs can be patented. We can avoid buying patented merchandise if we think it's too expensive and we'll suffer no harm. In contrast, we may die if we cannot afford to buy a patented life-saving drug. The right way to go with drugs is to abandon the current system and replace it by non-profit enterprises that invent, develop and bring new drugs to the market. Several capitalist countries have established state-owned drug companies,[39,40] and it was suggested in the UK in 1976 that the government should take over sections of the drug industry.[41] This didn't materialise, but in 2007, the Medical Research Council announced that it planned to do this to speed advances against rare diseases.[42]

As long as we continue to endure the for-profit model, we could introduce an award system, where drug companies, instead of patent monopoly, would receive a financial award when they have obtained marketing authorisation, the size of which could be related to the degree to which the invention represented a break-through. After that, the drugs could be licensed to multiple firms to manufacture and sell at generic prices, which would ensure that also many poor people and countries could afford to use the drugs. The WHO Global Strategy and Plan of Action on Public Health, Innovation and Intellectual Property (GSPoA) of May 2008, and the EU Council Conclusions on Global Health in May 2010 both called for needs-driven innovation and for further exploration of innovation models that de-link the cost of research and development from the price of medicines to encourage both needs-driven research and more affordable access to essential medical technologies.[43] Such de-linkage would address three weaknesses of the current model of medical innovation: unaffordability, unavailability and unsuitability. It would also dramatically reduce incentives for development of me-too products and the marketing and promotion of medicines that are used irrationally, or that are no better than the alternatives.

CLINICAL TRIALS

We cannot trust industry trials at all and the reason is simple. We don't trust a person who has lied to us repeatedly, even though that person might tell the truth sometimes. The industry has broken our trust and it has an enormous conflict of interest. Further, drug companies choose investigators that have long-standing relations with the drug industry and don't ask uncomfortable questions. To allow industry to do trials on their own drug is like allowing me to be my own judge in a court case. Imagine if I were accused of a crime and turned up in court with boxes containing 250 000 pages of evidence for my innocence that I had produced myself (which is about the volume of clinical documentation for a new drug), and that I told the judge this was the only evidence there was, on which he or she needed to make a verdict. I would be thrown out of court.

It's very strange that we have accepted a system where the industry is both

judge and defendant, as one of the most firm rules in laws of public administration is that no one can ever be allowed to be in a position where they shall
evaluate themselves. The fact that drug agencies will look at the submitted
material cannot compensate for this transgression, as the evidence has often
been deliberately distorted in ways that escape detection. The industry should
no longer be allowed to carry out clinical trials, but they could provide funds for
academic-led trials. That would be vastly cheaper for industry. The European
Society of Cardiology has estimated that university centres can perform drug
trials for about one-tenth to one-twentieth the cost of industry trials where there
are numerous for-profit middlemen who tack a hefty surcharge.[44] Similarly, the
National Cancer Institute has estimated that it can do trials for little more than
the usual drug cost.[40] The last trial I conducted was a multicentre trial of 112
patients with rheumatoid arthritis that were treated with disease-modifying
agents or placebo for 6 months,[45] and the budget for the trial was less than my
monthly salary. We bought the drugs and got the placebos free from the companies. This shows that trials can be done at almost no cost, if doctors want to
do them.

The premises for our current system are wrong. Capitalism operates on the principle that private risk yields either private loss or private wealth. But the idea
that public risk (patients participating in trials) is turned into private wealth is
a perversion of the capitalist ethic and an exploitation of patients.[38] We need
a major culture change where we see clinical trials as a public enterprise, done
for the public good, and performed by independent academic institutions.[1,46]
Academics can also be biased – or bribed by industry – but such problems can
be solved by ensuring effective blinding during data analysis and writing of
manuscripts. This was how I did randomised trials.[47] I analysed the data under
code and produced two different manuscripts. The code wasn't broken before
my co-authors had approved both manuscripts.

While we await a major system change that may never come, we may do our
own independent trials of new drugs before we decide whether or not to use them
or reimburse them. In the Netherlands, legislation in 1979 enabled the minister to
restrict certain technologies to certain hospitals while they were being evaluated
by systematic reviews of the literature.[48] A fund was created in 1986 of about
€16 million a year with the effect that new unevaluated technologies, including drugs, were reimbursed only when offered 'as part of a properly designed
research study to assess their effects', i.e. a randomised trial.

Funds for independent trials could be provided by taxes. The drug industry makes huge profits based on publicly funded research and reimbursement
of drugs, and it would therefore be reasonable if the industry was taxed to an
extent that allows academics to run the trials we need where we compare a new
drug against the best available treatment before we decide anything. If we taxed
prescriptions with as little as 2%, it would quickly create a large fund for such
research. The Italian drug agency requires drug companies to contribute 5% of
their promotional expenses apart from salaries, which has created a large fund
used partly for independent clinical research.[49,50] There are similar initiatives
in Spain.[50] Funds may also be provided from government or hospital budgets,

as independent trials could easily become a source of income rather than an expense. As long as we are running a trial where only half of the patients will get the new expensive drug, we will save half of the drug costs, and when we are done, we will more often than not discover that the new drug has nothing to offer.

The requirement of independent trials before we make decisions would have a tremendous impact not only on the public purse but also on public health. It would no longer be profitable to develop endless numbers of me-too and me-again drugs and the industry would be forced to do innovative research instead of spending its money on marketing. Revival of the Norwegian 'medical need' clause would also reduce the amount of me-too drugs. Norway had only seven NSAIDs on the market compared with 22 in the Netherlands, but its medical need clause was eliminated in 1996 when it harmonised its drug approval process with that in the EU.[51] As there isn't much price competition anyway, it wouldn't matter much for our drug expenses whether there were seven or 22 different drugs of the same type, but it could mean a lot for innovation.

Independent testing of drugs would also mean that we could compare new drugs with old, cheap ones under fair circumstances where the old drug is not given in a dose that is too high (so that the manufacturer can falsely claim that their drug is better tolerated), or a dose that is too low (so that the manufacturer can falsely claim that their drug is more effective). There are also far too few comparisons with non-pharmacological interventions. When a study found that a programme of exercise and weight loss was better for preventing type 2 diabetes than metformin (56% and 31% effect, respectively),[52] the only thing the *Wall Street Journal* wrote about was the effect of the drug!

We also need much better and honest reporting of harms, which we'll never get in industry trials. Although the first thing we know about any drug is that it may cause harm, a survey of 192 reports of trials of at least 100 patients showed that the space devoted to harms was 0.3 page, which was similar to the amount of space devoted to contributor names and their affiliations.[53]

Finally, the rationale for a proposed clinical trial must be based on a rigorous, recent systematic review of all previous trials with similar drugs, with meta-analysis if possible.[54] This will often tell us that what looked like 'conflicting' results in previous trials are not at all conflicting. If this isn't done, many unethical trials will be approved, as the type of drug might already have been shown – or could have been shown – to be either life-saving or harmful. Such a requirement was introduced in Denmark in 1997,[55] but for reasons unknown to me it was quietly taken out when the law about trials was revised. The research ethics committees have failed miserably to pay attention to what matters most to patients. They have done nothing to ensure that the trials they approve are ethical; that the informed consent forms accurately depicts the state of knowledge and uncertainty; and that the results of all trials become publicly available, although this was pointed out to them in a well-argued *BMJ* paper in 1996.[54]

We won't get rid of industry-conducted trials for a long time. But in the interim, we could decide to let the regulatory authorities select those clinicians who would be allowed to test drugs, instead of industry's picking of the most willing doctors,[41] who are also those that are easiest to corrupt and most likely to keep quiet about industry's manipulations of the evidence. Patients should know everything about money involved in trials and investigators' conflicts of interest. If doctors are uncomfortable about this, they have something to hide, which makes it even more pertinent to ensure transparency. Protocols and contracts with drug companies should be publicly available so that we can all see whether to trust our institutions. It's a sad fact that many still accept gagging clauses,[56] and also that when authors solemnly and routinely declare in journals that they had access to all the data, it is rarely true.[57,58]

Drug companies should be required by law to deliver placebos for independent research at no more than the manufacturing cost as a condition for having a product on the market. It should also be obligatory for companies to deliver the pure drug, e.g. in powder form, for independent research. If drug companies want to be a part of society, they must be willing to further public health by letting other researchers do research on their products.

Trials come to their full fruition when assembled in systematic reviews, and such reviews should always tell the readers how many trials, outcomes and results that might be missing, and also to which extent the reviewed trials were sponsored by the manufacturer. Here is a good example from a Cochrane review of hypertension, where the Plain Language Summary aimed at patients says:

> Most of the trials in this review were funded by companies that make ACE inhibitors and serious adverse effects were not reported by the authors of many of these trials. This could mean that the drug companies are withholding unfavorable findings related to their drugs ... Prescribing the least expensive ACE inhibitor in lower doses will lead to substantial cost savings, and possibly a reduction in dose-related adverse events.[59]

Finally, seeding trials should be made illegal, as they now are in the EU. The directive on pharmacovigilance (post-authorisation safety studies) was amended in 2010 to say 'Studies shall not be performed where the act of conducting the study promotes the use of a medicinal product.'[60]

DRUG REGULATORY AGENCIES

Drug agencies have a major responsibility for the many drug deaths. They approve many dangerous drugs and use fake fixes by issuing an enormous number of warnings and precautions, although they know perfectly well that they won't work.

We would never accept it if airlines crashed several times a day the year round because their construction made them too difficult for the pilots to fly.

We need a revolution in drug regulation. Drug agencies need to become evidence-based and realise that the current system isn't working and cannot work. They should reject far more drugs and require sufficient safety data.

Surrogate outcomes should not be accepted

I have given many examples earlier[61] and in this book how terribly misleading surrogates can be. The patients may be injured or die while their surrogate improves. Cancer drugs are such a disaster area. The regulatory requirements for cancer drugs are close to none. They are often approved based on single-arm studies that cannot say anything about whether the drug increases or lowers mortality.

Of 27 different indications in Europe, of which 14 were new applications and 13 extensions of earlier approvals, the clinical documentation consisted entirely of small single-arm studies in eight cases.[62] The total number of patients was small, a median of 238, and in half of the cases, only surrogate outcomes such as complete or partial tumour response were provided, although they are highly prone to biased assessment, particularly in single-arm studies. This is very worrying because most cancer drugs may cause both tumour shrinkage and increased mortality, e.g. if given in a too high dose. Those drug studies that did report on survival found a median difference of only 1 month.[62] Another study, of 12 new cancer drugs approved in Europe from 1995 to 2000, showed that none of them offered any significant progress and yet one cost 350 times more than the competitor.[63]

It's even worse at the FDA, which approves most cancer drugs (68%) based on outcomes other than survival. In addition, 35% of the drugs were granted a licence even without a single randomised trial.[62]

Based on published data, I have calculated that 33 years of randomised trials in solid tumours sponsored by the UK Medical Research Council hasn't led to any progress against cancer, on average.[64] It was a large material, 32 trials comparing one treatment with another, and 6500 deaths, and the mortality on the new treatment was the same as that on the control treatment. Other cancer surveys have confirmed this, e.g. for 57 trials of radiotherapy the relative risk was 1.01,[65] and for 126 trials in childhood cancer, the odds ratio was 0.96.[66]

Zero progress against cancer, on average, means that it is very difficult to find new treatments that are better than those we already have. Rarely, a new treatment is better, and rarely, it is worse. As long as our drug agencies don't require mortality data from randomised trials, they will allow harmful drugs to be introduced on the market without anybody knowing.

Relevant patient populations, comparators and outcomes

Patients above 65 years of age are routinely excluded from industry-sponsored trials,[67-69] e.g. only 2% of patients in NSAID trials were 65 years or older,[68] although these are the patients most likely to take drugs and most likely to be harmed. Exclusion of these age groups also makes it difficult to detect harms caused by the combined effects of taking many drugs (polypharmacy). The EMA recently announced that they will from now on expect the age distribution of patients to be representative in studies presented for marketing authorisation.[70]

This is good but still not good enough, as drug firms can still write in their protocols that a condition for participation is that the patients don't receive other drugs than the trial drugs, and don't have more than one disease. We need to ensure that drugs are tested in realistic settings, which isn't the case today. A survey showed that common medical conditions formed the basis for exclusion in 81% of the trials, and patients receiving commonly prescribed medicines were excluded in 54% of the trials.[69] Such exclusions were significantly more common in industry-sponsored trials.

According to the Helsinki Declaration, a new drug must be tested against those of the best current proven intervention, and placebo should only be used when no such intervention exists, or where there are compelling and scientifically sound methodological reasons for the use of placebo (e.g. when current treatments have doubtful effect).[71] I therefore believe drug agencies should require relevant head-to-head comparisons against commonly used drugs, and that, when placebo is needed, they require that some of the trials have used active placebos to reduce the risk that they approve useless drugs (*see* Chapter 4).[72]

Safety

The current practice, where drugs are approved based on only 500–3000 patients[73] in short-term trials, even when the drugs are to be used for decades, sets the stage for major drug disasters, which are very expensive because of legal fees and settlements. These costs are subsequently added to the price of other medicines.[74]

Apart from identical twins, people are genetically different, e.g. in how quickly they metabolise a drug or how susceptible they are to its effects. It is therefore expected that for most drugs, some people will react very badly. These reactions can only be detected reliably if many patients are studied in randomised trials. If, for example, a drug causes fatal liver failure in one patient out of 2000, even a trial of 20 000 patients may not detect it (since we would only expect to see five liver failures in the 10 000 randomised to the new drug, we might have seen none at all). If that drug is an analgesic to be used in, say, 50 million people, 25 000 of these will die of liver failure although they didn't need the drug, as there are so many other analgesics.

This won't happen in practice of course. The drug would be withdrawn long before the 25 000 liver failures, but if it had been an increase in heart attacks, we might never have found out, as so many will get a heart attack anyway.

Drug agencies should require much larger numbers of treated patients before they make any decisions, and they should also require trials that run over several years, if the drug is to be taken for years, as harms may take time to develop, e.g. if the drug causes cancer. The standard excuse that it would take too long to get valuable new drugs on the market, if requirements were tightened, doesn't hold. There are years between such an outstanding drug and the fact that drugs are the third most common cause of death says more than enough about the current system.

If post-marketing studies are required because of remaining safety concerns, it's essential that these be conducted by, and commissioned to, as part of the regulatory approval, independent investigators. Companies have every reason in the world to blindfold themselves by conducting poor studies, or fail to report them, or fail to even do them.

All clinical data must be publicly available

It's a terrible misconception that a company can own clinical trial data. According to the European ombudsman, data and results belong to society, for obvious reasons. Patients don't volunteer for trials and run a personal risk to benefit the shareholders of a particular company. They do so to contribute to science and help improve treatments for future patients. If we accept that companies can claim ownership to trial data, we also accept that it's legitimate to exploit patients for commercial benefit. It obviously isn't and would violate the Helsinki Declaration.[71] We should therefore force companies to make all their trial data available, including raw anonymised data in statistical programmes, which is what the EMA intends to do for new drugs (*see* Chapter 11).

We should also use our muscle, e.g. by deciding not to recommend drugs or not to buy them until all data have been made available. UK law makes it possible to take legal action without notice and to delay approving the company's pending drugs, or even to withdraw a marketed drug if the company refuses to provide all the data. Confiscation of the company's patents is another penalty that is under consideration. If a company abuses a patent by marketing a drug for a purpose it has not been approved or tested for, why should it then continue to benefit from the exclusivity?[75]

Health Technology Assessment agencies should follow the lead of the German agency IQWIG and refuse to assess a drug unless all data are provided from all trials without any conditions about confidentiality, so that the public can also see the data.

As suggested by the Danish drug agency,[76] there should be full public access to all documents in drug agencies, including data from toxicology studies.[49] Drug companies should be required to submit all documentation in easily searchable formats, e.g. as text-recognisable pdf files; the agencies should check that the files are complete and include all documents listed in indexes; and the files should be made publicly available. US legislation from 2007 ensured that the data bank at clinicaltrials.gov would be expanded to include all phase 2 and subsequent trials, and that results information would be added after the product has been approved for marketing.[77] The restriction to marketed drugs needs to be removed, however, as unknown harms of a drug might lead to unnecessary experimentation and additional harms of similar drugs in future. The six healthy volunteers in the United Kingdom who nearly died in a phase 1 trial is a case worth remembering.[78]

Above all, there should be no redactions, which will require changes of some national laws. We should not accept receiving documents from drug agencies that are so heavily censored that they look more like military intelligence documents than drug studies,[79] and where all the harms of the drug have been wiped out, which we experienced when we received study reports for a slimming pill from the Danish drug agency and on SSRIs from the Dutch agency. An additional problem is that redaction is arbitrary. Sidney Wolfe, director of the Public Citizen's Health Research Group, said, 'I've never been able to get any kind of protocol for what [FDA staff] are instructed to redact, but in general they redact way more than they should.'[79] He added, 'Of course, it's a catch-22, because if you don't know what they are redacting you can't argue that it should not have been redacted.' Alastair Wood, the head of the FDA's advisory committee on the safety of COX-2 inhibitors, insisted that there is no reason ever to redact clinical trial data. Absurdly, without knowing what information is being withheld or the rules guiding redaction, the interpretation of what constitutes a trade secret seems itself to be a trade secret.

We also need laws requiring firms to disclose all knowledge about their drugs and research data,[80] and that not only allow but require drug agencies to publish what they know. Currently, the companies may not disclose anything even when they know that their drugs are harmful.

Conflicts of interest

Drug agencies should be publicly funded, as user fees create competition between the agencies about becoming the fastest and therefore also the least critical agency. For example, it was a goal in the contract between the Danish drug agency and the Ministry of Health to be more attractive to the industry than other agencies.[81] Drummond Rennie believes that user fees are profoundly corrupting and that 'It is ludicrous to imagine that the FDA could truly work for the public interest if they continue to be paid not to.'[13]

Divisions in drug agencies that deal with harms of drugs should be separated from the divisions that approve drugs and should have their own authority, enabling them to remove drugs from the market. According to laws of public administration, a person or a body must never come in a position where it evaluates itself. For this reason alone, it's clear that the two functions must be separated. Alastair Wood, whose nomination as the new FDA commissioner was withdrawn in the last minute because he put too much emphasis on drug safety (*see* Chapter 10), has noted that 'When a plane crashes, we don't turn over the investigation to [the airline] and the air-traffic controllers. We get someone else to do it.'[82] The Danish drug agency understands this and has separated the two functions,[83] but the FDA won't.

Since our drugs kill us, drug agencies should be evaluated by how well they handle safety issues. Currently, however, the emphasis is on the speed with which new drugs are being approved,[1,84] with performance-based salaries to the top executives, e.g. in the Danish drug agency.[81] This incentive is not only perverse; it is lethal.

Labelling of drugs

If the drug agencies' clients were the people and not the industry, the label on drugs would look very different, somewhat like this (inspired by drug epidemiologist Jerry Avorn):[67]

> *This new drug hasn't been shown to be any better than currently available drugs, and we know much less about its harms, including the lethal ones, than we do for old drugs. There is no evidence that its higher price is accompanied by any therapeutic advantage. It's generally safer to take an old drug, as many new drugs come off the market later because of safety problems.*

Patients should be informed about what the drug does, with numbers they can understand for both the benefits and the harms. Researchers from Dartmouth showed that if patients are told the facts, they are much better at choosing the better drug and in knowing what the effect is.[85] If people knew that the effect of a sleeping pill is to make them fall asleep 15 minutes faster,[86] and could make them dizzy and drowsy the next day, they might be less interested in taking one, and if they also knew that the effect would disappear within 2 weeks if they take it every night, there would be few long-term users. The Dartmouth researchers convinced the FDA's Risk Communication Advisory Committee that the agency adopt their suggestions. However, after having thought about it for a year, the Department of Health and Human Services announced it needed at least three more years to come to a decision.[87] Of course they do. An initiative that indisputably helps patients to choose much more rationally between drugs, or even to say no to drugs, is almost like an attack on the state, as it could lead to loss of income for the drug industry.

DRUG FORMULARY AND GUIDELINE COMMITTEES

Doctors with financial ties to drug companies should not serve on drug or guideline committees, whether in drug agencies, hospitals, specialist societies or elsewhere.[88,89] A persistent argument put forward by conflicted doctors and those who use them is that the best people will produce the best decisions and guidelines, and that it's only to be expected that the best people collaborate with the industry for mutual benefit. This argument is amusing, as it's so obviously incorrect. As explained in Chapter 9, people on industry payroll tend to be irrational in their views on drugs and tend to prefer expensive drugs that are not any better than cheaper alternatives. Worse still, when it's discovered that widely used drugs are harmful, these experts are always the last to recommend against them. They find all sorts of excuses for not accepting the new evidence, no matter how strong it is.

This was, for example, very clear when it was shown that hormones given to women around menopause are harmful.[90,91] Unveiled court documents show that Wyeth ran a programme of ghostwritten review articles, which touted that hormones were good for all sorts of things, and which were published in high-impact journals such as *Archives of Internal Medicine* with expert authors who had done very little or nothing to qualify as authors.[92,93] None of the papers have been retracted although they are highly misleading. Here are some examples of titles:

- *Is there an association between hormone replacement therapy and breast cancer?* (yes, it causes breast cancer)
- *The role of hormone replacement therapy in the prevention of postmenopausal heart disease* (there is none, as hormones *cause* heart disease)
- *The role of hormone replacement therapy in the prevention of Alzheimer disease* (there is none, as hormones increase the risk of getting the disease).

Specialist denial of harms abounds everywhere, including in non-drug areas, e.g. when it became clear that mammography screening had doubtful benefit, whereas it leads to tremendous harm in terms of overdiagnosis and overtreat-ment of healthy women.[94]

We need people to guide us who are driven by the data and not for hire. Doctors with financial conflicts of interest are not best; they are not even second best. The best are those who are skilled methodologists who have some knowl-edge about the area in question, as they can – and are willing to – find the flaws in the scientific documentation. The second best are skilled methodologists. The third best could be those specialists on industry payroll who are also skilled methodologists.

Many people – particularly those doctors who cash the money – think that declarations about conflicts of interest by some magic will make the problem go away, but as Sheldon Krimsky has noted, 'we would not permit a judge ... to have equity in a for profit prison, even if the judge disclosed it'.[95] We would not accept either a judicial proceeding in which the judge was paid by one of the corporate litigants.[36] Doctors are their patients' advocates and their primary responsibility is to ensure they aren't harmed, as expressed in the Hippocratic oath: First, do no harm. It is therefore untenable that doctors won't accept a court case where the judge is paid by one of the sides whereas they willingly accept to be paid by the drug industry. Doctors suffer from this delusion to such a degree that it looks like a collective psychosis. When I lecture on this, I therefore sometimes provoke my colleagues in a desperate attempt to wake them up:

Judge Smith runs a court case against Cosa Nostra and before it starts, he declares that he:
- has received travel grants from Silvio Berlusconi
- is on the Advisory Board for Unmerciful Lone Sharks
- has received funds from Drug Pushers International
- has received unrestricted educational grants from La Camorra
- is on the speaker's bureau for Murder Incorporated.

The mob doesn't kill many people compared to what the drug industry know-ingly does, so why accept money from the industry if you aren't willing to accept money from the mob? According to medical ethicist Carl Elliott, 'Disclosure is an empty ritual designed to ease the consciences of academics unable to wean themselves from the industry payroll.'[96] Doctors are grasping at the straw of disclosure of their conflicts because it allows them to have their cake and eat it too.[14] They should ask themselves whether they would be willing to have their arrangements generally known, and if so, they should be happy for the informa-tion to be shared with their patients in their waiting room,[56] particularly since doctors believe they are immune to industry favours.

According to laws of public administration, it cannot be accepted that spe-cialists on advisory committees in drug agencies are paid consultants to the manufacturers, and it therefore defies reason that *most* such specialists are on industry payroll.[1,14,38,97] It is equally unacceptable that those who, in formulary or guideline writing committees, recommend which drugs to use receive industry money.[2] They often circumvent the problem by hiding it. We studied 45 Danish guidelines from 14 specialty societies from 2010 to 2012, and found that 43 of them (96%) had one or more authors with a conflict of interest, but only one guideline disclosed any conflict of interest.[98] About half of the authors had ties to drug companies.

The US Institute of Medicine issued a report about conflicts of interest in 2009, which called for exclusion of people with conflicts of interest from guideline panels and prohibition of industry funding of guidelines.[99] If, in exceptional cases, it was impossible to find experts who were not conflicted, such people should be excluded from deliberating, drafting or voting on specific recommendations. I would argue that there should be no 'exceptional cases'. Any little economic loophole offered to doctors always tends to become very wide. Furthermore, as it is considered very prestigious to be on guidelines committees, it should be easy to require that those who wish to be on them should get rid of their financial arrangements with the industry. Finally, about one-third of US professors don't collaborate with industry,[100] so what's the problem? Choose them instead.

In France, doctors with the non-profit organisation Formindep (Formation Indépendante) charged that guidelines issued by the French Health Authority should be withdrawn because they contravened national law on conflicts of interests and the agency's own internal rules.[101] The authority refused, although, for example, the chairpersons of the working groups on type 2 diabetes and Alzheimer's disease had major financial conflicts. Formindep went to court and the highest administrative court in France ruled that the guidelines must be withdrawn immediately because of potential bias and undeclared conflicts of interest among its authors. I regard this as a great victory for common sense, which is met with so much resistance in healthcare.

DRUG MARKETING

There is no need for drug marketing, as the products should speak for themselves. Marketing of drugs is similarly harmful as marketing of tobacco, and it should therefore be banned, just like marketing of tobacco is. What a victory for public health it would be if there would no longer be any ads for drugs, no salespeople, no seeding trials and no 'education' sponsored by industry. Try to imagine what a world that would be. People would be much healthier and richer.

We might never get there, but we can make progress within the system we have. It should be a crime for companies and doctors to participate in seeding trials and other studies of no scientific value, as it is a form of bribery, and sanctions should not be restricted to fines, but should also involve a period of quarantine where doctors and companies are banned from doing clinical research. Drug agencies – and research ethics committees, in case the studies are submitted to such committees – currently don't disapprove of such studies but they should.

Drug companies should be prohibited from financing continuing medical education,[89] as the purpose is to sell drugs and as it's harmful.[1] In the interim, speakers should declare their conflicts of interest and the size of their honorarium and other benefits, from all company-sponsored events within the last 3 years. If it became obligatory to list these in the advance programme, there would be fewer attenders and fewer events, as it would be easy to identify 'education whores' who are willing to say anything for money.

Fines for illegal marketing should be large enough to have a preventive effect. If fines for cheating the tax authorities were far smaller than the revenue from the cheating, there would be little incentive for honest declarations. Danish taxpayers get fined three times the amount they cheated for, even though the cheating doesn't harm other people directly, as drugs do. In 1979, a bill in the United States would have allowed judges to fine defendants twice the loss or gain resulting from their crimes, but Senator Edward Kennedy deleted this from the bill after pressure from corporations.[102] We need legislation that ensures that both companies' and top executives' earnings that are based on crimes will be fined at least thrice the gain from the crimes. Currently, the companies see even the large fines in the United States as a marketing cost. To deter bad behaviour, the fines would need to be so large that the companies would risk going bankrupt, but this is unlikely to happen. The largest companies earn so much money to their home country that the governments wouldn't dare run such a risk. In 2010, the 10 largest companies sold drugs for $303 billion,[103] which is more than the gross national product for all but the richest 34 countries in the world.[104] US federal law requires that any company found guilty of marketing fraud be automatically excluded from Medicare and Medicaid, but government prosecutors decided that this exclusion would lead to the collapse of 'too big to fail' Pfizer.[105] Exclusion from the Medicare and Medicaid programmes has occurred in only a handful of cases, and rarely in a case involving a major pharmaceutical company.[106]

Also in this way, the drug industry resembles other types of organised crime, which in some countries or cities have acquired so much influence on society that they have become 'too big to fail'. Another similarity relates to the behaviour at the top. Both in the mob and in big pharma, the top bosses prefer to be kept ignorant about the uncomfortable details of the trade, as long as the dirty work gets done and ensures a copious flow of money.[102]

To bring the crimes to light also outside the United States, we need laws that protect whistle-blowers and ensure they get a fair proportion of the fines. Fines of US size would ensure that it is cost-effective also in other countries to investigate the crimes and bring them to court. The US Justice Department has estimated that the prosecutions reap more than $15 in recoveries for every $1 spent.[106]

We need to avoid the situation that, by settling accusations of crimes, the drug companies can pretend they are innocent, claiming they have not been convicted of a crime.[106,107] By avoiding a verdict, companies furthermore get the advantage that there is no precedent next time they come under attack.

Top executives should be held personally accountable for the crimes so that they would need to pay attention to the risk of going to jail when they consider performing or acquiescing in crimes, and we need prison sentences as deterrents. Charges of involuntary manslaughter were raised against Grünenthal, the manufacturer of thalidomide, because the company had withheld data on the horrific harms of this drug.[39,108] Such charges could be raised against those who, by fraudulent research or marketing, or by withholding data on lethal harms of drugs, cause the deaths of patients, whether they are employed by industry, by drug agencies, or elsewhere. If someone kills a pedestrian in a street crossing through reckless driving, that person goes to jail. No question about it. Compare with top industry executives who kill many people through reckless and deliberate neglect. The only thing that happens to them is that they get rich. We need to prosecute corporate criminals with at least as much vigour as traditional criminals, and if we did, there might be more white-collar criminals in prison than blue-collar ones.[39] The industry is already prepared for this, as some companies hold the position of 'vice president responsible for going to jail'. This, however, cannot provide immunity for the CEO, as corporate ethics indisputably is determined by that person.[39]

In some countries, e.g. in the United States, drug firms can buy prescription data allowing them to spy on individual doctors.[12] This is highly unethical, as it so obviously invites corruption through 'rewards' to high-volume prescribers. It must be banned.

DOCTORS AND THEIR ORGANISATIONS

Physicians' organisations should declare that it's against the patients' interests that physicians participate in meetings or educational events sponsored by the industry, accept visits from drug salespeople, or accept donations from industry, including free travel and free samples of drugs (the delivery of which should be prohibited by law), as this has clear negative consequences for patients.[2,14,29,39,67,88,109-114] Some universities and hospitals have introduced policies that prevent this from occurring,[115] and for many years, the Danish Medical Association has refused to offer industry-sponsored 'education' to its members.

Doctors are delearning their bad habits, but slowly. A study of 105 residents at a university-based internal medicine residency programme showed that 61% believed that contact with industry didn't influence their own prescribing, while only 16% believed that other physicians were similarly unaffected.[116] Jerome Kassirer considers it one of the greatest scandals of our time that physicians are not held to the standards of journalists, attorneys and other professionals.[14] Physicians should live up to the same rules that apply to journalists. A journalist who writes press releases for Pfizer to supplement her income will not be allowed to write a story for the *New York Times* about new drugs for treating impotence.[117] Why have we accepted that this rule somehow shouldn't apply to doctors? Doctors' relationships with pharma don't even live up to the criteria for wine testing in the *Wall Street Journal*,[14] although doctors' choice of drugs, or no drugs at all, is far more important for people's health than the type of wine they drink: 'We do not accept free wine, free trips, or free meals ... We taste wines blind unless noted otherwise. We believe wines should speak for themselves.' So should drugs!

Doctors suffer from the delusion that their financial relationships with industry can be managed, and numerous foolish – so-called ethical – guidelines have been construed, which often speak about some cash amount below which there should be no problem. This is self-serving rationalisation.[117] The relationships cannot be managed; they should be avoided. Some sort of contact with the industry is of course needed, e.g. in relation to conducting important trials, but the knee-jerk reaction that this must involve exchange of financial benefits is simply wrong. Similarly, if a doctor is desperate to sit at a company's advisory board or give good advice in other ways, it can be done for free. *It takes two to tango and what we need more than anything else is for doctors to stay clean and say no to the money.* It should be illegal in all countries, like it is in Denmark, for a doctor to help a company in its marketing, although this is what many doctors actually do when they consult for the industry, sit on an advisory board, or 'educate', also in Denmark.

We have a very long way to go. A US survey found that a staggering 94% of a broad range of physicians had interacted with the drug industry within the last year.[118] Most of these interactions involved receiving food in the workplace (83%) and drug samples (78%), and 28% had been paid for consulting, lectures or enrolling patients in studies. The extent of these interactions are likely underestimated, as social desirability bias may have caused people to under-report what may be viewed as negative, and the survey wasn't anonymous.

When the American Medical Association in 2001 launched a campaign to convince physicians *not* to accept gifts from the industry, the campaign was funded by Eli Lilly, Bayer, GlaxoSmithKline, AstraZeneca, Merck, Pfizer and Wyeth-Ayerst,[14] which include some of the worst companies on earth whose ruthless actions have led to the deaths of thousands of patients.

The Association itself continued to accept gifts. When, in 2009, US senator Charles Grassley asked for financial information from 33 professional associations and groups that conduct research or promote disease awareness, the American Medical Association reported that 16 drug, device and communications companies donated nearly $5 million in 2007 for 'continuing medical education' programmes and 'communications conferences'.[119] It didn't respond to an inquiry by the *BMJ* regarding the issues. Manufacturers provided more than half of the total funding of the North American Spine Society and nearly half the funding of the Heart Rhythm Society and the American Academy of Allergy, Asthma and Immunology. Jerome Kassirer has given many egregious examples of academic prostitution in specialist societies.[14]

Restricted uneducational grants

There is a widespread form of 'collaboration' between academia and industry that doesn't require approval from an authority. It goes under various names and here is an example. A 2007 paper surveying US department chairs of medicine and psychiatry reported that 67% of them had received *discretionary funds* from industry within the last year.[120] This is likely an underestimate, as the survey was not anonymous. The donations to department chairs and other decision-makers are sometimes called *unrestricted educational grants*, although – as a witty person once put it – they are in reality restricted uneducational grants, as their purpose is to buy doctors.[39] In one case, such a grant was used for paying for a doctor's swimming pool.[16]

Industry is very careful about how it spends shareholders' money, and if it gives away some, it's not a sudden outburst of altruism but because it expects more in return than it spends. The purpose of discretionary funds, which the department may use for research, education or whatever its chair deems relevant, is to buy loyalty, and it works. Department chairs know all too well that if they start using cheap generics instead of the donor's expensive products, the funding stream will dry out. And the industry knows that if someone at the department finds serious harms with one of the company's drugs, the department chair will be more tempted to protect the drug than the whistle-blower. It's unbelievable that doctors cannot see that acceptance of money with 'no strings attached' is corruption. I believe everybody else can. Academic institutions should not accept financial support from industry.[39,97,121]

We are moving in the right direction but much too slowly and timidly. In 2009, the Association of American Medical Colleges urged all medical schools and teaching hospitals to adopt policies prohibiting physicians, faculty or staff members, residents and students from accepting any industry gifts, including industry-supplied food and meals unrelated to accredited continuing medical education programmes.[122] The same year, the US Institute of Medicine went one step further. It suggested that doctors should decline all gifts from industry, including meals; that product promotion among doctors by drug and device companies should be virtually eliminated; that doctors should refuse to participate in activities and publications where contents are controlled by the industry; and that professionals with conflicts of interest should not participate in writing practice guidelines.[123]

In 2012, the American Medical Association – at last – changed its pro-industry position and announced that 'when possible', CME activities should be developed without industry support and without the participation of teachers or programme planners who have financial interests in the subject matter.[124] The next step will be to close the foolish loophole that is a carte blanche to do business as usual. It is *always* possible to avoid industry influence.

Currently, we have a culture among doctors where accepting industry largesse and accepting 'authoring' highly flawed industry papers is not a career impediment; in fact, it seems to advance people's careers as they get many more publications and become known speakers. We need to reverse this culture into one of professional ostracism so that such a person would no longer show their face in places where their academic colleagues gathered.[117] Ghostwritten articles should be seen as scientific fraud, and the honorary authors should be treated like students who sign their names to papers they buy on the internet.[96] There should be substantial fines for concealing ghost authorship, as it erodes the trust that is so fundamental in medical publishing. Legislation is needed to hold physicians accountable when they contribute to illegal marketing with harmful consequences for patients – whether by 'authors' of ghost papers or in other ways – including the possibility of being struck off the medical register.

Doctors should decline to accept drug industry awards, and specialists societies should decline to offer them. The Danish Society of Clinical Microbiology handed out a Wyeth Prize for many years, worth €1300, but decided to stop this and pay for the award themselves through membership fees. That's the way to go.

All countries should have publicly accessible registers of doctors' collaboration with industry detailing the monetary amounts and other benefits. There is no disinfectant like sunshine, and in the United States, the Physician Payments Sunshine Act requires that pharmaceutical, medical device, biological and medical supply manufacturers report to the Department of Health and Human Services payments that are more than $10 to physicians and teaching hospitals.[125] The law requires reporting of stock options, royalties, consulting fees, honoraria, education, research grants, meals, gifts, entertainment and travel. The database provides information on the physicians receiving the payment, their address, payment date, and drug or device that the physician helped promote. There will be stiff penalties for both inadvertent lapses (up to $150 000 annually for failure to report) and intentional nondisclosure (up to $1 million annually).

One of the worst types of academic prostitution is when doctors contact politicians and pretend they are independent experts when in reality they are hired guns. Our societies build on trust and our politicians cannot rule our countries prudently when they are being misled. Understandably, they get very upset when they discover incidentally that they have been fooled.[126]

Last, but not least, doctors and their organisations should consider carefully whether they find it ethically acceptable to receive money that has been partly earned by crimes that have harmed their patients. As noted in Chapter 3 and elsewhere, many crimes would be impossible to carry out if doctors weren't willing to participate in them.

PATIENTS AND THEIR ORGANISATIONS

Patient organisations have the same problems as physician organisations. They are often sponsored by industry and often support industry's marketing goals rather than taking care of patients' interests. Patient organisations have done absolutely nothing to stop the blatant abuse of patients in industry-sponsored trials.[56] Many clinical trials are unethical because the patients don't know that they don't contribute to science but only to the income of the sponsoring company and because many trials or results never get published. According to the Helsinki Declaration, 'Authors have a duty to make publicly available the results of their research on human subjects and are accountable for the completeness and accuracy of their reports.'[71] When did we ever see a patient organisation take the industry to task for failing to do this?

Another example of the total failure of patient organisations is that they often complain loudly when national bodies have decided a drug is too expensive to be used compared to what it has to offer, whereas I have never heard any patient organisation complain that the price was too high and that the drug company should lower it. It seems to be a vicious circle: a lot of what we pay for drugs goes to marketing, which includes support to patient groups and physician experts, which in turn insist that we should pay very high prices for these drugs, undermining independent organisations like NICE that provide advice to our governments about which drugs to use.[56]

Patient organisations should warn their members not to get information from drug companies or from websites funded by drug companies. Companies have found out that they can circumvent the law forbidding direct-to-consumer advertising by selling diseases instead of drugs. This is highly lucrative,[2] and an overwhelming amount of disease websites are made up by drug companies, either directly or via some willing patient organisation.[127] Further, patient organisations supported by industry sometimes distribute marketing material from drug companies. The Danish ADHD Association visited schools and distributed leaflets written by a drug company alerting people that they might have ADHD, although this diagnosis is already widely overused. The only type of treatment that was discussed in the leaflets was drugs, and the director of the association was hired because of her 'commercial orientation', with a focus on establishing 'partnerships with private companies'.[128] It's disgusting.

Patient organisations are often set up by drug companies, although they hide this. Between 1996 and 1999, the US National Alliance for the Mentally Ill, 'a grassroots organisation of individuals with brain disorders and their family members', received almost $12 million from 18 drug companies, led by Eli Lilly.[129] It is hugely rewarding for companies to brainwash leaders of patient organisations, as they can allow themselves to be much more vocal and belligerent than the companies themselves. I have often witnessed this, and it's among my worst professional experiences. To hear leaders of such organisations crave drugs that I know are harmful and terribly expensive as well is just too much for me. Very often they start scare campaigns that push hundreds of thousands of patients into using drugs they don't need. In 2005, the Danish Heart Foundation announced that 30 000 people would die within 10 years if not an additional 900 000 started cholesterol-lowering drugs.[130] An additional nine hundred thousand? There are only about 5.4 million Danes!

I have a brief from 2005 with two logos at the top, one from The Oxford Health Alliance and one from Novo Nordisk. It says: 'The Oxford Dialogue on Patient Rights is being convened by Novo Nordisk Denmark under the umbrella of the Oxford Health Alliance Dialogues Program.' When the drug industry talks about ethics and patient rights, it is really time to wake up and say: 'That's none of your business. We doctors take care of this.'

Large international patient federations have successfully lobbied the European Commission to propose allowing industry to provide direct-to-consumer 'information' about prescription medicines, which would be immensely harmful for the patients. Luckily, the European Parliament has for many years fiercely opposed this proposal, which comes up again and again.

In 2011, there was no beating about the bush. The International Alliance of Patients' Organizations (IAPO) bills itself as the only global organisation promoting patient-centred healthcare around the world and representing patients of all nationalities across all disease areas, with more than 200 members in more than 50 countries, encompassing an estimated 365 million patients, their families, and carers.[131] Healthcare companies interested in becoming members of the alliance's 'Healthcare Industry Partners Framework' are invited to provide four levels of financial support: gold ($50 000 per year), silver ($25 000 per year), bronze ($10 000 per year) and standard ($5000 per year). And what's it all about? A guide funded by Novo Nordisk sets up tips on working with various stakeholders, including pharmaceutical companies; such businesses are key partners in improving patient health and quality of life and an excellent source of expertise, information and contacts. The benefits of working with the drugs and healthcare industry, according to the guide, include providing an additional voice for lobbying policy makers.

Have you had enough? Luckily, there are some broad consumer organisations that are radically different and actually do work for patients. I enjoy collaborating with several of these, e.g. Trans Atlantic Consumer Dialogue and one of its member organisations, Health Action International Europe.

In 2010, the Danish Association of the Pharmaceutical Industry published data showing that the industry had reported 163 cases of support to patient organisations.[132] There should be no support at all. When asked about gifts to physicians, half of the patients were against;[117] it's therefore not consistent to accept gifts to their own organisations. It should be made illegal for the industry to communicate with patients, e.g. through ads, disease awareness campaigns, and leaflets about diseases and their treatment.

Patient organisations generally believe they can enter into partnerships with the industry for mutual benefit, which is extremely naïve. Just like doctors should, patient organisations should also consider carefully whether they find it ethically acceptable to receive money that has been partly earned by crimes that are harmful to patients.

Here is what you can do:

- Withdraw your membership if your patient organisation accepts industry favours.
- Ask your doctor whether he or she receives money or other benefits from the industry, has shares in a company or is visited by drug salespeople, and if so, find yourself another doctor.
- Avoid taking drugs unless they are absolutely necessary, which they rarely are. Ask if there are other options and whether you'll be better also without treatment; remember that very few patients benefit from the drugs they take (*see* Chapter 4).
- Ask if there are cheaper drugs than the one your doctor suggests.
- Avoid taking new drugs the first 7 years they are on the market because, unless it is one of those very rare 'breakthrough' drugs that offers you a documented therapeutic advantage over older drugs, most drugs that are withdrawn for safety reasons get withdrawn within the first 7 years.[133]
- Remind yourself constantly that we cannot believe a word of what drug companies tell us, neither in their research nor in their marketing or information to patients.

MEDICAL JOURNALS

In 2011, *Emergency Medicine Australasia* announced that the journal would no longer publish ads because the prime aim of marketing of drugs is to bias readers towards prescribing a particular product, which is fundamentally at odds with the mission of medical journals.[134] The editors added that their move was a response to growing evidence about the detrimental effects of the drug industry in medicine, including claims that the industry distorts research findings and engages in dubious and unethical publishing practices.

Medical journals have generally failed us on this point. They should stop advertising drugs, just like all journals have stopped advertising tobacco, as both activities are very harmful for public health. Many medical journals might not survive without ads, but so be it. There are far too many anyway and most of them publish substandard research that merely contributes to the pollution of science. A biostatistician who was a consultant to the *BMJ* expressed this in the title of his editorial:[135]

> *The scandal of poor medical research: we need less research, better research, and research done for the right reasons.*

Medical journals have major conflicts of interest and they should publish the amount they get from sales of reprints, supplements and advertising,[136,137] and should check manuscripts about drugs or devices particularly carefully to ensure that they don't contribute to illegal marketing or ghost authorship. To mention just one example, editors should always ask what is behind 'editorial assistance' in an acknowledgment, as it usually means 'this person wrote the paper'.

As noted earlier, randomised trials are so important for all of us that they should not be hidden behind a paywall. Reports of drug trials should not be published in traditional subscription journals that have drug ads and sell reprints, but in electronically published, open-access journals or on the web, where the protocol, amendments to the protocol and the full dataset should also be posted.[138] It was a great leap forward when Harvard University in Boston in 2008 made a commitment to open-access publishing. The university forbids assigning exclusive copyright to the faculty's work to a scientific society or a commercial publisher.[139] Some journals, e.g. the *BMJ* and *Lancet*, already ask for the trial protocol, and the *BMJ* also asks authors if they are willing to share their data with other researchers.

Finally, journals should not accept editors that have conflicts of interest in relation to drug and device companies. There are very few journals that have such a requirement, e.g. *La Revue Prescrire*, which comes out in French and English. This journal aims at providing doctors unbiased information about interventions, it's a non-profit continuing education organisation committed to better patient care, and it doesn't accept advertising or other outside support. This is exactly the type of journal we need to help us decide what is right and what is wrong about healthcare interventions.

JOURNALISTS

Industry's long tentacles also reach healthcare journalists. It funds professorships and scholarships at US universities and offers awards to journalists that write about issues that may boost sales.[140] Eli Lilly and Boehringer Ingelheim have co-sponsored an award for reporting on urinary incontinence, Boehringer has an award for chronic obstructive pulmonary disease, Eli Lilly and AstraZeneca for cancer, Roche for obesity and Novo Nordisk for diabetes.[111,140] Sometimes, the relationship is not obvious, as awards can be sponsored by organisations that are themselves heavily funded by industry, such as the non-profit Mental Health America. Its 2007 annual report shows that almost half of its funds came from drug companies, including more than $1 million each from Bristol-Myers Squibb, Lilly and Wyeth.

Sponsored patient organisations can be particularly disruptive for rational priority setting in healthcare when they provide patients for journalists to interview to add a 'human dimension' to stories, which journalists love. The main problem with these compelling anecdotes of treatment success is that they represent the exception, rather than a more typical experience, misleading audiences. Since most patient organisations pocket industry money, they are not likely to provide patients for the 'human dimension' who have been harmed by drugs.

The way forward is simple.[140] Journalism educators should not accept funding from the healthcare and drug industries, journalists should not accept gifts, awards or any financial support from the industries they cover, and journalists should routinely disclose their own conflicts of interest and those of their sources. They should remember that they only get awards if they write stories that are good for drug sales. Further, the media should be less focused on a single murder here and there and more focused on drugs that kill thousands of patients. The public knows very little about this and virtually nothing about organised crime in the drug industry. Wake up, journalists!

REFERENCES

1 Angell M. *The Truth about the Drug Companies: how they deceive us and what to do about it.* New York: Random House; 2004.

2 Moynihan R, Cassels A. *Selling Sickness: how the world's biggest pharmaceutical companies are turning us all into patients.* New York: Nation Books; 2005.

3 Weingart SN, Wilson RM, Gibberd RW, *et al.* Epidemiology of medical error. *BMJ.* 2000; **320**: 774–7.

4 Starfield B. Is US health really the best in the world? *JAMA.* 2000; **284**: 483–5.

5 Lazarou J, Pomeranz BH, Corey PN. Incidence of adverse drug reactions in hospitalized patients: a meta-analysis of prospective studies. *JAMA.* 1998; **279**: 1200–5.

6 Ebbesen J, Buajordet I, Erikssen J, *et al.* Drug-related deaths in a department of internal medicine. *Arch Intern Med.* 2001; **161**: 2317–23.

7 Archibald K, Coleman R, Foster C. Open letter to UK Prime Minister David Cameron and Health Secretary Andrew Lansley on safety of medicines. *Lancet.* 2011; **377**: 1915.

8 Centers for Disease Control and Prevention. *Leading Causes of Death.* Available online at: www.cdc.gov/nchs/fastats/lcod.htm (accessed 5 February 2013).

9 Lenzer J. Anticoagulants cause the most serious adverse events, finds US analysis. *BMJ.* 2012; **344**: e3989.

10 Centers for Disease Control and Prevention. *Tobacco-Related Mortality.* Available online at: www.cdc.gov/tobacco/data_statistics/fact_sheets/health_effects/tobacco_related_mortality/ (accessed 2 February 2013).

11 Iyer S, Naganathan V, McLachlan AJ, *et al.* Medication withdrawal trials in people aged 65 years and older: a systematic review. *Drugs Aging.* 2008; **25**: 1021–31.

12 Petersen M. *Our Daily Meds.* New York: Sarah Crichton Books; 2008.

13 Rennie D. When evidence isn't: trials, drug companies and the FDA. *J Law Policy.* 2007 July: 991–1012.

14 Kassirer JP. *On the Take: how medicine's complicity with big business can endanger your health.* Oxford: Oxford University Press; 2005.

15 Smith R. *The Trouble with Medical Journals.* London: Royal Society of Medicine; 2006.

16 Brownlee S. *Overtreated: why too much medicine is making us sicker and poorer.* New York: Bloomsbury; 2007.

17 World Health Organization. *World Health Report 2003 – shaping the future.* 2003. Available online at: www.who.int/whr/2003/annex_4_en.xls (accessed 20 December 2012).

18 Reinhardt UE, Hussey PS, Anderson GF. U.S. health care spending in an international context. *Health Aff (Millwood).* 2004; **23**: 10–25.

19 Roehr B. Health care in US ranks lowest among developed countries, Commonwealth Fund study shows. *BMJ*. 2008; **337**: a889.

20 Starfield B, Shi L, Grover A, *et al*. The effects of specialist supply on populations' health: assessing the evidence. *Health Aff (Millwood)*. 2001 March 15. DOI: 10.1377/hlthaff.w5.97.

21 World Health Organization. *The World Medicines Situation*. Available online at: http://apps. who.int/medicinedocs/en/d/Js6160e/6.html#Js6160e.6 (accessed 6 February 2013).

22 Wealth but not health in the USA. *Lancet*. 2013; **381**: 177.

23 Nolte E, McKee CM. Measuring the health of nations: updating an earlier analysis. *Health Aff (Millwood)*. 2008; **27**: 58–71.

24 Avendano M, Glymour MM, Banks J, *et al*. Health disadvantage in US adults aged 50 to 74 years: a comparison of the health of rich and poor Americans with that of Europeans. *Am J Public Health*. 2009; **99**: 540–8.

25 Jachuck SJ, Brierley H, Jachuck S, *et al*. The effect of hypotensive drugs on the quality of life. *J R Coll Gen Pract*. 1982; **32**: 103–5.

26 Krogsbøll LT, Jørgensen KJ, Grønhøj Larsen C, *et al*. General health checks for reducing morbidity and mortality from disease. *Cochrane Database Syst Rev*. 2012; **10**: CD009009.

27 Johnston ME, Gibson ES, Terry CW, *et al*. Effects of labelling on income, work and social function among hypertensive employees. *J Chronic Dis*. 1984; **37**: 417–23.

28 Butt DA, Mamdani M, Austin PC, *et al*. The risk of hip fracture after initiating antihypertensive drugs in the elderly. *Arch Intern Med*. 2012; **172**: 1739–44.

29 Abramson J. *Overdo$ed America*. New York: HarperCollins; 2004.

30 Oliver M. Let's not turn elderly people into patients. *BMJ*. 2009; **338**: b873.

31 Cacciotti J, Clinton P. Pharm Exec 50: growth from the bottom up. *Pharmaceutical Executive*. 2012 May 1. Available online at: www.pharmexec.com/pharmexec/Noteworthy/Pharm-Exec-50-Growth-from-the-Bottom-Up/ArticleStandard/Article/detail/773562 (accessed 17 July 2013).

32 Berwick DM, Hackbarth, A. Eliminating waste in US health care. *JAMA*. 2012; **307**: 1513–16.

33 Liberati A, Magrini N. Information from drug companies and opinion leaders. *BMJ*. 2003; **326**: 1156–7.

34 Tanne JH. US healthcare executives hit pay jackpot. *BMJ*. 2011; **343**: d8330.

35 Whelton RS. *Effects of Excessive CEO Pay on U.S. Society*. Available online at: www.svsu.edu/emplibrary/Whelton%20article.pdf (accessed 6 November 2007).

36 Schafer A. Biomedical conflicts of interest: a defence of the sequestration thesis – learning from the cases of Nancy Olivieri and David Healy. *J Med Ethics*. 2004; **30**: 8–24.

37 Relman A. *A Second Opinion: rescuing America's health care*. New York: Public Affairs; 2007.

38 Krimsky S. *Science in the Private Interest: has the lure of profits corrupted biomedical research?* Lanham: Rowman & Littlefield; 2003.

39 Braithwaite J. *Corporate Crime in the Pharmaceutical Industry*. London: Routledge & Kegan Paul; 1984.

40 Goozner M. *The $800 Million Pill: the truth behind the cost of new drugs*. Berkeley: University of California Press; 2005.

41 Abraham J. *Science, Politics and the Pharmaceutical Industry*. London: UCL Press; 1995.

42 Day M. MRC says it will invent, develop, and market its own drugs. *BMJ*. 2007; **334**: 1025.

43 Bloemen S, Hammerstein D. Time for the EU to lead on innovation. *Health Action International Europe and Trans Atlantic Consumer Dialogue*. 2012 April.

44 Bassand J-P, Martin J, Rydén L, *et al*. The need for resources for clinical research: The European Society of Cardiology calls for European, international collaboration. *Lancet*. 2002; **360**: 1866–9.

45 Gøtzsche PC, Hansen M, Stoltenberg M, *et al*. Randomized, placebo controlled trial of withdrawal of slow-acting antirheumatic drugs and of observer bias in rheumatoid arthritis. *Scand J Rheumatol*. 1996; **25**: 194–9.

46 Relman AS, Angell M. America's other drug problem: how the drug industry distorts medicine and politics. *The New Republic*. 2002 Dec 16: 27–41.

47 Gøtzsche PC. Blinding during data analysis and writing of manuscripts. *Controlled Clin Trials*. 1996; **17**: 285–90.

48 Borst-Eilers E. Assessing hospital technology in the Netherlands: new treatments are paid for only if they are part of an evaluation. *BMJ*. 1993; **306**: 226.

49 Garattini S, Bertele V. How can we regulate medicines better? *BMJ*. 2007; **335**: 803–5.

50 Liberati A, Traversa G, Moja LP, *et al*. Feasibility and challenges of independent research on drugs: the Italian Medicines Agency (AIFA) experience. *Eur J Clin Invest*. 2010; **40**: 69–86.

51 Light DW, Lexchin JR. Pharmaceutical research and development: what do we get for all that money? *BMJ*. 2012; **344**: e4348.

52 Knowler WC, Barrett-Connor E, Fowler SE, *et al*. Reduction in the incidence of type 2 diabetes with lifestyle intervention or metformin. *N Engl J Med*. 2002; **346**: 393–403.

53 Ioannidis JP, Lau J. Completeness of safety reporting in randomized trials: an evaluation of 7 medical areas. *JAMA*. 2001; **285**: 437–43.

54 Savulescu J, Chalmers I, Blunt J. Are research ethics committees behaving unethically? Some suggestions for improving performance and accountability. *BMJ*. 1996; **313**: 1390–3.

55 Goldbeck-Wood S. Denmark takes a lead on research ethics. *BMJ*. 1998; **316**: 1189.

56 Goldacre B. *Bad Pharma*. London: Fourth Estate; 2012.

57 Lundh A, Krogsbøll LT, Gøtzsche PC. Access to data in industry-sponsored trials. *Lancet*. 2011; **378**: 1995–6.

58 Lundh A, Krogsbøll LT, Gøtzsche PC. Sponsors' participation in conduct and reporting of industry trials: a descriptive study. *Trials*. 2012; **13**: 146.

59 Heran BS, Wong MMY, Heran IK, *et al*. Blood pressure lowering efficacy of angiotensin converting enzyme (ACE) inhibitors for primary hypertension. *Cochrane Database Syst Rev*. 2008; **4**: CD003823.

60 *Directive 2010/84/EU of the European Parliament and of the Council*. 2010 Dec 15.

61 Gøtzsche PC, Liberati A, Luca P, *et al*. Beware of surrogate outcome measures. *Int J Technol Ass Health Care*. 1996; **12**: 238–46.

62 Apolone G, Joppi R, Bertele V, *et al*. Ten years of marketing approvals of anticancer drugs in Europe: regulatory policy and guidance documents need to find a balance between different pressures. *Br J Cancer*. 2005; **93**: 504–9.

63 Garattini S, Bertele V. Efficacy, safety, and cost of new anticancer drugs. *BMJ*. 2002; **325**: 269–71.

64 Machin D, Stenning SP, Parmar MKB, *et al*. Thirty years of Medical Research Council randomized trials in solid tumours. *Clin Oncol*. 1997; **9**: 100–14.

65 Soares HP, Kumar A, Daniels S, *et al*. Evaluation of new treatments in radiation oncology: are they better than standard treatments? *JAMA*. 2005; **293**: 970–8.

66 Kumar A, Soares H, Wells R, *et al*. Are experimental treatments for cancer in children superior to established treatments? Observational study of randomised controlled trials by the Children's Oncology Group. *BMJ*. 2005; **331**: 1295–8.

67 Avorn J. *Powerful Medicines: the benefits, risks, and costs of prescription drugs*. New York: Vintage Books; 2005.

68 Rochon PA, Fortin PR, Dear KB, *et al*. Reporting of age data in clinical trials of arthritis. Deficiencies and solutions. *Arch Intern Med*. 1993; **153**: 243–8.

69 Van Spall HG, Toren A, Kiss A, *et al*. Eligibility criteria of randomized controlled trials published in high-impact general medical journals: a systematic sampling review. *JAMA*. 2007; **297**: 1233–40.

70 Cerreta F, Eichler HG, Rasi G. Drug policy for an aging population – the European Medicines Agency's geriatric medicines strategy. *N Engl J Med*. 2012; **367**: 1972–4.

71 World Medical Association. *Ethical Principles for Medical Research Involving Human Subjects*. 2008. Available online at: www.wma.net/en/30publications/10policies/b3/ (accessed 17 July 2013).

72 Whitaker R. *Anatomy of an Epidemic*. New York: Random House; 2010.

73 Strom BL. How the US drug safety system should be changed. *JAMA*. 2006; **295**: 2072–5.

74 Ray WA, Stein CM. Reform of drug regulation – beyond an independent drug-safety board. *N Engl J Med*. 2006; **354**: 194–201.

75 Newman M. Bitter pills for drug companies. *BMJ*. 2010; **341**: c5095.

76 Alsman SW. [Hidden research led to wrong recommendations about happy pills]. *Økonomisk Ugebrev*. 2004 May 3.

77 Senate Republican Policy Committee. *Legislative Notice No. 13. S. 1082 – The FDA Revitalization*

Act. Available online at: http://rpc.senate.gov/_files/L13S1082FDARevitalizationAct043007KP. pdf (accessed 30 October 2007).

78 Suntharalingam G, Perry MR, Ward S, *et al*. Cytokine storm in a phase 1 trial of the anti-CD 28 monoclonal antibody TGN 1412. *N Engl J Med*. 2006; **355**: 1018–28.

79 Lenzer J, Brownlee S. An untold story? *BMJ*. 2008; **336**: 532–4.

80 Gøtzsche PC. Why we need easy access to all data from all clinical trials and how to accomplish it. *Trials*. 2011; **12**: 249.

81 Danish Medicines Agency. [*Danish Medicines Agency's Performance Contract 2007 – 2010*]. Available online at: www.laegemiddelstyrelsen.dk/db/filarkiv/6653/resultatkontrakt2007_2010. pdf (accessed 15 August 2008).

82 Okie S. Safety in numbers – monitoring risk in approved drugs. *N Engl J Med*. 2005; **352**: 1173–6.

83 Carlsen LT. [A difficult balance]. *Tænk + Test*. 2003; **32**: 30–3.

84 Mundy A. *Dispensing with the Truth*. New York: St. Martin's Press; 2001.

85 Schwartz LM, Woloshin S, Welch HG. Using a drug facts box to communicate drug benefits and harms: two randomized trials. *Ann Intern Med*. 2009; **150**: 516–27.

86 Woloshin S, Schwartz LM, Welch HG. *Know your Chances: understanding health statistics*. Berkely: University of California Press; 2008.

87 Woloshin S, Schwartz LM. Think inside the box. *New York Times*. 2011 July 4.

88 Chren MM, Landefeld CS. Physicians' behavior and their interactions with drug companies. A controlled study of physicians who requested additions to a hospital drug formulary. *JAMA*. 1994; **271**: 684–9.

89 Brennan TA, Rothman DJ, Blank L *et al*. Health industry practices that create conflicts of interest: a policy proposal for academic medical centers. *JAMA*. 2006; **295**: 429–33.

90 Tougaard H, Hundevadt K. [The golden promises of the gynaecologists]. *Jyllandsposten*. 2004 Jan 18.

91 Fugh-Berman A, McDonald CP, Bell AM, *et al*. Promotional tone in reviews of menopausal hormone therapy after the women's health initiative: an analysis of published articles. *PLoS Med*. 2011; **8**: e1000425.

92 Singer N. Medical papers by ghostwriters pushed therapy. *New York Times*. 2009 Aug 4.

93 Rosenberg M. Pfizer's ghostwritten journal articles are still standing, still bogus. *Online Journal*. 2010 Feb 23.

94 Gøtzsche PC. *Mammography Screening: truth, lies and controversy*. London: Radcliffe Publishing; 2012.

95 Conflicts of interest in biomedical research. *Canada's Voice for Academics*. 2003; **50**: Feb.

96 Elliott C. Pharma goes to the laundry: public relations and the business of medical education. *Hastings Cent Rep*. 2004; **34**: 18–23.

97 Willman D. How a new policy led to seven deadly drugs. *Los Angeles Times*. 2000 Dec 20.

98 Bindslev JB, Schroll J, Gøtzsche PC, *et al*. Underreporting of conflicts of interest in clinical practice guidelines: cross-sectional study. *BMC Med Ethics*. 2013; **14**: 19.

99 Steinbrook R. Controlling conflict of interest – proposals from the Institute of Medicine. *N Engl J Med*. 2009; **360**: 2160–3.

100 Zinner DE, Bolcic-Jankovic D, Clarridge B, *et al*. Participation of academic scientists in relationships with industry. *Health Aff*. 2009; **28**: 1814–25.

101 Lenzer J. French guidelines are pulled over potential bias among authors. *BMJ*. 2011; **342**: d4007.

102 Clinard MB, Yeager PC. *Corporate Crime*. New Brunswick: Transaction Publishers; 2006.

103 Reuters. *Factbox – The 20 largest pharmaceutical companies*. 2010 Mar 26. Available online at: www.reuters.com/article/2010/03/26/pharmaceutical-mergers-idUSN2612865020100326 (accessed 17 June 2012).

104 Wikipedia. List of countries by GDP (nominal). Available online at: http://en.wikipedia.org/ wiki/List_of_countries_by_GDP_(nominal) (accessed 30 June 2012).

105 Annas GJ. Corporations, profits, and public health. *Lancet*. 2010; **376**: 583–4.

106 Thomas K, Schmidt MS. Glaxo agrees to pay $3 billion in fraud settlement. *New York Times*. 2012 July 2.

107 Khan H, Thomas P. Drug giant AstraZeneca to pay $520 million to settle fraud case. *ABC News*. 2010 April 27.

108 Brynner R, Stephens T. *Dark Remedy: the impact of thalidomide and its revival as a vital medicine*. New York: Perseus Publishing; 2001.

109 House of Commons Health Committee. *The Influence of the Pharmaceutical Industry. Fourth Report of Session 2004–05*. Available online at: www.publications.parliament.uk/pa/cm200405/cmselect/cmhealth/42/42.pdf (accessed 26 April 2005).

110 Wazana A. Physicians and the pharmaceutical industry: is a gift ever just a gift? *JAMA*. 2000; **283**: 373–80.

111 Grill M. *Kranke Geschäfte: wie die Pharmaindustrie uns manipuliert*. Hamburg: Rowohlt Verlag; 2007.

112 Ziegler MG, Lew P, Singer BC. The accuracy of drug information from pharmaceutical sales representatives. *JAMA*. 1995; **273**: 1296–8.

113 Dana J, Loewenstein G. A social science perspective on gifts to physicians from industry. *JAMA*. 2003; **290**: 252–5.

114 Moynihan R, Heath I, Henry D. Selling sickness: the pharmaceutical industry and disease mongering. *BMJ*. 2002; **324**: 886–91.

115 Campbell EG. Doctors and drug companies: scrutinizing influential relationships. *N Engl J Med*. 2007; **357**: 1796–7.

116 Steinman MA, Shlipak MG, McPhee SJ. Of principles and pens: attitudes and practices of medicine housestaff toward pharmaceutical industry promotions. *Am J Med*. 2001; **110**: 551–7.

117 Brody H. *Hooked: ethics, the medical profession, and the pharmaceutical industry*. Lanham: Rowman & Littlefield; 2008.

118 Campbell EG, Gruen RL, Mountford J, *et al*. A national survey of physician-industry relationships. *N Engl J Med*. 2007; **356**: 1742–50.

119 Lenzer J. Many US medical associations and disease awareness groups depend heavily on funding by drug manufacturers. *BMJ*. 2011; **342**: d2929.

120 Campbell EG, Weissman JS, Ehringhaus S, *et al*. Institutional academic industry relationships. *JAMA*. 2007; **298**: 1779–86.

121 Revill J. Doctor accuses drug giant of 'unethical' secrecy. *Observer*. 2005 Dec 4.

122 Steinbrook R. Physician-industry relations – will fewer gifts make a difference? *N Engl J Med*. 2009; **360**: 557–9.

123 Roehr B. US Institute of Medicine report calls for an end to firms' drug and device promotion to doctors. *BMJ*. 2009; **338**: 1100.

124 Steinman MA, Landefeld CS, Baron RB. Industry support of CME – are we at the tipping point? *N Engl J Med*. 2012; **366**: 1069–71.

125 Norris SL, Holmer HK, Ogden LA, *et al*. Characteristics of physicians receiving large payments from pharmaceutical companies and the accuracy of their disclosures in publications: an observational study. *BMC Medical Ethics*. 2012; **13**: 24.

126 Arnfred CE, Pedersen LN, Agger C. [Politicians feel cheated by lobby-doctors]. *Jyllandsposten*. 2011 Aug 29.

127 Thirstrup S. [Can you sell diseases]? *Rationel Farmakoterapi*. 2010 Dec.

128 Borg O. [Pill ads are distributed in school yards]. *Jyllands-Posten*. 2011 Nov 1.

129 Herxheimer A. Relationships between the pharmaceutical industry and patients' organisations. *BMJ*. 2003; **326**: 1208–10.

130 Rathje M. [Heart Association scares the Danes]. *TV2 News*. 2012 April 20.

131 Cassidy J. The International Alliance of Patients' Organizations. *BMJ*. 2011; **342**: d3485.

132 [Danish Association of the Pharmaceutical Industry's collaboration with patient associations and others in 2010]. 2010. Available online at: www.lifdk.dk/graphics/Lif/Inside%20Lif/2011/09/Medlemmers%20samarbejde%20med%20patientforeninger%20m.v.%202010.pdf (accessed 28 June 2011).

133 Wolfe S. The seven-year rule for safer prescribing. *Aust Prescr*. 2012; **35**: 138–9.

134 Jelinek GA, Brown AF. A stand against drug company advertising. *Emergency Medicine Australasia*. 2011; **23**: 4–6.

135 Altman DG. The scandal of poor medical research: we need less research, better research, and research done for the right reasons. *BMJ*. 1994; **308**: 283–4.

136 Lexchin J, Light DW. Commercial influence and the content of medical journals. *BMJ*. 2006; **332**: 1444–7.

137 Lundh A, Barbateskovic M, Hróbjartsson A, *et al*. Conflicts of interest at medical journals: the influence of industry-supported randomised trials on journal impact factors and revenue – cohort study. *PLoS Med*. 2010; **7**: e1000354.

138 Smith R, Roberts I. Patient safety requires a new way to publish clinical trials. *PLoS Clin Trials*. 2006; **1**: e6.

139 Clinical knowledge: from access to action. *Lancet*. 2008; **371**: 785.

140 Schwartz L, Woloshin S, Moynihan R. Who's watching the watchdogs? *BMJ*. 2008; **337**: a2535.

Having the last laugh
at big pharma

What I have described in this book is so tragic that I felt it needed a good-humoured ending. I shall start with a tragicomic industry-sponsored meeting. In 2011, the vice-chairman of the Danish Medical Association, Yves Sales, and I were invited to give talks at a meeting arranged by the Danish Society for Rheumatology. The theme was: *Collaboration with the drug industry. Is it THAT harmful?*

A chief physician at my hospital had suggested the theme but was met with protests when he suggested the title, *Collaboration with the drug industry. Is it harmful?* Some of the members of the society's board were in the pocket of the industry, whereas the standard at his department was to have no contact with sales departments in companies. Opinions were divided about whether the society should continue to have industry-sponsored meetings, and they felt a need for information and provocation. The Danish Association of the Pharmaceutical Industry first declined to participate but sent its vice director, Henrik Vestergaard.

I was told that there would be industry people in the audience although they didn't appear in the list of 115 participants. Ah, well, of course. A society called Young Rheumatologists had just held a meeting with about 30 rheumatologists and about 60 people from the drug industry. Like the parents, so the children.

During a pre-meeting dinner, the chairman of the meeting asked me not to be too tough with the industry; I smiled and said it was too late to change my talk. I don't go to sponsored meetings, unless I have a chance of influencing the prevailing culture among doctors, which was the case here. In my talk, I took the five sponsors, Merck, Pfizer, UCB, Abbott and Roche, one by one, from the bottom up:

Roche was a drug pusher that had built its fortune on selling heroin illegally in the United States; made millions of people hooked on Librium and Valium while the company denied they caused dependence; and had lured European governments into buying Tamiflu for billions of Euros, which I considered the biggest theft in European history.

Abbott and its hired gun, a Danish cardiologist (*see* Chapter 11), blocked the access the Danish drug agency had granted us to unpublished trials of the slimming pill, sibutramine, which was later withdrawn from the market because of cardiovascular toxicity.

UCB in Belgium sent us a letter stating that UCB is an ethical company and that all data are proprietary solely to the UCB who has the exclusive right to make whatever it deems desirable.[1] I remarked that talking about being an ethical company and at the same time concealing trial data was bullshit.[2] We performed a meta-analysis of a natural hormone, somatostatin, used for stopping bleeding although the effect is doubtful,[1] and we discovered that the biggest trial ever done had not been published.

Pfizer lied at an FDA hearing about the cardiovascular harms of celecoxib; it agreed to pay a record fine of $2.3 billion for promotion of off-label use of four drugs; it entered a Corporate Integrity Agreement with the US Department of Health and Human Services, which probably wouldn't work, as Pfizer had entered three such agreements previously. I explained that the reason Pfizer was the world's biggest company might be that it was more criminal than other companies.

Merck had caused the unnecessary deaths of tens of thousands of patients with rheumatological problems through its ruthless behaviour; it selectively targeted doctors that raised critical questions about the drug; it concealed the cardiovascular risk both in publications and marketing; and the only thing that happened to its CEO, Raymond Gilmartin, was that he became immensely rich.

After this introduction, I fired some more torpedoes about habitual fraud and crimes in the drug industry with devastating consequences for the patients and ended my talk by quoting the *BMJ*'s editor, Fiona Godlee: 'Just say no.'[3] I also told the society that if they still couldn't see there was a problem in receiving money from activities that were partly criminal, then why not get a sponsorship from Hells Angels?

Yves Sales supported me in the discussion although he told me later that he felt my direct approach might have pushed some people away who were undetermined. The chairman of the society argued that their meetings would be very expensive without industry support, to which Sales bluntly replied that there was no reason to shed tears if industry sponsorship was banned, and that it wasn't correct that the society couldn't arrange meetings without such support. I drew attention to the fact that other academics educate themselves without industry support and noted that the general practitioners had observed that there was little difference in their costs after they had banned industry support of their annual gathering.

Henrik Vestergaard was very angry. He talked about my outrageous and insulting allegations, which is typical industry speak. How can facts be 'allegations'? The industry has committed the crimes themselves, and if it's insulting to tell the truth, then perhaps the industry should consider improving on its practices. Vestergaard was highly offended and refused to reply when I asked him if it wouldn't be in his organisation's interest if fines for illegal activities became so high that they were perceptible. This would force the companies to compete at a higher ethical level, which would also benefit those working in the industry, as it would become more attractive to work there. Vestergaard used the standard tactic, hinted at the lone bad apple, and said that *when the public purse wouldn't pay for postgraduate education, the industry had to do it.* This hypocrisy was too much for a rheumatologist who remarked that the industry did it because it paid off, not because of some humanistic motive.

The passions ran really high. Merete Hetland, a rheumatologist with many links to industry, claimed I was employed to quarrel, that I threw suspicion on the industry, and that we were able to collaborate with the Germans although they were Nazis during the Second World War. Industry speak again. To tell the facts about companies is not to throw suspicion, and industry routinely rejects uncomfortable facts by saying they are things of the past and that it has become much better, which it never has, as I had just demonstrated.

A year later, I looked at the society's homepage. It still had industry-sponsored meetings, and it was still possible for drug firms to become members. Provided they paid 10 times as much as a doctor. This was a bit depressing and another doctor who is against industry sponsorship accomplished greater change than I did:[4]

> The audience ... seemed immensely interested – and acutely aware of the rarity of an occasion in which the relationship between medicine and the drug industry was questioned ... Immediately after my talk, one pharmaceutical company representative announced to the organiser that her company would no longer support the annual conference. Another packed up his exhibit and walked out. Other drug representatives were observed muttering angrily into their cell phones, which may, or may not, have been related to the near total exhibitor boycott the next day. Only one exhibitor showed up, prompting a physician friend of mine to remark, 'Maybe he missed your talk.'

In 2010, the chairman for the Danish Society for Pulmonary Medicine invited speakers to introduce a round-table discussion about drug trials in Denmark, with an estimated 80 attendants. The meeting would last 75 minutes and was sponsored by GlaxoSmithKline. There was an honorarium of $1000 for a 5–10 minute introduction. The invitation noted that 'It is necessary to sign a contract before the meeting.' I asked Glaxo why they required a contract and asked to see it. They didn't send it but explained it was required according to the industry's guidelines when they hired a doctor as a consultant. But why sign a contract when hiring a person for 10 minutes and why were 80 people expected for a 1-hour meeting about drug trials? I suspect the real aim of the meeting was to help Glaxo market its asthma products. In fact, the inviting company person was a 'marketing coordinator' and the headline for the meeting was: 'Exclusive course, Respiratory Scientific Forum'. The invitation said that the meeting venue was about a 60 minutes' drive from Copenhagen, but nonetheless people could stay for the night at the hotel while Glaxo paid the expenses. For 80 people. What an expense for so little, unless the company was buying doctors. Doctors who participate in such arrangements bring shame on themselves.

In 2001, German doctors were invited to Bayern with a scientific programme that lasted 10 minutes, just after they had arrived.[5] The rest of the time was their own. Another option for German doctors was to start 20 patients on a certain company's drug, which would earn them what seemed to be an all-expenses paid 3-day trip to Paris that included the finals in the football world championship. This time the doctors didn't have to waste 10 minutes of their precious time listening to a lecture.

MONEY DOESN'T SMELL

I am not much exposed to advertisements for drugs, but twice a year a company sends me an envelope by mistake. And I mean by mistake, as I must be blacklisted in all drug companies. For example, I received an advertising circular from Meda that said that 'About 300 000 people in Denmark suffer from overactive bladder.' On the rear side, there was a reference to this statement, *Continence News no. 4 – 2010*. So much for the science behind a claim that 6% of the whole population, including children, suffer from peeing too often or too suddenly. The solution was trospium chloride (Sanctura, perhaps a sanctuary for hyper-urinators?), an anticholinergic drug, which would cost you the price of two beers a day, which, however, would only worsen your peeing problem.

Before smart marketing people dubbed it overactive bladder, we used to call it urge incontinence. It feels very intrusive that the industry doesn't even leave our disease names alone. It's none of their business to name diseases but, unfortunately, doctors now also call it overactive bladder.

Pfizer mingled with what we have called impotence for centuries. When it discovered that a drug developed to treat hypertension caused erection as a side effect, impotence was renamed erectile dysfunction, which sounds more socially acceptable than being impotent:

'I have a physiological dysfunction.'

'Oh, poor you, what's the problem?'

'I am not sure I want to tell you, but luckily, there is a drug that works.'

The poor guy's friend might think he suffers from thyroid disease, type 1 diabetes, chronic foul-smelling diarrhoea, or worse.

I don't deny that some people are troubled by peeing too often or too suddenly. But I have always known that the effect of anticholinergic drugs is highly doubtful. The Cochrane review confirms this. The effects are statistically significant, but as everything gets statistically significant, no matter how small the effect is, if only there are enough patients, we should always look at the data. The number of leakage episodes per 24 hours in the largest study was 3.2 on drug and 3.3 on placebo, and the number of pees (called micturitions in doctor's language) was 10 on drug and 11 on placebo in the two studies that reported on this.[6] That doesn't seem a worthwhile effect, does it? Particularly not when you consider that all drug have harms. Frequent and disturbing side effects are: dry mouth, blurred vision, constipation and confusion. These are just the common ones; there are many others, e.g. dry eyes, dry nose, headache and gas. Some harms can be serious and require you call your doctor immediately: difficulty urinating, rash, hives, itching and difficulty breathing or swallowing. Such information on drugs can be found on the homepage of the US National Library of Medicine:

www.nlm.nih.gov/medlineplus/druginfo

By the way, how does a patient decide whether a few drops of urine are a leakage or not? Given the conspicuous side effects of the drugs, it's likely that many patients on active drug have guessed they are on it, and such unblinding will be expected to lead to biased assessments in favour of the drug over placebo (*see* Chapter 4). Furthermore, a patient who knows she is on active drug might suppress the urge to go to the toilet, and if this happens one time more per day than for a patient treated with placebo, it corresponds to the difference seen in the trials. So maybe there is no effect at all of these drugs? I consider that quite likely.

When the Roman emperor Vespasian was criticised for the tax he imposed on public urinals, he replied that money doesn't smell. In our time, the way money is made on urine can smell so strongly that it comes close to scientific misconduct. Yamanouchi, which later became Astellas, submitted a comparative trial for publication in 2005 with a Danish professor's name, Gunnar Lose, on the paper, although he had never seen the manuscript, the raw data or the more extensive clinical study report, which wasn't written until months later.[7] The paper showed that Yamanouchi's drug was better than Pfizer's drug, but Lose didn't feel that the statistical analysis or the paper was fair and balanced, and he required it be retracted.

The company refused to retract the paper, refused to show Lose the data, and later also refused to show him the clinical study report, although the contract with the company specified that he would get access to the report. Lose found the data analysis so doubtful that he withdrew his contribution as author. The clinical study report was submitted to the Danish drug agency, as required by law, but the agency refused to check whether the published data were reliable and even refused to share the report with Lose.[8]

Lose was right. The published trial report is not only miserable, it is extremely miserable,[9] a school example of how one should *not* report a trial. It was appropriately criticised by other researchers,[10] and, to take just one example, percentages were given to two decimal places, e.g. 3.58%, whereas there were no standard deviations or other measures of uncertainty in the data. I have no doubt it was a seeding trial. Enrolling 1177 patients in a micturition trial is far over the top, and the trial involved 17 countries and 117 study sites, i.e. only 10 patients per site. If one wants reliable data, it is preferable to use a few large sites with skilled investigators.

These events also show that drug agencies don't prioritise. While the trial was running, Lose had been visited by a monitor from the agency who checked whether signatures corresponded to the correct dates. But whether the public was misinformed about the merits of a new drug didn't have the agency's interest. According to the European ombudsman, clinical study reports are not the property of the sponsoring firm, they belong to society, which means that the agency shouldn't have refused to give Lose the report. Further, it is absurd to deny Lose the report of a trial to which he had himself contributed.

CREATING DISEASES

What diseases could you have without knowing? A Danish newspaper did an amusing investigation. It collected news stories throughout 3 months about what Danes suffer from and came to the conclusion that, on average, each one of us suffers from two diseases.[11] In fact, it's much worse because the journalists searched on *Danes suffer from*, which means that a lot of diseases were overlooked. Maybe the reason that we Danes come out as the happiest people on earth in poll after poll is that we don't know we are terribly ill.

The 300 000 who were said to suffer from overactive bladder weren't on the list of 12 million diseases in Danes, so we should add these 300 000. It is good to know that we can reduce human suffering by *not* asking people whether they have peeing problems and by *not* treating them with sanctuary drugs.

In 2007, The Danish Association of the Pharmaceutical Industry had lobbied our politicians in Parliament and convinced some of them that regular health checks would be a good idea in order to prevent diseases. When asked by a journalist whether it wasn't more a matter of selling more drugs, e.g. against elevated blood pressure or cholesterol, the industry spokesman admitted that this was the case.[12]

In 2011, our new government had regular health checks on the menu, but I asked for a meeting with the minister of health where I told her that the Cochrane review we had just completed, and which includes 16 trials, almost 250 000 participants and almost 12 000 deaths, found no effect of health checks on total mortality, cancer deaths or cardiovascular deaths.[13,14] One of my colleagues told her about a large Danish trial he had just finished that also failed to find an effect.[15] Health checks lead to more diagnoses of diseases or risk factors, which lead to more drug use and more harms. Our conclusion was therefore very firm: health checks should not be used. The minister agreed and said it was the first time the new government had broken a pre-election promise in an evidence-based manner. Our review will save billions for taxpayers and a lot of suffering, too.

Here is an example of the misery that a seemingly innocuous health check could cause. A highly prolific writer had suddenly lost his appetite for his hectic life.[16] The days were endless and terrible to such an extent that he contemplated suicide as the only way out. He was convinced that he had become old and didn't have strength any more. After a month, it suddenly dawned on him that it could be the pills. These pills were a beta-blocker, and his doctors had forgotten to tell him that they could cause depression. He stopped taking them and became himself again.

This story didn't start with a health check, but it could have. Very often, it doesn't occur to the patients that their worsened condition might be caused by the pills they take. Unfortunately, their doctors may not recognise either that the new symptoms are side effects of the first pill and may therefore prescribe a second pill against the symptoms, and so on.

The drug industry and its paid doctors don't even leave young, strong people alone. Applying European guidelines for cardiovascular disease on a Norwegian population, researchers found that 86% of males were at high risk of cardiovascular disease at age 40.[17] The irony is that Norwegians are some of the most long-lived people in the world. In another study, the researchers found that 50% of Norwegians had a cholesterol or blood pressure level above the recommended cut-off for treatment at age 24![18]

Osteoporosis is similar. In 1994, a small study group associated with the WHO defined normal bone mineral density as that of young adult women.[19] Pretty foolish, as virtually everything in us deteriorates as we get older. We'll be off limits in all sorts of ways if we compare ourselves with young women. The group – completely arbitrarily – defined osteoporosis as present if the bone mineral density was 2.5 standard deviations below that in a young woman, and didn't even stop there, but defined osteopenia as present if the measurement lay between 1.0 and 2.5 standard deviations below. These criteria were intended for epidemiological research but were a bonanza for the drug industry, as they rendered half of all older women 'abnormal'. The drug industry sponsored the meeting where these definitions were created, so there might have been some influence.

A bone mineral density test can only predict one-sixth of future hip fractures,[20] but despite such sobering observations, the test has become the gold standard for deciding which people to treat. Consumer sites on the internet are usually industry sponsored and they say that the test is good and predicts the risk of fracture, whereas health technology assessment organisations say the opposite.[20] The effect of the drugs is small, even for women at high risk of fractures: If 100 women who have already had a vertebral fracture are treated, one hip fracture is perhaps prevented.[21] I say perhaps because several studies suggest that long-term treatment leads to the opposite effect, an increase in hip fractures,[22-24] which may be explained by the fact that the new bone induced by the drugs is not of the same type as bone formed naturally.

Moreover, people who are told they have brittle bones may stop exercising, which is a bad idea, as it strengthens the bones. A woman I knew who was perfectly healthy received a bone scan for no good reason and was told she had brittle bones. She was very fond of her sports, but stopped immediately, as she feared falling and breaking a bone. So, already the diagnosis pestered her life and it also increased her risk, as exercise prevents fractures. It's bad medicine to screen healthy people without knowing from randomised trials that screening does more good than harm. That's not the case for osteoporosis; there are no trials of screening. I don't say that no one should be treated; I am only saying that far too many are being treated. The industry must be immensely grateful for the WHO group's assistance, as the industry sells its drugs also for osteopenia, which is a market of around 400 million women.

The osteoporosis-osteopenia madness has been subject to many jokes. Should we also treat those at risk of being at risk (those with osteopenia who may cross the arbitrary border to osteoporosis when they get older)?[19] When a colleague of mine left his home for a skiing holiday, he remarked that he now suffered from a prefracture.

Another joke, which unfortunately is taken seriously, is that people hold conferences about prehypertension, which starts when your diastolic blood pressure climbs over 80 mm Hg. Here is a tragedy: the American Heart Association recommends to screen children for high blood pressure, starting at age three.[25]

We showed in our review of health checks that screening for hypertension (at any age) isn't beneficial.[13,14]

We also have prediabetes. Trials have been performed to demonstrate that by treating healthy people with a glucose-lowering drug, you can lower their risk of developing diabetes.[26] That is a marvellous joke. Since the diagnosis depends on the blood glucose level, it wasn't necessary to conduct trials, as the result was given, a sort of circular evidence. Therefore, once drug treatment stops, there isn't any difference in the incidence of diabetes, so the drug didn't prevent anything from happening. The whole exercise was one of boosting sales of drugs like rosiglitazone, which was investigated in such a trial, the DREAM trial.[26] The dream was a nightmare, as the drug kills people. A further point is: how would you find healthy people and start treatment? This cannot be done without screening and we showed in our review of health checks that screening for diabetes doesn't work. It doesn't reduce morbidity or mortality.[13,14]

It's seducingly easy to convince healthy people to take drugs they don't need for a disease they don't have. The Australian artist, Justine Cooper, invented a hilarious hoax,[27] which can be seen on YouTube.[28] It looks like a TV commercial and advertises Havidol (have it all), with the chemical name avafynetyme HCl (have a fine time plus hydrochloric acid). Havidol is good for those who suffer from dysphoric social attention consumption deficit anxiety disorder (DSACDAD). Feel empty after a full day of shopping? Enjoy new things more than old ones? Does life seem better when you have more than others? Then you may have the disorder, which more than 50% of adults have. The ad says that Havidol should be taken indefinitely, and that side effects include extraordinary thinking, dermal gloss, markedly delayed sexual climax, inter-species communication and terminal smile. 'Talk to your doctor about Havidol.' Some people believed it was for real and folded it into real websites for panic and anxiety disorder, or for depression.

An even more hilarious video on YouTube[29] featured Ray Moynihan as the victim,[27] the journalist who wrote *Selling Sickness* with Alan Cassels. It's about an epidemic – motivational deficiency disorder – first announced in the *BMJ*'s 1 April issue in 2006,[30] and like Havidol, it was believed by some people. In its mild form, people cannot get off the beach, or out of bed in the morning, and in its most severe form it can be lethal as the sufferer may lose the motivation to breathe. Moynihan says 'All my life people have called me lazy. But now I know I was sick.' The drug is Indolebant, and its champion, neuroscientist Leth Argos, reports how a patient's wife telephoned him and was in tears. She said that after using Indolebant, her husband had mowed the lawn, repaired the gutter and paid an electricity bill – all in one week.

I shall let big pharma get the last word in my book, so here is your final laugh, offered by Stephen Whitehead, chief executive of the Association of the British Pharmaceutical Industry, in the *BMJ* in October 2012 in response to an article that was critical of the drug industry. I bring it in its entirety:[31]

McCartney makes several disparate claims about the drug industry. She states that the financial relations between charities and the industry are 'unclear' and implies that this unduly influences the daily activities of the third sector. In reality, the Association of the British Pharmaceutical Industry's code of practice requires that companies publicly declare their financial transactions with charities and the nature of their relationship. Those who fail to meet their obligations are subject to sanctions of the Prescription Medicines Code of Practice Authority – the arm's length administrator of the code. Charities are protective of their independence and wholly committed to the patients they serve – any malign influence is fiercely resisted.

Secondly, medical representatives do seek to engage with clinicians to educate them on the latest available treatments. There are strict rules about how this is conducted. I think it is important that clinicians are offered the chance to learn about new and innovative drugs and make their own decisions about their suitability for patients.

Finally, cooperation and partnership between the drug industry and the wider health community are valuable, despite negative preconceptions. By working together we can improve health outcomes, drive innovation, and save the NHS time and money. This should be, and is, conducted within strict guidelines that ensure commercial interests are secondary to patients' needs. This drive towards closer working has not been pushed by the drug industry but by all healthcare stakeholders. Earlier this year a range of signatories, including the Department of Health and the medical royal colleges, approved principles for working in partnership with the life sciences sector for the good of patients.

It may be fashionable to criticise the drug industry, but we shouldn't be quick to criticise the good work done to help people live healthier lives.

What a level of irony at the highest levels in the drug industry. Talking about codes of practice, strict rules and strict guidelines as the panacea solution for an industry that is the worst of all industries in routinely breaking the law to such an extent that it is organised crime that results in the deaths of innocent people in huge numbers! It's not only fake fixes, it's the ultimate joke. After I had lectured at a Prescrire meeting in Paris in January 2013 about the pervasive crime in the drug industry,[32] I had a chat with Alain Braillon who inspired me to finish my book with a cartoon.

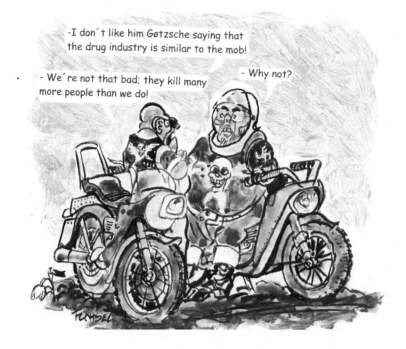

REFERENCES

1 Gøtzsche PC, Hróbjartsson A. Somatostatin analogues for acute bleeding oesophageal varices. *Cochrane Database Syst Rev.* 2008; **3**: CD000193.

2 Frankfurt H. *On Bullshit.* Princeton, NJ: Princeton University Press; 2005.

3 Godlee F. Editor's choice: say no to the free lunch. *BMJ.* 2005 Apr 16.

4 Fugh-Berman A. Doctors must not be lapdogs to drug firms. *BMJ.* 2006; **333**: 1027.

5 Grill M. *Kranke Geschäfte: wie die Pharmaindustrie uns manipuliert.* Hamburg: Rowohlt Verlag; 2007.

6 Nabi G, Cody JD, Ellis G, *et al.* Anticholinergic drugs versus placebo for overactive bladder syndrome in adults. *Cochrane Database Syst Rev.* 2006; **4**: CD003781.

7 Andersen NV. [Gunnar Lose vs. Yamanouchi]. *Ugeskr Læger.* 2006; **168**: 546–9.

8 Andersen NV. [Gunnar Lose considers the committee on scientific dishonesty]. *Ugeskr Læger.* 2006; **168**: 719–21.

9 Chapple CR, Martinez-Garcia R, Selvaggi L, *et al.* A comparison of the efficacy and tolerability of solifenacin succinate and extended release tolterodine at treating overactive bladder syndrome: results of the STAR trial. *Eur Urol.* 2005; **48**: 464–70.

10 Jonas U, Rackley RR. *Eur Urol.* 2006; **49**: 187–8; author reply 188–90.

11 Rasmussen LI. [Danes suffer from 12 million diseases]. *Ugeskr Læger.* 2011; **173**: 1767.

12 Andersen NV. [The drug industry increases lobbyism]. *Mandag Morgen.* 2007 Sep 3: 20–3.

13 Krogsbøll LT, Jørgensen KJ, Grønhøj Larsen C, *et al.* General health checks for reducing morbidity and mortality from disease. *Cochrane Database Syst Rev.* 2012; **10**: CD009009.

14 Krogsbøll LT, Jørgensen KJ, Grønhøj Larsen C, *et al.* General health checks in adults for reducing morbidity and mortality from disease: Cochrane systematic review and meta-analysis. *BMJ.* 2012; **345**: e7191.

15 Lifestyle intervention in a general population for prevention of ischaemic heart disease. Study record. Available online at: http://clinicaltrials.gov/ct2/results?term=inter99&Search=Search (accessed 3 June 2013).

16 Kvist J. [The possibility of suicide]. *Berlingske Tidende*. 2002 Nov 3.

17 Getz L, Sigurdsson JA, Hetlevik I, *et al*. Estimating the high risk group for cardiovascular disease in the Norwegian HUNT 2 population according to the 2003 European guidelines: modelling study. *BMJ*. 2005; **331**: 551.

18 Getz L, Kirkengen AL, Hetlevik I, *et al*. Ethical dilemmas arising from implementation of the European guidelines on cardiovascular disease prevention in clinical practice. A descriptive epidemiological study. *Scand J Prim Health Care*. 2004; **22**: 202–8.

19 Alonso-Coello P, García-Franco AL, Guyatt G, *et al*. Drugs for pre-osteoporosis: prevention or disease mongering? *BMJ*. 2008; **336**: 126–9.

20 Abramson J. *Overdo$ed America*. New York: HarperCollins; 2004.

21 Black DM, Cummings SR, Karpf DB, *et al*. Randomised trial of effect of alendronate on risk of fracture in women with existing vertebral fractures. Fracture Intervention Trial Research Group. *Lancet*. 1996; **348**: 1535–41.

22 Erviti J. Bisphosphonates: do they prevent or cause bone fractures? *Drug and Therapeutics Bulletin of Navarre*. 2009; **17**: 65–75.

23 Erviti J, Alonso Á, Oliva B, *et al*. Oral bisphosphonates are associated with increased risk of subtrochanteric and diaphyseal fractures in elderly women: a nested case-control study. *BMJ Open*. 2013; **3**: e002091.

24 Abrahamsen B, Eiken P, Eastell R. Cumulative alendronate dose and the long-term absolute risk of subtrochanteric and diaphyseal femur fractures: a register-based national cohort analysis. *J Clin Endocrinol Metab*. 2010; **95**: 5258–65.

25 Moynihan R, Cassels A. *Selling Sickness: how the world's biggest pharmaceutical companies are turning us all into patients*. New York: Nation Books; 2005.

26 Montori VM, Isley WL, Guyatt GH. Waking up from the DREAM of preventing diabetes with drugs. *BMJ*. 2007; **334**: 882–4.

27 Coombes R. Having the last laugh at big pharma. *BMJ*. 2007; **334**: 396–7.

28 HAVIDOL: female testimonial. Available online at: www.youtube.com/watch?v=sQw_cdhXGco.

29 A new epidemic (motivational deficiency disorder). Available online at: www.youtube.com/watch?v=RoppJOtRLe4.

30 Moynihan R. Scientists find new disease: motivational deficiency disorder. *BMJ* 2006; **332**: 745.

31 Whitehead S. Fashionable to criticise the drug industry? *BMJ*. 2012; **345**: e7089.

32 Gøtzsche PC. Lecture. Efficacité et effets indésirables des produits de santé: données confidentielles ou d'intérêt public? Available online at: www.prescrire.org/Docu/Archive/docus/PiluledOr2013_Conf_Gotzsche.pdf (accessed 8 Feb 2013).

Index